HOMEOPATHIC PHARMACY

TO BE
DISPOSED
BY
AUTHORITY

Dedication
This book is for
Calum, Eilidh, Tara and Alex.

For Elsevier:

Commissioning editor: Karen Morley
Development editor: Louise Allsop
Project manager: Emma Riley
Design direction: Jayne Jones

HOMEOPATHIC PHARMACY
Theory and Practice
Second Edition

Steven B Kayne

PhD MBA LLM MSc(Med Sci) DAgVetPharm FRPharmS FCPP FIPharmM FNZCP MPS(NZ) FFHom

Honorary Consultant Pharmacist to the Glasgow Homeopathic Hospital and Visiting Lecturer in Complementary Medicine at the School of Pharmacy, University of Strathclyde, Glasgow, UK

Foreword by
Ian M Caldwell

PhC MPhil FRPharmS MCPP

Retired Community Pharmacist from Larkhall, Lanarkshire, UK, and a former President of the Royal Pharmaceutical Society of Great Britain

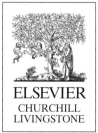

ELSEVIER
CHURCHILL
LIVINGSTONE

EDINBURGH LONDON NEW YORK OXFORD PHILADELPHIA ST LOUIS SYDNEY TORONTO 2006

ELSEVIER
CHURCHILL LIVINGSTONE

An imprint of Elsevier Limited

First edition 1997
Second edition 2006

ISBN 0 443 10160 4

British Library Cataloguing in Publication Data
A catalogue record for this book is available from the British Library.

Library of Congress Cataloging in Publication Data
A catalog record for this book is available from the Library of Congress.

Note

Knowledge and best practice in this field are constantly changing. As new research and experience broaden our knowledge, changes in practice, treatment and drug therapy may become necessary or appropriate. Readers are advised to check the most current information provided (i) on procedures featured or (ii) by the manufacturer of each product to be administered, to verify the recommended dose or formula, the method and duration of administration, and contraindications. It is the responsibility of the practitioner, relying on their own experience and knowledge of the patient, to make diagnoses, to determine dosages and the best treatment for each individual patient, and to take all appropriate safety precautions. To the fullest extent of the law, neither the publisher nor the author assumes any liability for any injury and/or damage to persons or property arising out of or related to any use of the material contained in this book.

The Publisher

Working together to grow
libraries in developing countries

www.elsevier.com | www.bookaid.org | www.sabre.org

ELSEVIER   BOOK AID International   Sabre Foundation

ELSEVIER SCIENCE   your source for books, journals and multimedia in the health sciences

www.elsevierhealth.com

Printed in China

The publisher's policy is to use paper manufactured from sustainable forests

Contents

Foreword to the 1st edition   vii
Foreword to the 2nd edition   ix
About the author   xi
Preface   xiii
Acknowledgments   xv

PART 1 Introduction

1. Introduction to complementary and
   alternative medicine   3
2. Historical background of homeopathy   39
3. The development of homeopathy
   around the world   59

PART 2 Procedures

4. Preparing the remedy   81
5. Supply of a named remedy   121
6. The provision of homeopathic
   treatment   137

PART 3 Clinical applications

7. The theory of disease and treatment   145
8. Choosing the remedy   167

PART 4 Homeopathic prescribing in practice

9. First aid and acute applications   213
10. Therapies allied to homeopathy   255

PART 5 Research and education

11. Homeopathic research   269
12. Education   321

PART 6 Reference section

13. Materia medica   337

Appendices

Appendix 1 Some useful addresses   357
Appendix 2 Further reading   361

Index of remedies   367

General index   373

Foreword to the first edition

Forewords to textbooks are usually written by the author or by an eminent supporter of the author's viewpoint. How, then, do you reply to someone who asks you to write a foreword to one of his books, knowing full well that the subject matter is that which occasioned a long, disputative correspondence in a learned journal? That you are flattered? That he has a funny sense of humour? In fact, you babble, "Yes, delighted, of course, only too pleased", and then you fret about what you have got yourself into. (Dr Kayne certainly has a sense of humour, as is evidenced by his inclusion on Box 4.1 on page 47 of 'P.C. Computeris'. This invitation could well be his revenge for the fact that my letter was the last one published in our long-running sequence.)

In spite of Hahnemann's dislike for the apothecaries of his time, it is understandable that some pharmacists now take an active interest in homoeopathy. Pharmacists of a certain age are well acquainted with the cultivation, preparation, action and uses of crude drugs and, although pharmacognosy (the study of medicinal plants) is no longer an important part of the pharmacy degree course, younger pharmacists are taking an interest in the field of naturally occurring medicines. This has been an area of expertise of the apothecary since antiquity when materials were drawn from all over the Old World, many of them travelling along the Spice Road from the East. Supply was necessarily sporadic and transport incredibly difficult so it is little wonder that drugs such as cardamom, myrrh, cinnamon, opium and rheum were valued on a par with precious metals. Few people could afford these exotica, nor were they widely available; consequently, herbals made much of native plants, the worts, belladonna, ergot, willow, feverfew and dandelion being only a tiny fraction of a comprehensive list of empirical treatments. The range available was further widened by imports from the New World and with the inclusion of metals and minerals. The British contribution was not without the bizarre since the *Pharmacopaeia Londonensis*, 1684, included moss scraped from a human skull (mucus crani humani); a rarity of unrecorded effect but one possibly contaminated with, dare I say it, subtherapeutic amounts of penicillin.

By the 18th century, the natural armamentarium was largely in place, human anatomy was extensively charted, and a start was being made towards an understanding of physiology. The challenge to surgeons, apothecaries and doctors was then to rationalise their knowledge and develop effective treatments. Even allowing for the imperfect knowledge of the time, some of the fashionable 18th and 19th century treatments, such as emetics, purges and bleeding, were baseless and of heroic proportions. Others were honest attempts to harness new facts with varying degrees of success. Lavoiser's experiments with oxygen gave rise to several 'pneumatic' theories, Jenner's vaccination came close to treating 'like with like', and Lister's use of phenols and cresols is credited with being the basis for the late 19th century popular treatment of croup and whooping cough in children, where the unfortunate infant was held in fumes rising from one of the tar boilers then used for street repair or shipyard caulking. Hahnemann's theories arose in this milieu and, whereas many of the other fashions in treatment evolved and faded, homeopathy persists. In the light of these changes, where does homoeopathy stand today? Both homoeopaths and allopaths can live comfortably with the use of natural medicines, herbal and inorganic, as proven agents in the treatment of symptoms and disease. It is certainly possible to accommodate the hypothesis of 'like treats like' as an empirically established approach to treatment. Modern practitioners would be brave indeed if they adopted a narrow, blinkered view of any condition presented by any patient, and this is underlined by the fact that government agencies and health insurers throughout the world are now increasingly demanding defined quality of outcome for all the treatments for which they pay. In doing so, these agencies are seeking a cost-efficient way of attaining the World Health Organization definition of health which Steven quotes later but which bears repetition here:

'A state of complete physical, mental and social well-being and not merely the absence of disease'

Best practice in health care has always tended towards consideration of the patient's circumstances as well as of the condition and, clearly, this 'holistic' attitude to care is now being adopted so enthusiastically that it is being made a condition of contract for practitioners.

Thus, three of the bases of homeopathy are commonly accepted which only leaves the contentious question of dilution. To make a reasoned decision on this requires an open mind, a preparedness to consider all the arguments. Steven Kayne has provided a wealth of well-documented information to enable you to reach your own conclusions. Steven and I obviously have divergent views on this topic but, having said that, I have always believed that having faith in the practitioner and in the treatment takes patients half way to winning the battle for health.

I.M.C. 1997.

Foreword to the second edition

It says much for the public thirst for information on health matters that Dr Kayne has brought forth a new edition of his original Introduction and Handbook. As humorous as he is erudite, Steven has sought to confuse me again by moving my favourite item 'P.C. Computeris' from the above quoted p 47 to Box 4.1 on page 89. Readers will no doubt be as relieved as I am to find that he continues to recommend the antidotes to this preparation, namely Maltus singlus major and Vinum rubrum, in allopathic form.

The new edition is much expanded but remains distinctly user friendly. The change in title to *Homeopathic Pharmacy – Theory and Practice* is no mere cosmetic change but denotes a determined attempt to consider both the educational and the research aspects of homoeopathy in detail. This is timely given the re-ignition of the debate on efficacy fired by the work of Aljing Shang et al. as reported in *Lancet* (26.8.05). Indeed, Steven goes so far as to seek valid 'gold standard' alternatives to existing clinical trial concepts. Whether this approach will ever bridge the gap between the entrenched positions of the protagonists in the dilution debate remains to be seen but it is a route worthy of scientific exploration.

I.M.C. September 2005.

About the author

Steven B. Kayne practised in Glasgow, UK, as a Community Pharmacist with an interest in homeopathy and other complementary disciplines for more than 30 years. He served terms on the councils of the British Homeopathic Association and the Faculty of Homeopathy and was the first Pharmacy Dean of the Faculty from 1999 to 2003. He was awarded an Honorary Fellowship of the Faculty in 2000. He now serves on several Government bodies in an advisory capacity and is Honorary Consultant Pharmacist at Glasgow Homeopathic Hospital and Visiting Lecturer in complementary medicine at the University of Strathclyde in Glasgow. He also writes and lectures widely in the UK and overseas on a variety of pharmacy and related healthcare topics.

Dr Kayne is a member of the Scottish Executive of the Royal Pharmaceutical Society of Great Britain and Chair of the College of Pharmacy Practice in Scotland.

Preface

This is a good time to publish a book on homeopathic pharmacy. Not only did we celebrate the 250th year of the birth of Samuel Hahnemann in 2005, but the opportunities for a proper integrative healthcare system have never been greater. When I was writing the first edition of this book, more than 10 years ago, healthcare delivery was taking place in a very different environment: general practitioners diagnosed and prescribed, pharmacists dispensed and counselled patients – albeit with some hesitation – and nurses looked after patients with the same traditional skills they had used for centuries. On a corporate level, none of us talked to our non-medically qualified practitioners. On a personal level, some of our best friends were professional homeopaths and we interacted frequently.

In the UK, the shift from a product-oriented health service to a patient-oriented service and the granting of NHS prescribing rights to healthcare professionals other than doctors have brought about a totally different situation. 'Fire-fighting' disease is no longer our main aim; instead this is merely one of many, situated half way along a continuum extending from the promotion and maintenance of good health at one end to ongoing support and rehabilitation at the other.

An integrative healthcare system and the creation of a team approach to patient care will offer real benefits both clinically and economically. Homeopathy has enjoyed a special status since the NHS was set up but it surely cannot be too long before other disciplines become equally valued. It is to be hoped that as current dialogue with professional homeopaths and fellow practitioners in other disciplines progresses, their potential contribution within an expanded NHS will be recognised too.

Evidence based medicine is an important issue and undoubtedly there are substantial gaps in our knowledge as far as homeopathy is concerned. In many instances we do not know how, why or even whether it works. Although we have moved on greatly in the past decade there is still much more to do before we can offer the sort of evidence that is acceptable to colleagues, patients and purchasing authorities. Despite this, people do appear to benefit from homeopathy and that is what really matters.

Now that homeopathic pharmacy has acquired a generic status (that is, it has become a subject in its own right and not just something pharmacists do) I have tried to make this second edition of *Homeopathic Pharmacy* more appealing to homeopathic practitioners in general. Chapters have been updated and in some cases expanded and reorganised. As in the first edition, some important material is repeated so that chapters may be read in isolation without the need to flick back and forth. Topics that appear in more than one chapter are cross-referenced. The main thrust of the book remains unchanged – it is intended to support the provision of homeopathic health-care by practitioners at preliminary and intermediate levels.

Finally, I offer my thanks to all those colleagues who have taken the time and trouble to contact me with helpful suggestions. Comments are always welcome.

Glasgow   Steven Kayne
August 2005   steven@scottish-saltire.com

Acknowledgements

I am indebted to a large number of colleagues and good friends who helped in the production of the first edition of this text. These included:

- Dr David Reilly, Consultant Physician at Glasgow Homeopathic Hospital and Director of the Academic Department of Homeopathic Medicine, Dr Neil Beattie, Dr Stuart Semple and Ms Felicity Lee, pharmacist and a former Director of the Society of Homeopaths, all of whom made useful comments on the manuscript
- Ms Mary Gooch and her staff at Glasgow Homeopathic Hospital
- Dr Ian Nash for help in interpreting the NMR trace
- Dana Ullman of California for permission to use material from his books
- Gregory Vlamis for sharing information on Bach remedies.

In addition I acknowledge contributions to the second edition from:

- Jay Borneman (USA), Ms Amanda Macrae (New Zealand) and Dr Ashley Ross and Dr David Naude of the Department of Homeopathy, Durban Institute of Technology in South Africa, for bringing me up to date with homeopathic developments in their respective countries
- Dr Peter Fisher, Clinical Director at the Royal London Homeopathic Hospital and Editor of *Homeopathy*, and Dr David Spence, Chairman of the British Homeopathic Association and Consultant Physician at Bristol Homeopathic Hospital, for information on their hospitals
- Dr Jeremy Swayne, former Academic Dean at the Faculty of Homeopathy, for his detailed review of the first edition
- Weleda (UK) for information on legislation

and last (but definitely not least) my elder son Dr Lee Kayne and his wife Rebecca for their help with Chapter 11 and the Appendices.

To you all – and to anybody whom I have inadvertently missed out – my sincere thanks.

PART 1

Introduction

PART CONTENTS

1. Introduction to complementary and
   alternative medicine   3

2. Historical background of homeopathy   39

3. The development of homeopathy
   around the world   59

Chapter 1

Introduction to complementary and alternative medicine

CHAPTER CONTENTS

Definition of CAM   4
Types of CAM   4
Classification of CAM   5
Classification by system of therapy   5
Classification based on the House of
    Lords' report (2000)   5
The NCCAM classification   6
Practising CAM   7
The holistic approach to health care   7
The alternative and complementary
    approaches to health care   12
Factors prompting the current
    interest in complementary and
    alternative therapies   14
The profile of CAM users   15
The profile of homeopathic consumers   16
The reasons for the demand for CAM   18
Push factors   18
    Perception of drug risks   18
    Disenchantment with orthodox
        medicine   18
    Reduced efficacy of existing
        medication   20
Pull factors   20
    Time to consider more than just
        symptoms   20

Financial reasons   20
The 'green' association   23
Encouragement by the media   23
Royal support   23
Cultural reasons   23
The most popular applications of CAM   24
The market for CAM   25
The homeopathic market   26
The integration of CAM into health
    care   27
The Foundation for Integrated Health
    (http://www.fihealth.org.uk/)   28
Sources of information for prospective
    CAM users   29
Safety issues   31
CAM research   31
Funding of research   32
Quality of research   32
Classification of research   32
    Randomised clinical trials and
        meta-analyses   32
    Objective outcome measurements   33
    Clinical audit   33
    Anecdotal evidence and case studies   33
Recent developments in CAM   34

DEFINITION OF CAM

Complementary and alternative medicine (CAM) is frequently defined by what it is not, rather than what it is. Thus, it may be described as being 'not taught formally to health professionals' or 'not scientifically tested'. Current definitions often obscure the debate about holism and integrative care and give therapies and therapists precedence over patients in the design of healthcare systems (Leckridge, 2004); for example:

> *CAM is a group of non orthodox and traditional therapies that may be used alone, or to complement orthodox or other non orthodox therapies, in the treatment and prevention of disease in human and veterinary patients.*

The Cochrane Collaboration (2000) offers a wider definition:

> *CAM is a broad domain of healing resources that encompasses all health systems, modalities and practices and their accompanying theories and beliefs, other than those intrinsic to the politically dominant health systems of a particular society or culture in a given historical period. CAM includes all such practices and ideas self-defined by their users as preventing or treating illnesses or promoting health and well-being. Boundaries within CAM and between the CAM domain and that of the dominant system are not always sharp or fixed.*

Health is defined in the preamble to the constitution of the World Health Organization as being 'a state of complete physical, mental and social well-being and not merely the absence of disease or infirmity' (WHO, 1946).

A distinction can be made between complementary and alternative medicine, for example herbalism and homeopathy, associated with the administration of medicines or 'remedies', and complementary and alternative therapies. The latter includes interventions that rely on procedures alone. In this book, however, the term CAM will be used to describe both applications.

TYPES OF CAM

Complementary and alternative medicine is a term applied to well over 700 different treatments and a large variety of diagnostic methods. It also includes an uncertain number of traditional therapies that are associated with particular ethnic groups or geographic locations (for example, Traditional Chinese, Indian, African or New Zealand Maori medicine). Some are well known, while others are exotic or mysterious and involve spiritualism. Some may even be dangerous.

The more commonly used disciplines include the following:

- Acupuncture: a Traditional Chinese discipline that involves the insertion of needles at predefined points on imaginary lines or 'meridians' on the body; it seeks to restore the balance of positive and negative (*yin* and *yang*) forces within the body.
- Aromatherapy: involves the use of essential oils, normally administered by inhalation or massage.

- Ayurveda: a therapy of Indian origin. It is based on principles derived from ancient Hindi scriptures, combining holistic therapies such as homeopathy, naturopathy and herbalism in the treatment of body, mind and spirit.
- Chiropractic: uses vertebral manipulation, massage and other techniques to treat musculoskeletal conditions.
- Medical herbalism: uses herbal remedies to strengthen and support body organs whose functions have become depleted.
- Homeopathy: characterised by the administration of small quantities of medicines that in much greater concentrations precipitate appearance of the symptoms of the disease being treated.
- Iridology (or iridiagnosis): a diagnostic method based on a detailed study of markings on the iris of the eyes and noting changes that are related to diseased organs.
- Massage: rubbing and kneading of the body, normally with the hands.
- Naturopathy: a complete system that uses diet and exercise together with non-orthodox therapies to improve all aspects of a person's health status.
- Osteopathy: uses various manipulative techniques to restore and maintain musculoskeletal function.
- Reflexology: a type of massage treatment where certain areas on the soles of the feet and the hands are compressed and massaged to stimulate the blood supply and relieve tension. These areas are associated with various organs or body functions.
- Shiatsu: a Japanese form of massage involving the stimulation of many different 'pressure points' in the body by finger pressure. It is often used on the face, in conjunction with aromatherapy or herbalism.

CLASSIFICATION OF CAM

There are several different methods of classifying CAM. The following are among those quoted most frequently in the literature:

Classification by system of therapy

Petroni presents a classification of the different approaches in CAM that has been in currency for many years (Petroni, 1986):

- Complete systems of healing including acupuncture, chiropractic, herbalism, homeopathy, naturopathy and osteopathy
- Specific therapeutic methods including aromatherapy, massage and reflexology
- Psychological approaches and self-help exercises including relaxation, meditation and exercise
- Diagnostic methods including hair analysis, iridology and kinesiology.

Classification based on the House of Lords' report (2000)

In a letter dated 28 July 1999, the UK House of Lords science and technology committee (sub-committee 111) issued a 'call for evidence' to numerous organisations and individuals related to complementary medicine. The request related to six areas – evidence, information, research, training, regulation and risk – as well as provision within the National Health Service (NHS). The 140-page report was published in November 2000 (House of Lords, 2000). It divided CAM into three groups and set out major recommendations for action on the development of integrated conventional and complementary health services in the UK.

- Group 1 embraces disciplines which have an individual diagnostic approach and well-developed self-regulation of practitioners. Research into their effectiveness has been established, and they are increasingly being provided within the National Health system. The report says that statutory regulation of practitioners of acupuncture and herbal medicine should be introduced quickly and that such regulation may soon become appropriate for homeopathy too.
- Group 2 covers therapies which do not purport to embrace diagnostic skills and which are not well regulated.
- Group 3 covers other disciplines which are either long established but indifferent to conventional scientific principles (3A), or which lack any credible evidence base (3B).

There have been criticisms of this classification. For example, the inclusion of Chinese Herbal Medicine in Group 3A would seem to ignore the existence of research that has shown this therapy's usefulness in many disorders and supports its provision in state hospitals throughout China, alongside conventional medicine (Dharmananda, 1997). Although the research is of variable quality, it should not be ignored. Promising trials have also been carried out in the West, on a Chinese formula for atopic eczema. It concluded that there was substantial clinical benefit to patients who had been unresponsive to conventional treatment (Sheehan et al., 1992).

The committee recommended the formation of a single, national regulatory body for each CAM modality (Section 5.5). In the fullness of time, every UK-based CAM practitioner should, ideally, become subject to a unitary regulatory authority (Clarke et al., 2004). This has already been accomplished for chiropractic and osteopathy, each of which has several practitioner associations but only one statutory regulator charged with enforcing the legal protection of title, maintaining a register of practitioners, and defining and defending nationally defined standards.

The NCCAM classification

The US National Center for Complementary and Alternative Medicine classifies CAM in five domains (www.nccam.nih.gov/health/whatiscam/):

- Alternative medical systems
- Mind–body interventions
- Biologically based therapies
- Manipulative and body based methods
- Energy therapies.

PRACTISING CAM

The holistic approach to health care

The origin of the word 'holism' is attributed to Jan Christian Smuts (1870–1950), a South African botanist and philosopher in whose memory the international airport at Johannesburg is named. Smuts, who was Prime Minister of his country after the First World War, wrote a book entitled *Holism and Evolution* in which he described holism as 'the principle which makes for the origin and progress of wholes in the universe' (Smuts, 1926).

He further explained his idea thus:

- Holistic tendency is fundamental in nature.
- It has a well marked ascertainable character.
- Evolution is nothing but the gradual development and stratification of progressive series of wholes, stretching from the inorganic beginnings to the highest levels of spiritual creation.

The concept of holism is a great deal older than the word we now use to describe it, dating back at least to Cicero (106BC–43BC), to whom the following opinion has been attributed: 'a careful prescriber, before he attempts to administer a remedy or treatment to a patient, must investigate not only the malady of the person he wishes to cure, but also his habits when in health, and his physical condition'.

The precise definition of what is now understood by a 'holistic approach' seems to vary between practitioners (Coward, 1989). Rosalind Coward found that some practitioners consider holism as the ability to integrate different treatments for different needs, such as using herbal medicine for a specific ailment, acupuncture for chronic pain or hypnosis to stop smoking. A small minority stressed that holism implied links between individual and environment and suggested treatments which would not only balance the internal parts of an individual but would also balance the relationship between the individual and the environment. More generally, however, practitioners and patients define holism as the treatment of the whole person, an approach that considers body, mind and spirit as a single unit.

When a person attends a homeopath for the first time to seek treatment for a longstanding or chronic condition, the consultation may last anything up to 2 hours, although 30–40 minutes is more usual. In the case of acute self-limiting conditions the consultation can be reduced to a few key questions (see Ch. 8).

The practitioner needs to obtain information on how a patient functions in a normal state of well-being – in short, what makes him or her tick. To do this, patients are asked a whole list of seemingly unrelated questions, for example:

- What sort of food do you like – sweet, salty, spicy or bland?
- What sort of weather do you prefer – hot, cold, windy, rainy?
- Do you like to be in company or alone?
- Are you an extrovert or an introvert?
- Do you normally fall asleep quickly and do you dream?
- If you dream, what do you usually dream about?
- Do you have a favoured sleeping posture?

It has even been suggested that handwriting and the patient's favourite colours could be useful in establishing various personality traits, and therefore in choosing an appropriate remedy (Mueller, 1993).

Having built a picture of the patient's normal state of wellness, the practitioner can begin to investigate the reason that prompted a visit. The aim is to treat people's ailments in such a way that each person can return to their own particular state of health or 'well-being', rather than to some average state based on the population as a whole. A good example of this might be a sportsperson who, having sustained an injury during a game, is carried off to hospital for treatment and then spends some time recovering. When is this patient better? When he or she is able to leave hospital? Return to work? Kick a ball around the garden with a son or daughter? It is now generally accepted by the medical professions that such a patient would only be considered better when able to regain their team position and play at the same level as before the injury.

Environmental and social factors have to be considered too. All diseases result from a combination of genetic and environmental factors, necessitating the adoption of a more individualistic approach to treatment in many instances. For example, some farmers suffer symptoms of poisoning after dipping sheep with insecticides containing organophosphates while others do not. These compounds act by inhibiting acetyl-cholinesterase, an enzyme that can vary widely in its activity within the population. If exposure to the organophosphate is relatively minor there could be sufficient excess activity of the enzyme present to accommodate some reduction in activity without the effects being noticed. If, however, enzyme activity is at a critical level the slightest exposure to the organophosphate will cause symptoms of poisoning.

Lifestyle and family status may also affect a person's ability to combat disease. A degree of anaemia that was unnoticeable to an inactive person might be seriously incapacitating to an energetic person playing sport at altitude.

Pain thresholds, like other aspects of the person, can vary widely with age and gender.

It may be necessary to involve more than one health professional to treat all aspects of a disease. This idea is being slowly accepted by orthodox practitioners and it is becoming more common for physicians to involve, for example, social workers and others in constructing an individualised treatment plan.

It might help to understand the holistic approach better if we consider for a moment two different ways of treating the following (hypothetical) case:

A foreign tourist is knocked down by a cyclist while crossing the road and looking the wrong way to check for oncoming traffic. He sustains a number of lacerations to his arm but does not seek medical help and the wound subsequently becomes infected. This unfortunate person then contracts septicaemia and eventually dies. The series of events can be represented in a linear fashion, as shown in Figure 1.1.

There is a clear link here between the fall and the injury, the injury and the infection, and so on. The link between the fall and death is rather more

Figure 1.1   The linear approach to treatment

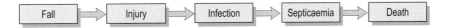

Figure 1.2   The holistic approach to treatment

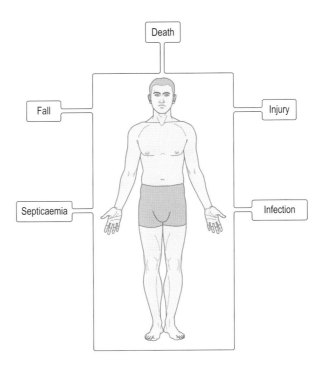

tenuous. This means that each episode is treated in isolation, when in fact they are all interrelated. If we now look at the scenario in a holistic way we see an altogether different approach. Here we relate each of the medical states back to the patient individually and look at treating each one (Fig. 1.2).

The holistic practitioner thus needs to know the answers to a number of questions; for example:

- Why didn't the tourist hear the cyclist? Perhaps he was deaf, or inebriated?
- Why didn't he bother to have the lacerations treated?
- What were the environmental factors that caused his wounds to become infected?

In this way a complete picture of the patient can be painted and an individualised treatment plan designed, though in this case the patient outcome could not have been improved without earlier intervention – once septicaemia had set in it was too late. Of course there is also a linear relationship between the sequence of events, but the 'systems approach' just outlined adds to and complements the healing process.

The holistic approach may be demonstrated by the following two cases:

Case Study: 40-year-old patient

Mr J, aged 40, requests something to treat spasmodic diarrhoea. You note that he is wearing protective clothing that has paint splattered on it and he walks with a pronounced limp.

Conventional thinking might lead you to offer an antidiarrhoeal drug. If a closer look is taken, however, additional facts emerge. As well as the normal questions that a medicines' assistant or a pharmacist might ask in an OTC situation involving a request for a diarrhoea remedy, the following would be important to consider:

1. His clothing suggests that he might be a painter.
2. The spasmodic nature of the condition might indicate association with a particular work procedure.
3. The limp might be important.

It transpires that Mr J is in fact a painter and decorator with an allergy that is worse when he works indoors and the paint fumes are confined. He confirms that this is precisely when his diarrhoea is at its most troublesome. When he last went to his GP he was prescribed an antihistamine, but it made him drowsy and he fell off his ladder – hence the limp. In the light of this information the patient might be counselled to help him manage the problem more efficiently. He could be offered a more appropriate antihistamine (so he does not fall off his ladder again!) or a homeopathic remedy, either alone or on a complementary basis.

Case Study: 20-year-old patient

Ms L is a 20-year-old woman with red rings around her eyes who asks in a soft voice for something to stop diarrhoea. Half way through the conversation she yawns and apologises profusely. The following can be determined without asking any questions:

1. The red eyes may signify that she has been crying.
2. The yawn might indicate a lack of sleep.

3. The general appearance is possibly consistent with Ms L being a student.

Ms L is indeed a student, who has been studying all night and is extremely anxious about her forthcoming examinations. Here a homeopathic remedy for anxiety – Argent nitricum (Argent nit) – would be appropriate. This remedy also has antidiarrhoeal properties.

Thus, by adopting a holistic approach, we reveal that two apparently similar cases of diarrhoea require quite different approaches.

Another feature that is taken into consideration in applying the holistic concept is the patient's personality. This is not totally foreign to orthodox practice. It is often the case that patients seeking treatment for various minor conditions are advised differently according to their attitude or demeanour. A loud, bombastic person is likely to be treated rather less sympathetically than a quiet mild-mannered one, and may even be offered a different medicine. This approach is typically carried out in a rather covert manner; in a pharmacy it may follow a whispered consultation among staff in the back of the premises. In one American study, medical staff were found to have given placebos to unpopular patients who were suspected of exaggerating their pain or had failed to respond to traditional medication (Goodwin et al., 1979). The holistic practitioner fully acknowledges that people have different personalities and overtly treats them while taking this fact into consideration. Thus people suffering from similar symptoms may be subject to very different interventions; similarly, a particular intervention may be used to treat an array of different symptoms in different people.

The question as to how GPs and non-medically qualified trained professional practitioners (see Ch. 12) describe their homeopathic treatment models for asthma and allergy has been investigated (Launsø and Rieper, 2005). Six GPs and 11 professional homeopaths participated in semi-structured interviews. The main difference was in the descriptions of the purpose of treatment. While GPs understood asthma and allergy as independent entities in reference to physiological reactions and conditions, the professional homeopaths understood asthma and allergy as symptoms of something underlying. However, the GPs developed, on the basis of their clinical experience, a more multifactorial explanation of asthma and allergy. Further, the professional homeopaths did not consider it entirely necessary to make a diagnosis before treatment was initiated. A working hypothesis or assumptions can be disproved or confirmed by the effect of medicine. It was not the asthma or allergy that determined which homeopathic medicine was chosen, but the person's overall symptom or reaction pattern. The purpose of the interview was to identify the homeopathic medicine and not the disease.

Obviously it is impossible to spend the time necessary for a full CAM consultation in a busy healthcare environment such as in a pharmacy. In homeopathy there is a range of homeopathic remedies, known as polychrests, which have a wide spectrum of activity (see Ch. 8). Experience over many years has shown that they can be used to treat a large number of simple, self-limiting conditions without the need for the protracted investigations implied above. There are also remedies that are considered to be specific for a given condition. This book concentrates mainly on specifics and polychrests, and how they can be used in the treatment of acute problems, although chronic disease and other remedies will be mentioned as well.

Many manufacturers also have 'specialities' – herbal and aromatherapy products and also mixtures of homeopathic polychrests and other remedies (known as complexes) that give specific indications for use: 'for rheumatic pain', 'for colds and flu', etc. (see Ch. 4). Homeopathic complexes are extremely popular in many countries: in the USA for example, almost 90% of all health food outlets keep them (see Ch. 8).

The holistic approach to treating patients using interdisciplinary care is being increasingly embraced in modern orthodox medicine. In a study carried out among elderly patients in Airedale, England (Aveyard, 1995), nearly 76% of respondents were considered to be in need of help or complete supervision with medicine administration. The author concluded that there was a definite need for a pharmaceutical contribution to 'the multidisciplinary assessment of such people' (Aveyard, 1995). The healthcare strategy documents issued by the health authorities of all four countries in the UK in the period 2001–2004 were based on putting patients at the core of the healthcare system. In Scotland, the pharmaceutical community has embraced care, a holistic culture involving interdisciplinary cooperation was quickly established.

Not all members of professions making a contribution to the health team are in accord with the concept of holistic therapy (McKee, 1988). The sociological literature often highlights the fact that in concentrating on individuals, the needs of the wider community may be overlooked. When responsibility for maintaining a healthy lifestyle is shifted to a single person, the social structures that constrain individual behaviour and lifestyle choices may thereby be obscured (Labonte and Penfold, 1981). It has been suggested that this emphasis on such apparent weaknesses in the holistic view may be the reason for its lack of acceptance in the past.

The alternative and complementary approaches to health care

Some years ago the following tragic headline appeared in a newspaper: 'Child killed by homeopathic remedy'. The story related the case of an infant who had died from meningitis, having been given homeopathic medicines (or 'remedies' as they are often called) by her parents in place of the antibiotics prescribed by their family doctor. A far more accurate heading would have been 'Child dies through lack of antibiotics'. More recently there have been reports in the pharmaceutical press of a patient trying to treat insulin-dependent diabetes with homeopathy.

These cases demonstrate the unfortunate approach adopted by some people who believe they must have homeopathy or nothing. This idea has been refuted since the earliest days of homeopathy. As an example, in his address to the first annual meeting of the British Homeopathic Society, held in August 1846, Dr F. H. Quin, generally credited with introducing homeopathy to Britain, counselled against rejecting orthodox medicine out of hand:

> In order to build a temple to Hahnemann it is not necessary to endeavour to destroy that raised to Hippocrates ... Let us admire and do justice to their [here he was referring to his allopathic colleagues] learning and honourable conduct, whilst we lament their blindness to the great truths contained in our doctrines. (Quin, 1862)

This was, however, a rather different view to that expressed by Hahnemann, the founder of homeopathy, who disliked the idea of 'half homeopaths', as he called homeopathic colleagues who also used non-homeopathic medicines in their practice.

The words 'complementary' and 'alternative' are often used interchangeably (please note the spelling 'complementary' – with an 'e' in the middle; 'complimentary' has quite a different meaning). In the past, UK health professionals tended to use the former term only, because it implied an ability to complement, or complete, other treatments. It was believed that CAM was more likely to be used concurrently with other therapies rather than in isolation (Sharma, 1992). It is not unusual for homeopathic physicians in the UK to prescribe an antimicrobial and a homeopathic remedy (e.g. Belladonna) on the same prescription form. Further, in some cases CAM practitioners may use more than one complementary discipline in a treatment schedule. For example, asthma may be treated by a whole range of therapies including relaxation, breathing exercises, hypnosis, chiropractic, homeopathy and massage (Ernst, 1998).

As noted above, the terms 'alternative' and 'complementary' are often used interchangeably to describe a large number of holistic therapies. 'Alternative', however, implies that one must choose between two courses of action, for example, whether to treat a patient with orthodox medicine alone (sometimes called *allopathy*, a term that implies the use of drugs that have opposite effects to the symptoms) or with homeopathy alone. In fact, as described, there are many instances when patients can enjoy the best of both worlds by using homeopathy to support other medical disciplines. Further examples might include:

- In both the meningitis and diabetes examples given above, homeopathy could have been used alongside orthodox medication.
- Homeopathy provides a method of treating minor conditions suffered by HIV-positive and AIDS patients where orthodox medication is likely to interact with existing drug regimens. Some workers even think that certain aspects of AIDS might be treated successfully with homeopathy (Rastogi et al., 1993), although there is no clear-cut evidence that this is so. Silver (1993) has reported the use of different mother tinctures and nosodes (see Ch. 8) during inert phases of the disease and claims that the use of potentised drugs can be of major importance where patients take prescribed medicines such as AZT and fluconazole, to reduce or neutralise side-effects. Homeopathy also provides a method of addressing psycho-emotional factors.
- Drug abuse is another example of the complementary applications of homeopathy. There has been increasing recognition that the problems of drug abuse are not homogeneous, but are symptoms associated with a wide variety of social and environmental problems. Treatment for individuals abusing drugs needs to offer different approaches to deal with the physical craving, but also medicines geared to their highly individual needs. Remedies can be used to treat nervous excitement and sleeplessness, persistent nausea, vomiting and colic without interfering with the detoxification programme. In an Indian study, homeopathic treatment is reported to have been successful in supporting a group of 30 addicts undergoing opiate withdrawal (Bakshi and Singhal, 1993).
- The successful treatment of gum disease should include a consideration of the patient's resistance to the problem. Homeopathy can help greatly by complementing orthodox therapy in providing support for lowered resistance to dental problems (Stevenson, 1994).

These examples all demonstrate how homeopathy can assume a complementary role, supporting a course of orthodox treatment rather than replacing it. There are occasions – for instance where the body needs relatively large amounts of vitamins, minerals or hormones to correct some deficiency – when homeopathy cannot be used alone. Thus, there are no homeopathic iron tablets, HRT drugs or oral contraceptives. Having said that, the remedy Medorrhinum has been reported as curing iron deficiency anaemia (Schore, 1993), and some homeopaths claim success in treating conditions that would normally require hormone replacement therapy (HRT) but where the patients concerned are unsuitable for HRT because they have had hysterectomies for malignancy.

There are, in addition, conditions for which we do not have any suitable orthodox medicines. For instance, complementary medicines can offer a solution for morning sickness in pregnancy, or anxiety prior to examinations.

The term 'complementary', since it implies a degree of flexibility, is to be preferred to 'alternative' in the healthcare environment. A similar shift in attitude towards a complementary approach has recently been adopted by the British Medical Association (BMA, 1993). Not all homeopaths agree with the distinction between the two terms, however, believing that we should not use either, and that the use of such terms will lead to a marginalisation of homeopathy and a tendency by colleagues to equate allopathy with medicine or pharmacy in total.

In recent years there has been a move towards using the term 'complementary and alternative medicine' (CAM), a designation popular in North America. Certainly there is evidence that clients purchasing homeopathic medicines over the counter in a pharmacy do so *instead of*, rather than in addition to, orthodox medicines (Kayne et al., 1999).

According to Guajardo et al. (1994), we should be campaigning to have homeopathy viewed as a specialty. Like other specialties, homeopathy (or 'homeotherapeutics') depends on a broad scope of application, a depth of expertise and a research programme for its survival and growth. These elements should be encouraged.

FACTORS PROMPTING THE CURRENT INTEREST IN COMPLEMENTARY AND ALTERNATIVE THERAPIES

The most significant factor leading to the re-emergence of complementary and alternative medicine in modern times was the events surrounding the use in pregnancy of the drug thalidomide to treat morning sickness. Soon after the drug was introduced in Europe in 1956 a shocked public became acutely aware of the risks associated with the administration of medicines, for within 5 years more than 8000 deformed children had been born to mothers who had taken the drug during the first trimester of their pregnancy. From these tragic occurrences regulatory authorities all over the world learnt of the dangers of drug approval without proper testing programmes (BMA, 1990).

With gathering intensity, consumers began asking searching questions about the use of prescribed medication and the issue of accountability became a much more important one for major pharmaceutical producers. By 1981, awareness of adverse drug reactions was such that 36% of all patients admitted to a hospital in Boston were identified as suffering from iatrogenic symptoms (Steele et al., 1981). In consequence patients began seeking alternative unorthodox treatments and the demand for complementary medicine took off, alongside the so-called 'green revolution'. The principle of choice has created a new market-led environment rather than the previous product-led situation where relatively uninformed patients were treated as their doctor or pharmacist decided and had little input into the management of their own condition. These changes have meant that the way healthcare providers practise has had to change as well, with a requirement to provide better patient service in terms of facilities and advice. The demand for complementary medicine is one result of this changing scenario.

In recent years other factors have changed the whole process of healthcare delivery in the UK, facilitating the uptake of CAM. These include:

- The development of a healthcare system that puts patients at its core and respects individual choice.
- The increasing numbers of drugs removed from the market due to adverse reactions.
- The wider availability of diagnostic screening, placing emphasis on prophylaxis.
- The opening up of prescribing under the UK National Health Service to professions allied to medicine and professional and non-medically qualified therapists.

THE PROFILE OF CAM USERS

Increasingly research has begun to investigate the prevalence of CAM use and the profile of CAM users. Users are more likely to be female, be better educated, have a higher income, and be employed (MacLennan et al., 2002). Research also reveals that users tend to employ CAM alongside conventional health services, are more likely to be married than not, to be aged between 35 and 49 and to have poorer health status than non-CAM users (Adams et al., 2003). They are more likely to have used CAM before their current illness than non-users (Harris et al., 2003).

The majority of CAM profile work has been undertaken in North America (Russell, 2004), with research by Eisenberg et al. (1998) being widely quoted in the literature. According to a US nationwide survey, 36% of US adults used some form of CAM during the previous 12 months (CDC, 2004). And when prayer specifically for health reasons is included in the definition of CAM, the percentage of US adults using some form of CAM rose to 62%. The survey was developed by the National Center for Complementary and Alternative Medicine (NCCAM) (http://nccam.nih.gov) and the CDC's (Centers for Disease Control and Prevention) National Center for Health Statistics (NCHS) and included interviews from 31 044 adults aged 18 years or more.

Survey results indicated that CAM was most often used to treat back pain or back problems, head or chest colds, neck pain or neck problems, joint pain or stiffness, and anxiety or depression. The 10 most commonly used CAM therapies and the percentage of US adults using each therapy are: prayer for own health (43%); prayer by others for the respondent's health (24%); natural products such as herbs, other botanicals and enzymes (19%); deep breathing exercises (12%); participation in prayer group for own health

(10%); meditation (8%); chiropractic care (8%); yoga (5%); massage (5%); and diet-based therapies.

The profile of homeopathic consumers

In a study carried out between December 1996 and March 1998, 120 community pharmacies were selected randomly from the British Homeopathic Association's list of independent and small chain (less than five outlets) pharmacies known to sell homeopathic remedies (Kayne et al., 1999). Of these 120 pharmacies, which were located across England, Scotland and Wales, 109 (91% of the total) agreed to participate in the study. Questionnaire cards were offered to buyers of homeopathic remedies on a first-come first-served basis. The questionnaire covered five main areas: (a) personal information about the buyer; (b) information about the remedy (for whom it was bought? what it was for? how often and for how long it was taken?); (c) reasons for buying a homeopathic remedy; (d) whether or not the remedy was considered effective; and (e) what other complementary treatments were used on a regular basis or whether they were taken as monotherapy.

The survey showed that it is generally the higher socio-economic groups who buy OTC homeopathic medicines. With frequently higher discretionary incomes, these groups may also be less price sensitive than other groups. This may mean that pharmacies can use more flexible pricing policies. It may also suggest that buyers of OTC homeopathic medicines are intelligent enough to become well-informed about their purchases and be in a position to make a sensible assessment of the products.

However, there is some recent evidence to suggest that the market is developing and the use of CAM may now be wider than found in this survey and no longer confined to any circumscribed socio-economic group (Wolsko et al., 2000). A Norwegian study found considerable differences in the homeopathic consumer profile over a 13-year period between 1985 and 1998 (Steinbekk and Fønnebø, 2003). The authors concluded that patients visiting homeopaths in 1998 differed in age and in diseases treated compared to previous users of homeopathy and general practice patients.

There was a predominance of polychrest homeopathic medicines bought by respondents. This is understandable for they are the type of remedies best suited to the OTC environment. With polychrests buyers can readily equate remedies with ailments and so buy the medicine most likely to be effective for their particular condition. Retailers also benefit by not having to offer what can be lengthy and complex advice to buyers. Point-of-sale materials such as charts and leaflets available in some of the multiples largely obviate the need for advice from the pharmacy staff which can be very costly in terms of staff time. They may also reduce the need for extensive training for staff in homeopathy. However, the very large number of homeopathic medicines available and the complexity of matching remedies and ailments may still be confusing to some patients who will seek advice from the staff. One problem is that there may be several remedies for the same ailment. Some patients also like the comfort of a confirmatory word from the pharmacist or another member of staff when buying untried medicines.

Most of the buyers of homeopathic medicines in this study had bought them before, though they were not asked how many times or for how long they had been buying them. The authors suspected that many respondents had bought them for many years and that any advertising that does take place is not very effective in bringing new buyers into the market and generating sales.

Concern was expressed at the excessive length of time for which some respondents had taken their remedies; this ranged from a few days to several years. Most homeopathic remedies offered for sale over the counter are designed for short-term administration. Long-term chronic conditions are best treated under the guidance of a practitioner. While taking homeopathic medicines for long periods should not do any harm, since the medicines are not in themselves harmful, patients may suffer because they may not be receiving appropriate treatment for their condition. On the other hand, there are many skilled and knowledgeable people who may be self-treating effectively over longer periods of time, so no firm conclusions can be drawn. Another factor which allows patients to continue to use the medicines longer than advised is the number of tablets in a typical container, namely 125. Taken at a rate of three tablets per day, a single container will last well over a month, which could be too long for an acute condition.

Almost all homeopathic medicines are classed as GSL (general sales list) in the UK and may thus be distributed through health stores and groceries as well as pharmacies. Homeopathic remedies are considered to be medicines under UK law and there is a feeling among many health professionals that sales of all medicinal products should be restricted to places where professional advice is available. In fact, some studies have shown that staff in health stores are often better trained than staff in pharmacies and the major pharmacy groups are working to rectify this by improving the training given to pharmacy staff on homeopathy and other complementary treatments.

A further issue is that of licensing regulations. EU Directive 92/73/EEC presently precludes claims of efficacy on newly registered remedies, although this does not prevent the formulation of local national rules to allow restricted claims in the future. At the time of writing there is discussion concerning the formulation of a scheme that will allow products not covered by the European Directive (e.g. injections) to be licensed and make limited claims of therapeutic benefit (see Ch. 2).

It is thus important for unskilled purchasers to be able to obtain advice from a source other than the product label and this is often achieved by point-of-sale materials, specifically charts and leaflets. In fact some remedies do have claims of efficacy on the label. These are products with product licences of right (PLR); these were granted to all products on the market at the time of the Medicines Act 1968. As yet there are no plans to require PLR to be converted to full product licences.

A study was carried out in Manchester on a sample of health store clients (Reid, 2002). Results were largely similar to those obtained by Kayne et al. (1999). In addition, Reid found 13% of respondents were using homeopathy concurrently with prescription drugs.

THE REASONS FOR THE DEMAND FOR CAM

The demand for CAM is in part a search for a broader range of therapies, but is also a call for a different approach to care, with less emphasis on drugs and a more 'whole person' approach (Reilly, 2001). Mostly, people look to CAM when orthodoxy has failed. But CAM is also increasingly becoming a first-line intervention for some, because of the worry about the side-effects of conventional treatments and a perception that orthodoxy has become dehumanised.

Vincent and Furnham (1996) divided the reasons into 'push' and 'pull' factors. *Push factors* relate to the perceived dangers of using conventional medicines, such as drug toxicity and invasive techniques, which encourage patients to seek safer alternatives. *Pull factors* are those that encourage people to use complementary treatments (usually for particular complaints) while at the same time continuing to use orthodox treatments for other complaints. There are several reasons why people choose to use homeopathic medicines. These reasons can be expressed in terms of Vincent and Furnham's push and pull categories:

Push factors

Perception of drug risks

Perceptions of drug risks have been found likely to influence patients' treatment choices (Von Wartburg, 1984). The attitudes and perceptions of a representative sample of Swedish adults with respect to a number of common risks have been studied by Slovic et al. (1989). Respondents characterised themselves as people who disliked taking risks and who resisted taking medicines unless forced to do so. Evidence for safety and efficacy appeared to make people much more tolerant of any risks. Prescription drugs (except for sleeping pills and antidepressants) were perceived to be high in benefit and low in risk. Homeopathic remedies were not included in the study, but the results for herbal medicines showed an extremely low perceived risk, only slightly higher than vitamin pills, and a perceived benefit approximately equal to vitamin pills, contraceptives and aspirin. The distinction between homeopathic and herbal preparations is not always readily appreciated by the general public (Kayne, 2005). For the purposes of this discussion a parallel will be drawn between the two as far as patients' perceptions are concerned. Homeopathy and the other related therapies that collectively make up complementary medicine are considered by many people to be attractive because they have acceptable risk:benefit ratios.

Disenchantment with orthodox medicine

It has been suggested that people who choose complementary medicine may do so from disenchantment with, and bad experiences of, orthodox medical practitioners, rather than a belief that traditional medicine is ineffective (Furnham and Smith, 1988). It is known that several factors affect the length and quality of a consultation in orthodox medicine (OM), including: the socio-economic status of the patient, the gender of the practitioner and the gender of the patient (Saxena et al., 1995; Howie et al., 1999: Deveugele et al., 2002).

Bakx (1991) has summarised some of the possible reasons for the development of widespread discontent with OM amongst users of CAM. OM has:

- culturally distanced itself from the consumers of its services
- failed to match its promises with real breakthroughs in combating disease created by modern lifestyles
- alienated patients through unsympathetic or ineffectual practitioner–patient interaction.

With the advent of healthcare consumerism, and as a result of a finite health budget, people are now encouraged to be largely responsible for their own health. And that does not apply only to self-treating trivial ailments. It means having a 'responsible' lifestyle too.

Balint and co-workers have reported a series of investigations based on the analysis of doctor–patient consultations to answer the question: 'Why does it happen so often, that, in spite of earnest efforts on both sides, the relationship between patient and doctor is unsatisfactory and even unhappy?' (Balint, 1971). Balint pointed out that these situations can be truly unfortunate; the patient is desperately in need of help and the doctor tries his or her hardest, but still, despite sincere efforts on both sides, things go wrong. One conclusion reached by the researchers was that the doctor should arrive at a diagnosis not on the basis of physical signs and symptoms alone, but also from a consideration of the so-called 'neurotic' symptoms. It is likely that many doctors' beliefs, personality and behavioural standards affect the way in which patients are treated. This means that the management of a patient's disease may vary widely according to the practitioner consulted. Time is an important factor. In one large English survey 12% of patients complained about having insufficient time with their general practitioner, but this figure rose to 30% when patients were seen for 5 minutes or less (Department of Health, 1998).

With CAM a diagnosis is not necessarily required as a prelude to a prescription. The intervention is based on symptomatology and the individual's characteristics and though the consultation takes longer it involves a higher degree of patient interaction and may therefore be perceived as more sympathetic.

Furnham et al. (1995) asked three groups of CAM patients and an OM group to compare the consultation styles of GPs and CAM practitioners. CAM practitioners were generally perceived as having more time to listen. Ernst et al. (1997) tested the hypothesis that patients judge the manner of non-medically trained complementary practitioners more favourably than that of their GPs.

It may be that the discontent is due not just to the failings of conventional medicine itself, but to a new consciousness of the value of involving the individual in his or her well-being and a new sense of the value of being 'natural'. Patients are no longer willing to be treated in a paternalistic 'I know best' manner with standardised medication. They want a sensitive recognition of themselves as an unwell person, rather than accept treatment for a disease in isolation.

Reduced efficacy of existing medication

Some patients are thought have turned to homeopathy as a result of a dissatisfaction with the efficacy of allopathic medicine (Avina and Schneiderman, 1978). This has, rather unkindly, been called the 'Have you got something else?' syndrome. Skin conditions treated with steroids fall into this category; as time proceeds, patients often claim that the efficacy of the various topical preparations available lessens.

Pull factors

Time to consider more than just symptoms

It has been suggested that homeopathy appeals to patients who like the feeling that attention is being paid to more aspects of themselves than just the symptoms (English, 1986). In a survey of 161 CAM practioners carried out by White et al. (1997) it was found that the mean time spent with patients for a first consultation was 75 minutes (Acupuncture), 90 minutes (Homeopathy) and 40 minutes (Chiropractic). Subsequent consultations were between a third and a half less. There is substantial interpractice variation in consultation length of allopathic GPs in the Uk, from a mean of 5.7 minutes to one of 8.5 minutes (Carr-Hill et al., 1998). In some practices the longest average GP consultation time is about twice that of the shortest. However, correlational analysis of patients from nine GP practices was used to test the hypothesis that patients' perceptions of consultation length are influenced not just by actual consultation length, but by other aspects of their experience of consultations (Cape, 2002). Patient concerns about time may be as much about quality time as about actual time.

Financial reasons

National Health prescribing. In the UK homeopathic remedies may be prescribed on GP10/FP10/WP10 forms (and also on doctors' stock forms in Scotland). The net ingredient cost is, on average, substantially less than the cost of the newer orthodox medicines for a similar course of treatment, although this figure does not take into account the longer consultation times and does vary widely. In the case of older non-proprietary allopathic drugs the costs may be lower than homeopathic remedies.

A comparison of prescribing costs is presented in Table 1.1. The allopathic drugs are examples of those frequently prescribed within each therapeutic group. The homeopathic remedies are not direct equivalent medications to the allopathic drugs, but are merely given as examples of the type of remedies that might be considered for symptomatic treatment.

Apart from Jeremy Swayne (1992) who carried out a study on the prescribing costs of 21 doctors, there has been relatively little economic evaluation work to examine the cost-effectiveness of homeopathy. The results

Table 1.1 Comparison of costs of allopathic and homeopathic treatment

Therapeutic group	Allopathic drug	Cost (£)	Example of homeopathic symptomatic drug	Cost (£)
Analgesics	Co-dydramol	1.75	Belladonna	2.20
	Paracetamol	0.75		
Antiasthmatic	Salbutamol inhaler	1.78	Ipecacuanha	2.20
	Beclometasone	8.24		
Antirheumatics	Diclofenac retard	12.72	Rhus tox	2.20
	Ibuprofen 400 mg	2.46		
	Piroxicam 20 mg	3.13		
Cardiovascular	Propranolol	0.54	Baryta mur	2.20
	Nifedipine retard	8.50		
Diuretics	Amiloride	1.51	Apis	2.20
	Co-amilofruse	2.58		
	Furosemide	0.64		
GI tract	Famotidine	9.80	Arsen alb	2.20
	Ranitidine	5.13		
Hypnotics	Temazepam	0.62	Coffea, Passiflora	2.20
	Zopiclone	3.26		
Laxatives	Ispaghula	4.24	Nux vomica	2.20
	Lactulose	2.00		
	Senna	0.86		

suggested that doctors practising homeopathic medicine issue fewer prescriptions and at a lower cost than their colleagues. Unfortunately, there were several serious limitations to the study, not the least being that the sample was too small to allow generalisations to be made. As with the comparisons above, no account was taken of the extended consultation times involved. When it was published the survey gained widespread attention in the press and the results have certainly contributed to discussions on widening the availability of homeopathy in the health service. Similar cost advantages have been identified amongst German dental surgeons (Feldhaus, 1993).

Jain (2003) collected data for 4 years on 100 patients treated homeopathically. Costs of homeopathic remedies and costs of conventional drugs that otherwise would be prescribed for these patients was calculated for the total duration of treatment. Average cost savings per patient was £60.40 As with Swayne's study, no allowance was made for the prescribers' consultation time and there is the possibility that patients were chosen according to the potential likelihood of savings being made rather than at random.

Slade et al. (2004) claimed an annual saving of £2807.30 in a study that evaluated the effect of a GP led practice-based homeopathy service on symptoms, activity, well-being, general practice consultation rate and the use of conventional medication. A limitation of this result was the absence of a control group.

A study was carried out in 80 general medical practices in Belgium where physicians were members of the Unio Homeopathica Belgica. All patients and their physicians visiting the practices on a specified day completed a questionnaire (Van Wassenhoven and Ives, 2004). A total of 782 patients presented with diseases of all major organ systems Patients were very satisfied with their homeopathic treatment, both they and their physicians recorded significant improvement. Costs of homeopathic treatment were significantly lower than conventional treatment, and many previously prescribed drugs were discontinued.

Trichard et al. (2005) carried out a pharmacoeconomic comparison between homeopathic and antibiotic treatment strategies in recurrent acute rhinopharyngitis in children and concluded that the former could a offer cost-effective alternative.

A report commissioned by the Prince of Wales into the cost of complementary medicines sparked controversy in August 2005 even before its scheduled publication later in the year (Henderson and Pierce, 2005). Prince Charles asked an independent economist to work out how much such therapies could save the UK National Health Service. A draft of the report was sent to Professor Ernst in Exeter who criticised it publicly, saying that the conclusions were 'outrageous and deeply flawed' and there was a danger that 'unproved treatments could be integrated into the NHS at the expense of other treatments'.

There is also some advantage to the patient of having prescribed homeopathic remedies, because in nearly all cases the cost of the remedy will be less than the UK prescription tax and pharmacists will generally invite patients who are subject to it to buy the remedies OTC at the lower retail price (see below).

OTC purchases. In the UK most homeopathic remedies retail at about half the cost of an average OTC sale for a similar course of treatment, making them an attractive buy for customers.

Ernst and White (2000) have reported that, on average, British CAM users spent approximately £13.62 on CAM per month, which extrapolates to an annual expenditure of £1.6 billion for the whole nation. There is some evidence that the price may be rising; in a survey carried out in a health authority area in Wales 3 years later (Harris et al., 2003), 49.6% of the respondents (534 people) reported using at least one type of CAM during the past 12 months: 16.4% (221) said they had consulted a CAM practitioner (average cost per person, £28 per month); 15.4% (166) indicated using CAM techniques (average cost per person, £16 per month), and 42.3% (456) reported using OTC diets, remedies or supplements at an average cost of £10 per month per person.

In Australia a rising trend has also been identified: a 120% and a 62% increase in the cost of alternative medicines and therapists, respectively, between 1993 and 2000. In 2000 expenditure on alternative therapies was nearly four times the public contribution to all pharmaceuticals (MacLennan et al., 2002).

The 'green' association

Complementary medicine is often portrayed as being 'natural' by the media and this approach appeals to the fads and fashions of the 'green' lobby. We will see the importance of media exposure shortly. Together with a significant spin-off from royal interest, this has had the effect of making more people aware of the potential advantages of homeopathy and of stimulating demand.

Encouragement by the media

There is no doubt that patients are being encouraged to question the suitability of existing treatments. For instance, in her book entitled *Controversies in Health Care Policies*, the celebrated English Rabbi Julia Neuberger states that patients should ask their family doctor a series of questions, including the following:

- What is the likely outcome if I do not have the treatment you are offering?
- What alternative treatments are available?
- What are the most common side-effects?
- Would you use this treatment?

Newspapers are also encouraging patients to ask questions about their treatment and so make doctors accountable. 'Patient power makes the doctor think twice' stated the *Glasgow Herald* on 9 December 1994. Such a trend has not gone unnoticed by the medical profession, as the following comment from a *British Medical Journal* leader shows: 'Patients are sophisticated consumers who are challenging the unique authority of doctors.' Such developments are affecting all health professionals, not just our medical colleagues.

Royal support

The Royal Family have always been keen proponents of homeopathy. In particular, Prince Charles' patronage of homeopathy is well documented and it is thought that this has encouraged many people to try the remedies. His grandmother, the late Queen Mother, was patron of the British Homeopathic Association for many years.

Cultural reasons

Increased demand has been generated by mobility across national borders of people whose cultural backgrounds emphasise the use of holistic forms of medicine. Thus, migrants from the Indian subcontinent, and from China, take their customs with them when they migrate. Either from an inherent mistrust of Western medicine or from a misunderstanding of what it can achieve, such people prefer to continue using traditional methods that have proved successful over many centuries.

For all the above reasons there has been a significant and steady increase in the number of requests for homeopathic medicines in pharmacies and health stores over the past 15 years, and this has been matched closely by a similar trend with requests for homeopathic veterinary preparations for the treatment of both domestic and farm animals.

THE MOST POPULAR APPLICATIONS OF CAM

Perceptions are notoriously fickle and are often based on misconceptions. Knowing what our patients think about holistic treatments and where they obtain their information is important in designing education programmes and introducing the disciplines to new patients. Vincent and Furnham (1994) have examined the perceived efficacy of acupuncture, herbalism, homeopathy, hypnosis and osteopathy. They showed that conventional medicine was clearly seen by the majority of respondents as being more effective in the treatment of most complaints. Complementary medicine, on the other hand, was seen as being most useful in specific conditions, including depression, stress and smoking cessation (where hypnosis was superior to conventional medicine), and in the treatment of common colds and skin problems. Among those with a strong belief in complementary medicine, homeopathy and herbalism were also seen as valuable in chronic and psychological conditions. Overall, for all conditions, herbalism appeared slightly more popular than homeopathy and acupuncture, but homeopathy was favoured in the treatment of allergies.

A telephone survey at the end of 2000 carried out by the University of Exeter for BBC Radio revealed that 20% of people contacted in the UK had used some form of CAM in that year, with herbalism, aromatherapy, homeopathy, acupuncture, massage and reflexology proving the most popular therapies (Ernst and White, 2000). This compares with the 1991 figure of 26% quoted by Fisher and Ward (1994) and the figure of 10.5% derived from a pilot random study by Vickers (1994). Among patient populations there is a variability in the usage of CAM ranging from 17% in diabetic patients (Leese et al., 1997) to 69% of patients with psoriasis (Clark et al., 1998). CAM therapies are popular with patients who are HIV seropositive despite effective drug treatments, potential drug interactions and overlapping toxicities (Bica et al., 2003). If potential clients can be directed towards homeopathy with its positive risk:benefit ratio potential adverse reactions can be avoided. Sparber et al. (2000) have identified and characterised patterns of use of CAM by HIV/AIDS patients participating in clinical trials in a research setting. A total of 91% of the cohort ($n = 100$) had used at least one CAM therapy to treat dermatological problems, nausea, depression, insomnia or weakness.

UK regional usage was shown by Ernst and White to be highest in Wales (32%), and south-east England (23%) and lowest in the west midlands (16%) and northern England (13%). The main reasons for trying CAM were its perceived effectiveness, a positive inclination towards it, and its relaxing effects. Rates in the UK are appreciably lower than in many other European countries. For example, in Germany up to 65% of respondents may now use CAM, in the Netherlands 50–60% and in France 50%.

Table 1.2   Comparative usage of complementary medicine (Fisher and Ward, 1994)

% of population using:	Complementary medicine	Acupuncture	Homeopathy	Osteopathy chiropractic	Herbal medicine
Belgium	31	19	56	19	31
Denmark	23	12	28	23	No info
France	49	21	32	7	12
Germany	46	No info	No info	No info	No info
Netherlands	20	16	31	No info	No info
Spain	25	12	15	48	No info
UK	26	16	16	36	24
USA	34	3	3	30	9

If one compares the popularity of examples of complementary medicine across several countries some interesting idiosyncrasies emerge with respect to individual preferences and the estimated percentage of the population using complementary medicine. Table 1.2 shows that consumer surveys demonstrate positive public attitudes to complementary disciplines in many countries, with France and Germany leading the way. In Spain and the UK the most popular treatments appear to be the manipulative disciplines. Herbal medicine is more popular than homeopathy in the UK.

THE MARKET FOR CAM

The retail market for herbal, homeopathic remedies and aromatherapy oils, taken or used independently or in conjunction with therapy, is believed to have shown growth of 10–15% per year throughout much of the 1990s, although it fell to 7.3% in 2002 and to 5% in 2003. It is expected to rise to over 6.9% in 2006 and 6.5% by 2007. These variations in market value are largely the result of regulatory activity in herbal products, and of certain reports regarding safety and efficacy (Keynote Publications, 2003).

The major retail outlets for herbal and homeopathic remedies remain pharmacies and drugstores, followed by health-food stores. The removal of the final part of resale price maintenance, on OTC medicines, has also allowed grocery multiples to expand their medicines shelf space significantly (as well as open in-store pharmacies), which has indirectly boosted their sales share for alternative remedies.

Aromatherapy oils, however, are sold through a much wider selection of retail outlets, although sales through chemists and drugstores account for 57% of the total (Keynote Publications, 2003).

A report from the US Institute of Medicine, prepared at the request of the National Institutes of Health and the Agency for Healthcare Research and

Quality, has assessed what is known about Americans' reliance on complementary and alternative medicine (Marwick, 2005). It estimated that more than a third of American adults routinely use CAM, spending in excess of $27 billion a year.

The homeopathic market

Following heightened interest in the risk:benefit ratios of medicines in the 1960s and 1970s, homeopathy enjoyed a spectacular revival, growing steadily to an annual market value of around £29 million (Mintel, 2003), of which about half is likely to be OTC with the remainder being prescribed by homeopathic practitioners (Abecassis, 1997). The UK market for all OTC pharmaceuticals in 2002 was £1.73 billion and in 2003 it was estimated at £1.77 billion. These figures represent approximately 16% of the total UK pharmaceutical market of £10.29 billion and £11.27 billion respectively (ABPI, 2003). Thus, the OTC market for homeopathic remedies is very small, accounting for less than 1% of the UK pharmaceutical market. Yet, despite its small size, it is still significant for a number of reasons. These include:

- the growing acceptance of complementary treatments by health professionals and the public
- the large number of people now using such treatments on a regular basis
- the effect of complementary treatments on health status
- the confounding effect on clinical trials because many people are unwilling to admit using such treatments, for fear of admonishment (Vickers, 1994)
- the high usage by older people, females and health practitioners.

In the USA, a survey of 1600 natural foods retailers chosen at random revealed a 23% increase in homeopathic sales between 1991 and 1992, according to a review (Borneman, 1994). Industry sources are currently quoting an aggregate growth rate of 10–14% (Borneman, personal communication, June 2004). The 2002 estimate of the American Homeopathic Pharmaceutical Association showed sales in the USA to be approximately $400 million. Furthermore, while sales to the traditional markets of practitioners and natural food stores remain strong, particular growth is being seen in sales to drug store chains and mass merchandisers. It is estimated that 94% of natural food stores, 50% of independent pharmacies and 95% of chain pharmacies and mass merchandisers (e.g. Wal-Mart) now carry at least one homeopathic pharmaceutical product. Independent and chain groceries have also entered the field. The most typical medicines sold are for teething, leg cramps, coughs, colds and flu, allergies, sinus congestion, muscle soreness, stress and insomnia. Top-selling products include Cold-Eze and Zicam (cough/cold), the Boiron product Oscillococcinum (influenza), Hyland's Teething Tablets (paediatric dentition) and Hyland's Leg Cramps (analgesic). Arnica is reported to be the best-selling single remedy. As in other countries, the increasing demand by consumers is stimulating a reactive response from the market. This social trend is anticipated to support growth in the immediate future (Borneman, personal communication, November 2004). In Borneman's 1994 review, an estimate of the value of the world market for homeopathy was stated as being around US\$1.15 billion. Several important markets were omitted from this estimate; the true figure is probably nearer \$3–4 billion.

THE INTEGRATION OF CAM INTO HEALTH CARE

The rapid rise in demand for homeopathy and other CAM disciplines has largely occurred outside the auspices of conventional medical practice and comparatively little is known about how CAM may be integrated into mainstream care.

In the US, the term 'integrative medicine' is considered to mean more than simply combining conventional medicine and CAM; it is a whole system that includes the patient–practitioner relationship, multiple conventional and CAM treatments and the philosophical context of care (Bell et al., 2002). The dynamics of relationships between practitioners and clients are critical to the effectiveness of healing as a process of transformation (Bolles and Maley, 2004). Conscious examination of practitioners' emotional availability in relationship-centred care may be important in determining primary roles in delivering care. Bolles and Maley also suggest that the relationship between the healers involved in patient care is also of importance All these factors, together with the characteristics of the physical space in which healing is practised (including light, music, architecture and colour), contribute to the establishment of an optimal healing environment (Jonas and Chez, 2004).

A successful integrated healthcare system has been developing since the mid-1980s at Marylebone Health Centre in London and the personnel involved have written a guide to help clinicians, therapists and other health professionals discover their own best approach to integrate CAM into their existing practice (Chaitow et al., 2002). In 1995 Paterson and Peacock described an urban NHS practice in the west of England where four general practitioners worked closely with nine complementary therapists (Paterson and Peacock, 1995). This model was still working well 5 years later (Paterson, 2000). Working in a primary care setting, Riley et al. (2001) found that homeopathy ($n = 281$) appeared to be at least as effective as orthodox medical care ($n = 175$) in the treatment of patients with the following problems: upper respiratory tract complaints including allergies, lower respiratory complaints including allergies, and ear complaints.

In a questionnaire survey of primary healthcare workers in north-west London, general practitioners were targeted in a postal survey; other members of the primary care team, such as district and practice nurses, were targeted via colleagues (Van Haselen et al., 2004). The questionnaire assessed healthcare professionals' perspective on complementary medicine, referrals, ways to integrate complementary medicine into primary care and interest in research on CAM. The results demonstrated considerable interest in CAM among primary care professionals, and many are already referring or suggesting referral. Such referrals are driven mainly by patient demand and by dissatisfaction with the results of conventional medicine. Most of the respondents were in favour of integrating at least some types of CAM in mainstream primary care. There is an urgent need to further educate/inform primary care health professionals about CAM.

Evidence from the US suggests that once set up, integrative medicine clinics are effective (Scherwitz et al., 2004). Fifteen months after opening a clinic in San Francisco, the authors evaluated patient satisfaction from 146 patients after they visited with one of four healing clinic physicians. The results showed a high degree of satisfaction. Patients were also found to have been able to recall and follow a complex treatment regimen.

There is claimed to be evidence in Australia of widespread acceptance of acupuncture, meditation, hypnosis and chiropractic by GPs and lesser acceptance of homeopathy and other therapies (Pirotta et al., 2000). Barrett (2003) predicts that some degree of integration will occur throughout much of the United States. In his paper Barrett identifies potential barriers and facilitators to potential integration of medical disciplines and argues for an accessible multidisciplinary and evidence based approach.

It has been shown that education at medical school does appear to influence attitudes to CAM (Furnham, 2003). As their orthodox medical training proceeds, medical students seem to increase their scepticism about CAM. This could affect their later willingness to integrate CAM into orthodox practice.

Leckridge (2004) has proposed four models of delivery of CAM and biomedical care. These are:

- the market model in which there is no regulation or other state involvement
- the regulated model in which there are regulations to protect consumers
- the assimilated model in which CAM is no longer complementary but integrated in practice
- the patient-centred model which emphasises team working and full integrative care pathways across professional healthcare boundaries, producing a system designed for the benefit of the patient rather than for therapists or industries.

Leckridge suggests that only the patient-oriented model is likely to support the development of truly integrated medicine.

The Foundation for Integrated Health (http://www.fihealth.org.uk/)

In 1997 the Prince of Wales was responsible for an initiative that resulted in the establishment of the Foundation for Integrated Health. The Foundation's activities include the following:

- it encourages the complementary healthcare professions to develop and maintain statutory or voluntary systems of self-regulation
- it encourages the complementary healthcare professions to develop nationally recognised standards of education and training
- it is increasing access to integrated health care
- it is making information about integrated health care available to patients, practitioners, press and the public through its website, quarterly newsletter, publications, news releases and seminars
- it is actively raising additional funds which will enable it to expand the above programmes in order to facilitate integrated health care in the UK.

SOURCES OF INFORMATION FOR PROSPECTIVE CAM USERS

In a survey of 52 customers attending a Manchester pharmacy (Alton and Kayne, 1992) it was found that the biggest proportion of respondents claimed to obtain their information from the media and their friends or relatives (Fig. 1.3).

Of those people who said they asked a health professional for help, more people asked their pharmacist about homeopathy than all other professionals added together. Unfortunately, in another study by Davies and Kayne (1992), although 96% of a sample of pharmacists and their staff had heard about homeopathy, most were unable to identify the main features of the discipline (Table 1.3). Similar results were found by other researchers (Vincent and Furnham, 1994).

Figure 1.3 Sources of information on homeopathy

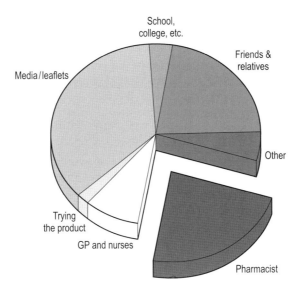

Table 1.3 Perceptions among pharmacy staff as to why homeopathy is effective

Reason for homeopathy being effective (more than one answer possible)	Pharmacists n = 17	Technicians n = 20	Assistants n = 38	All n = 75
Contains herbal ingredients	18%	50%	60%	47%
Because of 'like to treat like' concept	35%	25%	20%	25%
Because people have 'faith' in it	77%	30%	48%	50%
Because very small dose involved	0	10%	11%	8%
Because of the preparation method	0	0	0	0
Other reasons	18%	15%	3%	10%

Most of the respondents thought homeopathy worked either by faith alone or because it was herbal in nature, neither of which is entirely true. There is considerable evidence to show that a placebo effect is not the only thing responsible for the apparent efficacy of homeopathy, and only about 60% of the source material is herbal. These results cast doubt on the ability of the pharmacist to give accurate advice. It was thought that pharmacists working for multiples were likely to be more knowledgeable than their independent colleagues, due to the provision of in-house training (Islam, 1996). However, with the availability of continuing professional development resources by the relevant authorities in the four UK home countries, all pharmacists are able to obtain information much more readily than in past years.

The results on awareness in the UK compare favourably with those in the USA. In a study by Nelson et al. (1990) 86.4% of a sample of 434 British pharmacists said they knew 'something about' or 'a lot about' homeopathy. In contrast, only 55.8% of a sample of 197 American pharmacists claimed a similar amount of knowledge. The authors point out though that the results may not have been representative of the profession because the US response rate was only 19.7%, compared with 63% for the UK. Interestingly, acupuncture was thought to be the most useful complementary discipline by a majority of both nationalities of pharmacists, despite the fact that osteopathy and chiropractic are more popular disciplines in both countries (see Table 1.1).

Another source of information is the CAM practitioner. In a survey by Long et al. (2001) questionnaires were sent out to CAM organisations representing a single CAM therapy. The primary aim of the survey was to determine which complementary therapies were believed by their respective representing professional organisations to be suited for which medical conditions. The respondents were asked to list the 15 conditions they felt benefited most from their CAM therapy, the 15 most important contra-indications, the typical costs of initial and any subsequent treatments and the average length of training required to become a fully qualified practitioner. The conditions and contraindications quoted by responding CAM organisations were recorded and the top five of each were determined. Two or more responses were received from CAM organisations representing twelve therapies, including aromatherapy, Bach flower remedies, homeopathy, hypnotherapy, magnet therapy, massage, nutrition, reflexology, Reiki and yoga. The top seven common conditions deemed to benefit by all twelve therapies, in order of frequency, were: stress/anxiety, headaches/migraine, back pain, respiratory problems (including asthma), insomnia, cardiovascular problems and musculoskeletal problems. Aromatherapy, Bach flower remedies, hypnotherapy, massage, nutrition, reflexology, Reiki and yoga were all recommended as suitable treatments for stress/anxiety.

A questionnaire mailed to a random survey of Californian physicians has revealed that 61% of the respondents did not feel sufficiently knowledgeable about CAM safety or efficacy, and 81% wanted to receive more education on CAM modalities. The authors conclude that these findings raise important issues for medical education and patient care (Milden and Stokols, 2004).

At the World Pharmacy Conference (FIP) in Singapore in 2002, a survey was carried out among participants to determine the patterns of use, knowledge and attitudes toward CAM (Hwee-Ling et al., 2003). A total of 27.4% of the sample ($n = 420$) said they were interested in attending talks and seminars on homeopathy; more than half the sample agreed that it was important to have a basic understanding of CAM. Only 8.3% had used homeopathy themselves during the past 12 months.

Safety issues

No formal dedicated system exists for health professionals to report adverse reactions to CAM, although in some instances orthodox reporting systems are available and can be amended as appropriate. The difficulty here is that mechanisms do not usually exist to act on these data.

The public generally perceive that CAM is entirely safe, whereas in fact some disciplines (e.g. herbalism) have some remedies which are potentially toxic if they are not used according to instructions. Contraindications and interactions with orthodox drugs being taken concurrently may also be potentially dangerous (Brinker, 1998). More needs to be done to assess the composite effects of many herbal remedies. An important part of the assessment of CAM modalities is the therapeutic–toxicologic safety profile (risk:benefit ratio), and further research evaluating the clinical efficacy and mechanism of action of various CAM interventions for asthma is greatly needed (Bielory et al., 2004). Certain manipulative therapies can also cause damage if not performed correctly. Specific safety issues as far as homeopathy is concerned will be dealt with in Chapter 8.

CAM RESEARCH

The position with regard to research in homeopathy is discussed at length in Chapter 11. Here a brief review of CAM research in general is given.

Many – if not all – CAM disciplines suffer greatly from an inability to provide robust evidence acceptable to orthodox observers. It is important that CAM practitioners adopt the principle of evidence based medicine sooner rather than later. It promotes the idea that for each form of treatment the evidence regarding clinical effectiveness should be systematically reviewed and the results implemented into practice.

Giovannini et al. (2004) have analysed the diversity of CAM research across seven European countries (Germany, UK, Italy, France, Spain, Netherlands, Belgium) and the USA. In total, 652 abstracts of articles were assessed (Germany, 137; UK, 183; Italy, 39; France, 47; Spain, 24; Netherlands, 17; Belgium, 22; US, 183). The vast majority of CAM research was of a medical nature and published in medical journals. The majority of articles were non-systematic reviews and comments, analytical studies and surveys. The UK carried out more surveys than any of the other countries and also published the largest number of systematic reviews. Germany, the UK and the US covered the widest range of interests across various CAM modalities and investigated the safety of CAM.

The following are some of the difficulties associated with providing the necessary evidence:

Funding of research

A major problem relates to the availability of research funding although this situation has improved in recent years (Bensoussan and Lewith, 2004). The House of Lords report on CAM (House of Lords, 2000) recommended that the UK government should provide seed funding for research. Dedicated research funding (an estimated £5 million over 3 years) was to be provided to create centres of excellence and develop the infrastructure for high quality research. The focus of this programme is on research capacity building. Host institutions have been identified to give methodological advice, help develop appropriate skills, provide research support, and house post-doctoral and doctoral research awards. This process creates a supportive environment that allows for mentoring, appropriate review and the generation of high quality proposals. Before this, less than one-tenth of 1% of the NHS research budget went towards CAM research. This dedicated seed funding more than doubles previous allocations. Research funding from UK medical charities has also increased from £70 000 (0.05% of the research budget) in 1999 to more than £400 000 (0.31%) in 2002 (Wider and Ernst, 2003). Ernst (2005) described these amounts as 'dismal'. In the USA, the US Senate has set aside money for CAM research. The Office of Complementary Medicine, established in 1992, has grown to become the National Center for Complementary and Alternative Medicine (NCCAM), the 27th Institute of the NIH (National Institutes of Health), with a research budget of about US$113 million in 2003 (see Appendix 1 for address).

Quality of research

In the past, the evidence available has been sparse. In a review of recent advances in the status of CAM, Vickers (2000) states that the quantity of applied health research is growing rapidly and the quality is also improving. Following an evaluation of the quality of randomised controlled trials (RCTs) of CAM interventions for specific diagnoses to inform clinical decision making Bloom et al. (2000) also concluded that the overall quality of evidence for CAM RCTs was improving slowly.

Classification of research

A full review of research into CAM is beyond the scope of this introductory chapter. The following will illustrate some of the work that has been carried out under four headings:

Randomised clinical trials and meta-analyses

The number of randomised trials of CAM has approximately doubled every 5 years and the Cochrane Library (www.cochrane.org/index0.htm) now includes over 60 systematic reviews of CAM interventions. RCTs with varying degrees of quality of methodology exist in many disciplines includ-ing herbalism, homeopathy and acupuncture, some testing the therapy itself and others applied to individual interventions (Kayne, 2002).

It has been observed that the RCT does not always fit well with the under-lying principles of disease causation and treatment of CAM (Hilsden and Verhoef, 1998). Many forms of CAM take a holistic approach to the diagno-sis and treatment of disease, where the patient plays an active and key role in healing and treatments are often highly individualised. Therefore, the use of placebos, blinding and random allocation to structured treatment proto-cols in an RCT setting is often contradictory to the principles of CAM. There are other problems with RCTs (see Ch. 11). Nonetheless, such research is necessary to satisfy the provision of an evidence base acceptable to the scientific community.

Objective outcome measurements

These measurements have been developed to obtain some idea of the extent of positive or negative outcome. Examples include the Visual Analogue Scale, the Overall Progress Interactive Chart and the Glasgow Homeopathic Hospital Outcome Scale. These measures were developed for use in study-ing outcomes resulting from homeopathic treatment and are covered in Chapter 11.

Clinical audit

Abbot and Ernst (1997) quote three examples of what they consider to be good CAM audit studies:

- The first was an audit of acupuncture practice in a rheumatology unit that arose from a need to improve and standardise treatment, ensure that patient referrals were appropriate and that measurements of outcome were sensitive and meaningful (Camp, 1994).
- The second described how a service offering osteopathy for back pain was rapidly adapted to meet the requirements of local GPs (Peters and Davies, 1994).
- The third, involving an extensive audit of a German hospital specialising in Chinese medicine, resulted in improvements in the hospital's efficiency (Melchart et al., 1997).

Anecdotal evidence and case studies

This type of evidence is the basis of many CAM procedures. It usually refers to a collection of single episode reports collected in the literature over many years. This traditional bibliographical evidence is acceptable to regulatory authorities for certain licensing procedures. To be acceptable to orthodox colleagues, anecdotal reports must be well documented and outline new findings in a defined setting. CAM reports rarely include this detail and tend to be statistically non-significant because of the small sample size. Of course if one had enough anecdotal reports then the probability of success might be more predictable, but one is still faced with an inability to answer the question 'Would they have responded positively without treatment?' One often hears patients saying 'Yes, I got better, but I don't know if it was the treatment that did it or whether I got better on my own'.

RECENT DEVELOPMENTS IN CAM

Vickers (2000) has noted the following recent advances in CAM:

- There is now good evidence supporting the use of some complementary medicine treatments.
- Guidelines and consensus statements have been issued by conventional medical bodies.
- Organisations have recommended some complementary medicine treatments.
- Complementary medicine is increasingly practised in conventional medical settings, particularly acupuncture for pain, and massage, music therapy and relaxation techniques for mild anxiety and depression.
- There is a more open attitude to complementary medicine among conventional health professionals; this is partly explained by the rise of evidence based medicine.

REFERENCES

Abecassis, J (1997) The market for homeopathic medicines. Proceedings of the 1st International Conference on Homeopathy. Faculty of Homeopathy, London.

Abbot, NC and Ernst, E (1997) Clinical audit, outcomes and complementary medicine. *Res Complement Med*, 4: 229–234.

ABPI Annual Review 2003 http://www.abpi.org.uk/publications/publication_details/annualReview2003/ar2003_35-facts.asp. (Accessed 12 November 2004.)

Adams, J, Easthope, G and Sibbritt, D (2003) Exploring the relationship between women's health and the use of complementary and alternative medicine. *Complement Ther Med*, 11: 156–158.

Alton, S and Kayne, S (1992) A pilot study of the attitudes and awareness of homeopathy shown by patients in three Manchester pharmacies. *Br Homeopath J*, 81: 189–193.

Aveyard, K (1995) Pharmacist contribution to multidisciplinary assessments of vulnerable clients. *Pharm J*, 255: 302–304.

Avina, RL and Schneiderman, LJ (1978) Why patients choose homeopathy. *West J Med*, 128: 366–369.

Bakshi, JPS and Singhal, A (1993) Potentised street heroin/smack trials in post detox phase while detoxifying with homeopathic medicines. *J Organisation Médicale Homéopathique Int*, 6(2): 24–32.

Bakx, K (1991) The 'eclipse' of folk medicine in Western society. *Society of Health and Illness*, 13: 17–24.

Balint, M (1971) *The Doctor, his Patient and the Illness*, 2nd edn. Pitman Paperbacks, London.

Barrett, B (2003) Alternative, complementary and conventional medicine: is integration upon us? *J Alt Conventional Med*, 9: 417–427.

Bell, IR, Caspi, O, Schwartz, G et al. (2002) Integrative medicine and systematic outcomes research. *Arch Intern Med*, 162: 133–140.

Bensoussan, A and Lewith, GT (2004) Complementary medicine research in Australia: a strategy for the future. *Med J Aust*, 181: 331–333.

Bica, J, Tang, A, Skinner, S et al. (2003) Use of complementary and alternative therapies by patients with human immunodeficiency virus disease in the era of highly active antiretroviral therapy. *J Alt Comp Med*, 9: 65–76.

Bielory, L, Russin, J and Zuckerman, GB (2004) Clinical efficacy, mechanisms of action, and adverse effects of complementary and alternative medicine therapies for asthma. *Allergy Asthma Proc*, 25: 283–291.

Bloom, BS, Retbi, A, Dahan, S and Jonsson, E (2000) Evaluation of randomized controlled trials on complementary and alternative medicine. *Int J Technol Assess Health Care*, 16: 13–21.

Bolles, S and Maley, M (2004) Designing relational models of collaborative integrative medicine that support the healing process. *J Alt Comp Med*, 10(Suppl. 1): S61–S69.

Borneman, JP (1994) The state of the homeopathic industry. *Resonance*, 16(3): 23.

Brinker, F (1998) *Herb Contra-indications and Drug Interactions*, 2nd edn. Eclectic Medical Publications, Sandy, Oregon.

British Medical Association (1990) *Living with Risk*. BMA/Penguin, London, pp 195–196.

British Medical Association (1993) *Complementary Medicine: New Approaches to Good Practice*. British Medical Association/OUP, Oxford.

Camp, AV (1994) Acupuncture audit in rheumatology. *Acupunct Med*: 12: 47–50. Cited in: Abbot, NC, Ernst, E (1997) Clinical audit, outcomes and complementary medicine. *Res Complement Med*, 4: 229–234.

Cape, J (2002) Consultation length, patient-estimated consultation length, and satisfaction with the consultation. *Br J Gen Pract*, 52: 1004–1006.

Carr-Hill, R, Jenkins-Clarke, S, Dixon, P and Pringle, M (1998) Do minutes count? Consultation lengths in general practice. *J Health Serv Res Policy*, 3: 207–213.

CDC (2004) Centers for Disease Control and Prevention (CDC) 2002 National Health Interview Survey (NHIS), Washington DC National Center for Complementary and Alternative Medicine 2004 http://nccam.nih.gov/news/2004/052704.htm. (Accessed 13 November 2004.)

Chaitow, L, Harris, G and Morrison, S (2002) *Integrating Complementary Therapies in Primary Care: A Practical Guide for Health Professionals*. Churchill Livingstone/Harcourt, London.

Clark, CM, McKay, RA, Fortune, DG and Griffiths, CEM (1998) Use of alternative treatments by patients with psoriasis. *Br J Gen Pract*, 48: 1873–1874. (Cited in: Ernst, E and White, A (2000) The BBC survey of complementary medicine use in the UK. *Complement Ther Med*, 8: 32–36.)

Clarke, DB, Doel, MA and Segrott, J (2004) No alternative? The regulation and professionalization of complementary and alternative medicine in the United Kingdom. *Health Place*, 10: 329–338.

Cochrane Collaboration (2000) Complementary medicine information pack for primary care groups. Department of Health/MHS Alliance, London.

Coward, R (1989) *The Whole Truth: The Myth of Alternative Health*. Faber and Faber, London.

Davies, M and Kayne, SB (1992) Homeopathy – a pilot study of the attitudes and awareness of pharmacy staff in the Stoke-on-Trent area. *Br Homeopath J*, 81: 194–198.

Department of Health (1998) The national survey of NHS patients: general practice. http://www.dh.gov.uk/PublicationsAndStatistics/PressReleases/PressReleasesNotices/fs/en?CONTENT_ID=4080484&chk=F61f5g. (Accessed 21 January 2005.)

Deveugele, M, Derese, A, van den Brink-Muinen, A, Bensing, J and De Maeseneer, J (2002) Consultation length in general practice: cross sectional study in six European countries. *BMJ*, 325: 472.

Dharmananda, S (1997) *Controlled Clinical Trials of Chinese Herbal Medicine: A Review*. Institute for Traditional Medicine, Oregon.

Eisenberg, D, Davis, R, Ettner, S, Appel, S, Wilkey, S, Van Rompay, M and Kessler, R (1998) Trends in alternative medicine use in the United States, 1990–1997: results of a follow-up national survey. *J Am Med Assoc*, 280: 1569–1575.

English, JM (1986) Homeopathy. *The Practitioner*, 230: 1067–1071.

Ernst, E (1998) Complementary therapies for asthma: what patients use. *J Asthma*, 35: 667–671.

Ernst, E (2005) Why looking at complementary medicine receives so little funding. *Pharm J*, 274: 557.

Ernst, E and White, A (2000) The BBC survey of complementary medicine use in the UK. *Complement Ther Med*, 8: 32–36.

Ernst, E, Resch, KL and Hill, S (1997) Do complementary medicine practitioners have a better bedside manner? *J R Soc Med*, 80: 118–119.

Feldhaus, H-W (1993) Cost-effectiveness of homeopathic treatment in a dental practice. *Br Homeopath J*, 82: 22–28.

Fisher, P and Ward, A (1994) Complementary medicine in Europe. Report from Complementary research: an international perspective. COST and RCCM Conference London 1994. EU Science, Research and Development Directorate, Luxembourg, pp 29–43.

Furnham, A (2003) Medical students' attitudes about complementary and alternative medicine. *J Alt Comp Med*, 9: 275–284.

Furnham, A and Smith, C (1988) Choosing alternative medicine: a comparison of the beliefs of patients visiting a general practitioner and a homoeopath. *Soc Sci Med*, 26(7): 685–689.

Furnham, A, Vincent, C and Wood, R (1995) The health beliefs and behaviours of three groups of complementary medicine and a general practice group of patients. *J Alt Comp Med*, 1: 347–359.

Giovannini, P, Schmidt, K, Canter, PH and Ernst, E (2004) Research into complementary and alternative medicine across Europe and the United States. *Forsch Komplementarmed Klass Naturheilkd*, 11(4): 224–230.

Goodwin, JS, Goodwin, JM and Vogel, AV (1979) Knowledge and use of placebos by house officers and nurses. *Ann Intern Med*, 91: 112–118. (Cited in Comment – A place for placebos? *Br J Pharm Pract*, July 1990: 228.)

Guajardo, G, Searcy, R and Reyes, O (1994) The semantics of homeopathy. *Br Homeopath J*, 83: 34–37.

Harris, P, Finlay, HG, Cook, A, Thomas, KJ and Hood, K (2003) Complementary and alternative medicine use by patients with cancer in Wales: a cross-sectional survey. *Complement Ther Med*, 11: 249–253.

Henderson, M and Pierce, A (2005) Prince plots alternative treatments for the NHS. *The Times*, August 24.

Hilsden, RJ and Verhoef, MJ (1998) Complementary and alternative medicine: evaluating its effectiveness in inflammatory bowel disease. *Inflamm Bowel Dis*, 4: 318–323.

House of Lords (2000) *Report on Complementary and Alternative Medicine*. House of Lords Select Committee on Science and Technology, 6th report, 1999–2000 [HL123]. The Stationery Office, London. www.parliament.the-stationery-office.co.uk/pa/ld199900/ldselect/ldsctech/123/12301.htm. (Accessed February 2005.)

Howie, JGR, Heaney, DJ, Maxwell, M, Walker, JJ, Freeman, GK and Rai, H (1999) Quality at general practice consultations: cross sectional survey. *BMJ*, 319: 738–743.

Hwee-Ling, K, Hsia-Huei, T and Hui-Ling, N (2003) Pharmacists' patterns of use, knowledge and attitudes toward complementary and alternative medicine. *J Alt Comp Med*, 9: 51–63.

Islam, J (1996) An investigation into complementary medicine. BSc dissertation, School of Pharmacy, University of Portsmouth, Portsmouth, UK.

Jain, A (2003) Does homeopathy reduce the cost of conventional drug prescribing? A study of comparative prescribing costs in general practice. *Homeopathy*, 92: 71–76.

Jonas, WB and Chez, RA (2004) Toward optimal healing environments in health care. *J Alt Comp Med*, 10(Suppl. 1): S1–S6.

Kayne, SB (2005) Personal unpublished observations, 1975–2005.

Kayne, SB (1995) Negligence and the Practice of Pharmacy. LLM Dissertation, University of Cardiff Law School.

Kayne, SB (2002) *Complementary Therapies for Pharmacists*. Pharmaceutical Press, London.

Kayne, SB, Beattie, N and Reeves, A (1999) Buyer characteristics in the homeopathic OTC market. *Pharm J*, 263: 210–212.

Keynote Publications Ltd (2003) http://www.marketresearch.com/map/prod/867094.html. (Accessed February 2005.)

Labonte, RN and Penfold, PS (1981) *Health Promotion Philosophy: From Victim Blaming to Social Responsibility*. Western Region Office, Health and Welfare Canada, Vancouver, Canada, p 7.

Launsø, L and Rieper, J (2005) General practitioners and classical homeopaths treatment models for asthma and allergy. *Homeopathy*, 94(1): 17–25.

Leckridge, B (2004) The future of complementary and alternative medicine – models of integration. *J Alt Comp Med*, 10: 413–416.

Leese, GP, Gill, GV and Houghton, GM (1997) Prevalence of complementary medicine usage within a diabetic clinic. *Practical Diabetes Int*, 14: 207–208. (Cited in Ernst, E and White, A (2000) The BBC survey of complementary medicine use in the UK. *Complement Ther Med*, 8: 32–36.)

Long, L, Huntley, A and Ernst, E (2001) Which complementary and alternative therapies benefit which conditions? A survey of the opinions of 223 professional organizations. *Complement Ther Med*, 9: 178–185.

McKee, J (1988) Holistic health and the critique of western medicine. *Soc Sci Med*, 26(8): 775–784.

MacLennan, AH, Wilson, DH and Taylor, AW (2002) The escalating cost and prevalence of alternative medicine. *Prev Med*, 35: 166–173.

Marwick, C (2005) Complementary medicine must prove its worth. *BMJ*, 330: 166.

Melchart, D, Linde, K, Liao, JZ, Hager S and Weidenhammer, W (1997) Systematic clinical auditing in complementary medicine: rationale, concept, and a pilot study. *Altern Ther Health Med*, 3: 33–39.

Milden, SP and Stokols, D (2004) Physicians' attitudes and practices regarding complementary and alternative medicine. *Behav Med*, 30: 73–82.

Mintel Report (2003) *Complementary Medicines – UK – April, 2003*. Mintel International Group Limited, London.

Mueller, HV (1993) Handwriting as a symptom. *Allgemeine Homöopathische Zeitung*, 238: 60–63.

Nelson, MV, Bailie, GR and Areny, H (1990) Pharmacists' perceptions of alternative health approaches – a comparison between US and British pharmacists. *J Clin Pharm Ther*, 15: 141–146.

Neuberger, J (1994) *Controversies in Health Care Policies*. BMJ Books, London.

Paterson, C (2000) Primary health care transformed: complementary and orthodox medicine complementing each other. *Complement Ther Med*, 8: 47–49.

Paterson, C and Peacock, W (1995) Complementary practitioners as part of the primary health care team: evaluation of one model. *Br J Gen Pract*, 45: 255–258.

Peters, D and Davies, P (1994) Audit of changes in the management of back pain in general practice resulting from access to osteopathy. Executive summary. South and West RHA report of workshop on Research and Development in Complementary Medicine, 12 July, 1994, Winchester, UK. (Cited in Abbot, NC and Ernst, E (1997) Clinical audit, outcomes and complementary medicine. *Res Complement Med*, 4: 229–234.)

Petroni, PC (1986) Alternative medicine. *Practitioner*, 230: 1053–1054.

Pirotta, MV, Cohen, MM, Kotsirilos, V and Farish, SJ (2000) Complementary therapies: have they become accepted in general practice? *Med J Aust*, 172: 105–109.

Quin, FH (1862) Address of the President to the first annual meeting of the British Homeopathic Society. *Annals and Transactions of the British Homeopathic Society*, 1: 3–13.

Rastogi, DP, Singh, VP, Singh, V et al. (1993) Evaluation of homeopathic therapy in 129 asymptomatic HIV carriers. *Br Homeopath J*, 82: 4–8.

Reid, S (2002) A survey of the use of over-the-counter homeopathic medicines purchased in health stores in central Manchester. *Homeopathy*, 91: 225–229.

Reilly, D (2001) Comments on complementary and alternative medicine in Europe. *J Alt Comp Med*, 7(Suppl. 1): S23–31.

Riley, D, Fischer, M, Singh, B, Haidvogel, M and Heger, M (2001) Homeopathy and conventional medicine: an outcomes study comparing effectiveness in a primary care setting. *J Alt Comp Med*, 7: 449–459.

Russell, S (2004) San Francisco Chronicle, 28 May 2004, reproduced in ANMP Newsletter July 2004, http://anmp.org/newsl/NL43jul04w.htm. (Accessed 11 November 2004.)

Saxena, S, Majeed, A and Jones, M (1995) Socioeconomic differences in childhood consultation rates in general practice in England and Wales: prospective cohort study. *BMJ*, 318: 642–646.

Scherwitz, LW, Cantwell, MC, McHenry, P, Wood, CMT and Stewart, W (2004) A descriptive analysis of an integrative medicine clinic. *J Alt Comp Med*, 4: 651–659.

Schore, A (1993) A patient with iron deficiency anaemia. *J Am Inst Homeopath*, 86: 41–49.

Sharma, U (1992) *Complementary Medicine Today: Practitioners and Patients*. Routledge, London.

Sheehan, MP, Rustin, MHA, Atherton, DJ et al. (1992) Efficacy of Traditional Chinese herbal therapy in adult atopic dermatitis. *Lancet*, 340: 13–17.

Silver, S (1993) Homeopathy in the treatment of AIDS and HIV related illness. *J Soc Homoeopaths*, 51: 96–99.

Slade, K, Cloham, BPS and Barker, P (2004) Evaluation of a GP practice based homeopathy service. *Homeopathy*, 93: 67–70.

Slovic, P, Kraus, N, Lappe, H and Major, M (1989) Risk perception of prescription drugs: report on a survey in Sweden. *Pharm Med*, 4: 43–65.

Smuts, JC (1926) *Holism and Evolution*. Macmillan, New York.

Sparber, A, Wootten, J, Bauer, L, Curt, G et al. (2000) Use of complementary medicine by adult patients participating in HIV/AIDS clinical trials. *J Alt Comp Med*, 5: 415–422.

Steele, K, Gertman, PM, Crescenzi, C and Anderson, J (1981) Iatrogenic illness on a general medical service at a university hospital. *N Engl J Med*, 304: 638–642.

Steinbekk, A and Fønnebø, V (2003) Users of homeopaths in Norway in 1998 compared to previous users and GP patients. *Homeopathy*, 92: 3–10.

Stevenson, D (1994) So you have gum problems. *Resonance*, 16(4): 26–28.

Swayne, J (1992) The cost and effectiveness of homeopathy. *Br Homeopath J*, 81: 148–150.

Trichard, M, Chaufferin, G and Nicoloyannis, N (2005) Pharmacoeconomic comparison between homeopathic and antibiotic treatment strategies in recurrent acute rhinopharyngitis in children. *Homeopathy*, 94: 3–9.

Van Haselen, RA, Reiber, U, Nickel, I, Jakob, A and Fisher, PA (2004) Providing complementary and alternative medicine in primary care: the primary care workers' perspective. *Complement Ther Med*, 12(1): 6–16.

Van Wassenhoven, M and Ives, G (2003) An observational study of patients receiving homeopathic treatment. *Homeopathy*, 93: 3–11.

Vickers, A (1994) Use of complementary therapies. *BMJ*, 309: 1161.

Vickers, A (2000) Recent advances – complementary medicine. *BMJ*, 321: 683–686.

Vincent, C and Furnham, A (1994) The perceived efficacy of complementary and orthodox medicine: preliminary findings and development of a questionnaire. *Complement Ther Med*, 2: 128–134.

Vincent, CA and Furnham, A (1996) Why do patients turn to complementary medicine? An empirical study. *Br J Clin Psychol*, 35: 37–48.

Von Wartburg, WP (1984) Drugs and perception of risks. *Swiss Pharmaceuticals*, 6(11a): 21–23.

White, AR, Resch, KR and Ernst, E (1997) A survey of complementary practitioners' fees, practice, and attitudes to working within the National Health Service. *Complement Ther Med*, 5: 210–214.

WHO (1946) Preamble to the Constitution of the World Health Organization as adopted by the International Health Conference, New York, 19–22 June, 1946; signed on 22 July 1946 by the representatives of 61 States (Official Records of the World Health Organization, no. 2, p 100) and entered into force on 7 April 1948. http://www.who.int/about/definition/en/. (Accessed February 2005.)

Wider, B and Ernst, E (2003) CAM research funding in the UK 2003. Surveys of medical charities in 1999 and 2002. *Complement Ther Med*, 11: 165–167.

Wolsko, P, Ware, L, Kutner, J, Chen-Tan, L et al. (2000) Alternative/complementary medicine wider usage than generally appreciated. *J Alt Comp Med*, 4: 321–326.

olies of the Apothecaries' Guilds to prepare and dispense medicines. He had particular distaste for the complicated mixtures of drugs being offered to the public, the high prices charged and the practice of adulterating raw materials by unscrupulous members of the profession. Statutes were being drawn up to regulate these matters, but progress was slow. Not surprisingly, the apothecaries saw an erosion of their profits on the horizon, and resisted the measures strongly. Hahnemann was beginning to use ever decreasing amounts of medicine, and believed in the power of 'simplexes' or individual medicines, rather than complex mixtures. He maintained that no licensed apothecary could be trusted to adopt the correct technique in preparing his remedies and suggested that his medical colleagues produce their own remedies – and all this despite the fact that his brother, Samuel August, and his father-in-law, Herr Küchler, had both received an apothecary's training. In 1793, Hahnemann published his *Apothecaries' Lexicon* in four volumes. It was described by one reviewer as 'an excellent work that every apothecary should procure'. The book outlined the procedures (and precautions) that should be observed in an ideal pharmacy.

Another example of Hahnemann's work during this period was a report on a new wine test that was subsequently adopted officially in Prussia. This test allowed the wine trade to differentiate between wine adulterated with a solution of lead salt by dealers anxious to sweeten it (a criminal offence) and wine containing iron. His work *Poisoning by Arsenic* was dedicated to 'Good Kaiser Joseph' and led to the development of a method for detecting arsenic in the stomach contents of poison victims.

Hahnemann took up residence as Court Physician in a modest corner house in the small town of Köthen (see Fig. 2.1) situated at 270 (later 47) Mauerstraße ('Wall Street'). The house was described by Stephen Hobhouse (1933) following his visit in 1931 as being of two stories, quite picturesque with a wooden balcony, and situated close to the city wall. In 1991, when I visited, the area was in disrepair but the house was subsequently restored in the late 1990s and served for a time as a homeopathic resource centre.

Homeopathy – and Hahnemann – gained much popularity following the terrible winter of 1812 that took its toll of Napoleon's soldiers fighting in Russia. Following the defeat of the 'Grande Armée' in a 3-day battle in Leipzig in 1813, a fearful epidemic of typhoid broke out. Hahnemann treated 180 cases with homeopathy and lost only one patient. His fame rapidly spread throughout Europe.

Hahnemann's last important medical work was entitled *Chronic Diseases, their Nature and Homeopathic Treatment*. The book was initially published in Dresden in 1828 and eventually ran to 1600 pages and five volumes. It attracted considerable criticism among homeopaths as well as allopaths, owing to statements to the effect that seven-eighths of all chronic diseases were due to a hereditary or acquired 'taint' or miasm, called the psora. Many of his critics interpreted this hypothesis as blaming all such chronic conditions on the skin condition scabies. However, Hahnemann had in fact intended the term 'psora' to include a much wider class of diseases than just scabies or psoriasis (Mitchell, 1975). The subject of miasms will be dealt with in greater detail in Chapter 8.

In 1831–1832 an epidemic of cholera spread across Europe, causing many deaths. Hahnemann issued several pamphlets on the subject, advocating the use of the single medicine Camphor. As he had not treated, or even seen, one single cholera patient the depth of his belief in the efficacy of a single medicine was quite remarkable. Hahnemann postulated that cholera could be attributed to an organism (or 'miasm') and that the disease could be propagated by personal contact. This led him to demand isolation and disinfection – and also to the suggestion that medical staff were the most likely source of infection. Following this success an increasing number of doctors from all over Germany and beyond came to seek advice.

Johanna Hahnemann died in 1830, having borne eight daughters and two sons, and although Samuel was well looked after by his family, he was rather lonely. In his 80th year, a 34-year-old Parisienne requested a consultation. The woman was Melanie D'Hervilly-Gohier, the adopted daughter of the French Minister of Justice. One report suggests that she alighted from a mail coach outside the local inn dressed in man's clothing and gave instructions for two heavy trunks to be taken up to her bedroom. When the hairdresser appeared next morning in accordance with local custom to shave the young man he was surprised to find a lady who was lacing up her stays. Showing no sign of embarrassment Melanie invited the perplexed hairdresser into her room and explained how she would like her hair curled (Hunt, 1993). She succeeded in fascinating Hahnemann by her intelligence, her unusual degree of culture and her natural grace, much to the chagrin of his daughters. Despite Melanie being less than half his age, Samuel Hahnemann married her on 28 January 1835, in a union said to be based on an enthusiasm for the new form of healing. The newlyweds moved to Paris where Melanie secured permission for her husband to practise in the city through her influence with King Louis Philippe, a concession which was initially refused by the medical faculty. Now that he was living in a major metropolis the old doctor, who had only recently announced his wish to retire from practice, was far more accessible. He became surrounded by adoring clientele, not just from his adopted homeland, but from abroad as well.

On one occasion a poor lad of 12 years named John Young was brought from Scotland by a wealthy benefactor. The boy had been ill for 2 years and his own doctors had abandoned hope. After an examination lasting an hour and a half, Hahnemann declared himself able to help and the boy subsequently recovered. Unfortunately the literature does not record exactly what was wrong with John.

On his 86th birthday the town council of Meissen conferred the freedom of the city on Hahnemann, a gesture that he appreciated very much. A couple of days after his 88th birthday, on which Hahnemann was in great health and spirit, he became affected with bronchial catarrh, a condition to which he had been prone every spring for about 20 years. This time the illness was more protracted, lasting for 10 weeks. Hahnemann prescribed for himself, but seemed to know that the end was drawing close. At 5 a.m. on 2 July 1843, Hahnemann died. Melanie Hahnemann had her husband embalmed, and requested police permission to keep him unburied for 20 days. She spent much of the time before the secret funeral in the early hours of 11 July weeping beside the body. Hahnemann's third daughter, Amalie, her son Leopold (who practised homeopathy in London) and three servants were the only mourners present.

Mitchell (1975) writes that Leopold said later that Melanie berated the bearers for scraping the walls of the hallway as his grandfather's coffin was being carried out the house, not out of respect for her husband but on account of the expense of repairing the wall!

In 1898 the authorities in Paris sanctioned an exhumation from the small Montmartre grave where Hahnemann was initially buried, and he was finally laid to rest in the beautiful Père Lachaise cemetery close to the graves of Rossini, Molière and Gay-Lussac. The ceremony was attended by representatives of the medical profession from all over Europe.

In 1900 a monument of Scottish granite was erected and later the following inscription chosen by Hahnemann was added:

Non inutilis vixi (I have not lived in vain)

As Dr Margery Blackie wrote in her book *The Patient Not the Cure* (Blackie, 1976):

Hahnemann was not alone in recognising the shortcomings of medical practice and theory in his time; but he was in the forefront of those who, in a society plagued with epidemic, sought the swiftest, gentlest and most permanent means for the restoration and preservation of health.

The Faculty of Homeopathy possesses a number of interesting pieces of Hahnemannian memorabilia at their Hahnemann House headquarters in Luton, including a case of Hahnemann's remedies, his caps (Fig. 2.5), pipes, desk and an original photograph of him taken on 30 September 1841 by H. Foucault of Paris (Fig 2.6).

The photograph was originally the property of the Revd T. Everest, who recorded:

It was a dark rainy day, with violent gusts of wind, all which circumstances by increasing the difficulty of taking the photograph, have given the countenance of Hahnemann an air of stiffness. Hahnemann was, moreover, rather unwell that day.

The founder was also prone to presenting locks of his long, flowing grey hair to admirers, and several samples have survived.

Figure 2.5 Two silk and velvet caps belonging to Samuel Hahnemann (courtesy of the Faculty of Homeopathy)

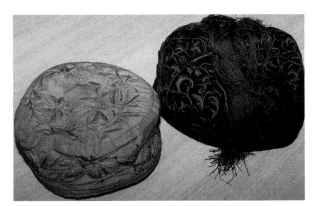

Figure 2.6 Samuel Hahnemann in 1841 (courtesy of the Faculty of Homeopathy)

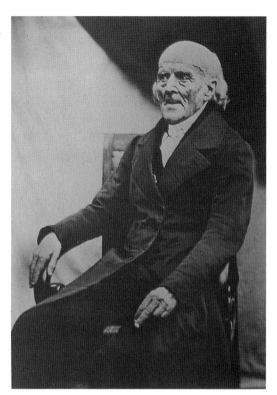

THE BIRTH OF HOMEOPATHY

In 1790, Hahnemann translated and annotated a materia medica by the great Scottish physician William Cullen (1710–1790). Cullen, who was respected for his innovative teaching methods throughout Europe, was the first Professor of Medicine at Glasgow University, subsequently moving to Edinburgh University in 1755. His procedures for treating disease, together with those of his pupil John Brown (1735–1788), were based on blood-letting or the administration of antispasmodics and stimulants. Cullen's work had been first published in London some 17 years earlier, with a reprint appearing in 1789. In this second edition Dr Cullen devoted 20 pages to Peruvian bark, also known as Cinchona after the Duchess of Cinchon, for whose benefit the medicine had been used. The drug was brought to Spain in 1640 by missionaries and has been used widely ever since for the treatment of a condition then known as the ague or marsh fever but now called malaria. It was suggested by Cullen that Cinchona was effective because of its astringent properties.

During his time with the Governor of Transylvania, Hahnemann had spent almost 2 years in the marshy lands of lower Hungary, where a substantial number of people suffered from marsh fever. He was thus able to acquire a thorough knowledge of the condition, so his interest in Cullen's statements was intense. Hahnemann knew of many other astringents that were not antimalarials and so he decided to test the drug on his own body, a practice that was not unusual in his time. He consequently took substantial doses of the medicine, carefully noting down all the physical and mental symptoms that occurred, reporting the following experiences:

> I took by way of experiment twice a day four drachms of good China [the Latin name for Cinchona bark] for several days. My feet, finger ends etc. at first became cold; I grew languid and drowsy; then my heart began to palpitate and my pulse grew hard and small; intolerable anxiety, trembling, prostration throughout all my limbs; then pulsation in the head, redness of my cheeks, thirst, and in short, all these symptoms which are ordinarily characteristic of intermittent fever made their appearance, one after the other, yet without the peculiar chilly shivering rigor. Briefly even those symptoms which are of regular occurrence and especially characteristic – as the stupidity of mind, the kind of rigidity in all the limbs, but above all the numb, disagreeable sensation which seems to have its seat in the periosteum, over every bone in the body – all these made their appearance. This paroxysm lasted two or three hours each time and recurred if I repeated this dose, not otherwise. I discontinued it and was in good health (Bradford, 1895).

Hahnemann found that the toxicity reflected in the above drug picture of Cinchona (now more usually known as China) mirrored closely the symptoms that could be found in a person suffering from marsh fever.

A year before his experiment, Hahnemann had noted that syphilis was cured by mercury not, as was popularly supposed, because it aroused salivation, perspiration, diarrhoea and increased urination, but because it awakened what he termed 'mercurial fever', a fever which resembled in some ways the disease it was capable of curing. Thus at the time of the Cinchona experiment he had already noted at least one other instance of an apparent similarity between a drug's curative and its poisoning symptoms (Mitchell, 1975).

Through his discovery of the power of Cinchona bark and mercury to produce the symptoms of disease, as well as an ability to cure that disease, Hahnemann had caught sight – albeit briefly – of what can be described as a 'law of cure'. To him the observations on Cinchona matched in importance Archimedes' bath water and Newton's falling apple.

These remarkable observations were not entirely novel, for similar phenomena had been made before by at least two workers. Hippocrates writing in the 4th century BC recommended treating vomiting with emetics. Almost 300 years before Hahnemann's observations, Paracelsus had declared that, if given in small doses, 'what makes a man ill also cures him'. Paracelsus was the adopted name of Philippus Aureolus Theophrastus Bombastus von Hohenheim, an itinerant physician and alchemist born in Switzerland in 1493. He was reputed to have cured many persons of the plague in the summer of 1534 by administering orally a pill made of bread containing a minute amount of the patient's excreta he had removed on a needle point. Elizabeth Danciger (1987) points out in her book *The Emergence of Homeopathy* that various people have tried to link the work of Paracelsus to that of Hahnemann, and certainly there appear to be many similarities. Hahnemann is said to have refuted any connection when asked by his followers, but with the extensive study of the medical literature he carried out it is inconceivable that he was unaware of the work of Paracelsus (Haehl, 1922).

Two further pieces of evidence supporting Hahnemann's embryonic law of cure may be related. The first concerned the treatment of scarlet fever in children, a disease that was endemic in Hahnemann's time. The toxic symptoms of Belladonna ingestion were well known, usually as a result of deliberate criminal acts of poisoning. Hahnemann had long established a close link between these toxic effects and the clinically recorded symptoms of scarlet fever, both of them producing a reddish skin eruption. He postulated that the drug could be used as a prophylactic to the disease as well as a treatment. It was not until 1812 that steps were taken by Hahnemann's colleagues to test this idea, when a fatal epidemic of scarlet fever prompted requests for help to stem the rapidly escalating mortality rate. Hahnemann sent three grains of carefully prepared extract of Belladonna that were to be triturated in a small mortar with an ounce of distilled water. To this an ounce of distilled water and an equal quantity of alcohol was to be added. A drop of this was to be added to 3 ounces of distilled water and an ounce of alcohol. In this form it was to be given, the dose being one drop to children under 9 years, two drops to those above that age, every 3 or 4 days. There were numerous reports from grateful colleagues convinced that the administration of Belladonna had minimised the effects of the disease (Black, 1843). A second piece of evidence that cannot be easily corroborated, but makes a good story, concerns the adoption of Sepia as a homeopathic remedy. Hahnemann was having his portrait painted by an artist in Leipzig. The man complained incessantly about a condition that might well be described as 'depression' in modern terms. He was using Sepia derived from the ink of the cuttlefish as his paint, and Hahnemann noticed that after dipping his paintbrush in the ink the artist licked it to bring the bristles to a sharp point. Hahnemann thought that the artist might be suffering ill effects from this procedure, so he took a sample of the paint. This was made into a homeopathic remedy and administered to the artist, whose mental symptoms were resolved rapidly.

Hahnemann then tried a number of active substances singly on himself, on his family and on healthy volunteers to obtain evidence to substantiate his findings. In each case he found that the remedies brought on the symptoms of diseases for which they were being used as a treatment. He called the systematic procedure of testing substances on healthy human beings in order to elucidate the symptoms reflecting the use of the medicine a proving, from the German *Pruefung*, meaning a test or trial. Each 'prover' had to be a healthy person who was not allowed to smoke, drink brandy, wine, tea or coffee or eat spicy foods. To ensure that all the symptoms were accurately recorded, distractions such as playing billiards, cards or chess were also banned. The provers were told to carry a notebook at all times so that any reactions could be recorded whenever they were experienced. Hahnemann examined the provers' reports closely to ensure that the results were not exaggerated. He adopted a cautious approach to his exciting discovery.

The proving was not only a practical method for determining the curative powers of medicines, but was also of great theoretical importance to the empirical view of medicine where experience rather than deduction was used as a guide to therapeutic procedures. The other view of medicine was known as the 'rationalist tradition', and derived its models for treating disease from a consideration of body systems and the application of various accepted paradigms – what might be called a 'scientific approach' in modern terms.

Empirics maintained that the physician could not possibly know with accuracy what was going on inside any particular body, and should not base treatment on assumptions. The medicinal use of a substance was based on its physical form or colour. Thus, red coral was used for haemorrhages and walnuts for brain diseases. This traditional interpretation of similarity was applied to medicine through the Doctrine of Signatures. After Hahnemann's provings the term 'similarity' became associated with individual symptoms rather than global physical characteristics. Further, the provers revealed mental and emotional symptoms as well as physical ones, and this was also highly significant because it led to a narrowing of the qualitative gap between physical and mental disease. Homeopathic prescribers began to use the same medicines to treat both; it was to be almost 150 years before a similar approach was adopted by all orthodox practitioners.

For the next 6 years Hahnemann tested the hypothesis gained through the experimentation with Cinchona until he was satisfied that he had identified a reliable method of selecting medicines based on the concept of like to treat like, expressed as the Law of Similars. He realised the need for individualising treatments, accepting that not all patients would react to treatments in the same way. The method of prescribing according to the Law of Similars he called 'homeopathy', from the Greek words *homoios* (similar) and *pathos* (disease or suffering). The term first appeared in writing in 1807. All treatment by the then universally accepted Law of Contraries he termed 'allopathy' from *alloios*, meaning contrary. This term is now used inaccurately to describe the whole practice of non-homeopathic medicine; it implies that orthodox practitioners prescribe only medicines that act as direct opposites in all cases, and this of course is not so. It takes no account of such treatments as replacement therapy, correction of hormone imbalances or the support given to malfunctioning organs.

Hahnemann had also noticed in his practice that most medicines appeared to have two actions – a primary (or direct) action and a secondary (or indirect) action. He stated that both the primary and secondary actions of a drug can be detected in every part of the body; additionally every medicine is associated with both mental and emotional symptoms. Significant doses of medicines elicit a powerful primary action followed by an equally strong secondary action, while homeopathic doses normally yield only primary actions.

A good illustration is offered by the action of Opium. This medicine first produces a fearless elevation of spirit, a sensation of strength and high courage, etc. After some hours, however, the patient becomes relaxed, dejected and confused. Hahnemann therefore welcomed as a first action some exacerbation (or aggravation) of the patient's symptoms. I will return to the practical implications of aggravation in Chapters 5 and 8.

THE PRINCIPLES OF HOMEOPATHY

The *Organon*

Hahnemann's most famous work was the *Organon of the Rational Art of Healing* (1810), also translated as the *Organon of a Rational Approach to Practical Medicine* and the *Organon of the Medical Art*. It ran to five editions during Hahnemann's lifetime, each of them revised by the author and some being prefixed with the motto *Sempere aude* ('Dare to be wise'). Although criticised by many colleagues, the work is often referred to in modern writings. A year before he died, Hahnemann completed the manuscript for a sixth edition (Hahnemann, 1842) but this remained unpublished for 79 years until Richard Haehl (1921) and William Boericke (1922) produced German and English versions respectively. Hahnemann's original manuscript of the *Organon* is now in the library of the University of California at San Francisco.

In spite of its centrality to homeopathic practice, the *Organon* remains difficult, obtuse and remote to many practitioners. At the level of the individual paragraphs, this is due largely to the cumbersome German sentence structure (Singer and Oberbaum, 2004).

The *Organon* comprises a preface, an introduction and 291 numbered paragraphs, termed aphorisms (denoted by the symbol §). There is no table of contents and there are no chapter headings. Hahnemann provided a synopsis of the *Organon* including a list of the aphorisms in abbreviated form. Unfortunately, this did little to elucidate the document's structure. This unhelpful presentation, generally maintained by subsequent translations, has tended to obscure the highly structured argument inherent in Hahnemann's treatise.

A translation by O'Reilly (1996) has made the work far more accessible. It includes a table of contents that offers a grouping of the aphorisms by subject:

Mission, (§1–2). This is a statement of the physician's mission and the highest ideal of cure.

Plan, (§3–5). In this short section Hahnemann details the three prerequisites to fulfilling the stated mission, i.e. ascertaining: (1) what is to be cured in the patient, (2) what is curative in medicines and (3) how to adapt the medicines to the patient.

Premise, (§6–8). Hahnemann felt it necessary to assert the philosophical premise upon which the ensuing argument, and indeed homeopathy, is based. Hahnemann places homeopathy firmly within the realm of empirical medicine.

Principles, (§9–27). In this section, Hahnemann develops the argument for treatment based upon the Law of Similars.

Mechanism, (§28–70). Hahnemann digresses to discuss the mechanism and its underlying science, a comparison with the allopathic method of cure and a summary of the principles of homeopathy.

Practice, (§71–285). This section discusses in depth the three prerequisites to homeopathic practice, according to the plan laid out in the Plan.

Appendix. This brief section is really an appendix on other modes of non-conventional medicine common in Hahnemann's time including 'the dynamic power of magnets, electricity, mesmerism and baths of pure water'.

The three important principles of homeopathy outlined in the *Organon* are considered below:

Like cures like

This principle first appeared in an 'Essay on a new principle for ascertaining the curative power of drugs', published in *Hufeland's Journal* in 1796:

> *One should proceed as rationally as possible by experiments of the medicines on the human body. Only by this means can the true nature, the real effect of the medicinal substance be discovered. One should apply in the disease to be healed, particularly if chronic, that remedy which is liable to stimulate another artificially produced disease as similar as possible; and the former will be healed* – similia similibus – *like with likes. That is, in order to cure disease, we must seek medicines that can excite similar symptoms in the healthy human body.*

This statement has been formalised in the Law of Similars, and we look at this in more detail on page 151. The Law of Similars implies a match between the primary symptoms of the remedy and the symptoms of the patient (Coulter, 1994). Examples of such treatment might be the use of Coffea (from the green coffee bean) to treat insomnia or Apis (from the bee) to treat stings and histamine type reactions. A remedy to treat alcoholism is obtained from the succulent used to make tequila; and Lactrodectus is a spider whose venom causes symptoms similar to angina and is therefore used to treat the condition. At first sight, this is rather different from the allopathic approach, when the use of a laxative to treat diarrhoea might be viewed rather strangely! However, there are many examples of this practice in orthodox pharmacy (Townsend and Luckey, 1960; Anon., 1987). Above a threshold dose, digoxin causes many of the arrhythmias for which it is a conventional treatment, aspirin in large doses causes headaches and several powerful chemotherapeutic agents are actually carcinogenic themselves. This may be a convenient analogy, but it must be acknowledged that, although these orthodox medicines appear to follow the Law of Similars, they are not prescribed holistically.

A further example, referred to by Medhurst (1995) in an article describing a rational approach to homeopathy, is the ongoing discussion on the protective effects of low doses of ionising radiation against the cumulative toxic effects of radiation. Therapeutic developments are now being planned as a result of this initiative.

The term 'hormesis' describes the notion that small doses of a toxin can be helpful. It has been used to describe the stimulatory effect of homeopathic doses of toxins upon in vitro and in vivo biological systems.

Provings

All remedies have a 'drug picture', a written survey of the symptoms noted when the drug was given to healthy volunteers, a process known as 'proving' the drug (see Ch. 1).

Theoretically, the proving of a substance refers to all the symptoms induced by the substance in healthy people. According to Belon (1995), these symptoms come from three sources:

- *Experimental provings* (or experimental pathogenesis): these are carried out using various non-toxic doses on subjects of different ages and gender, hence of unequal receptivity. They mainly cause 'changes in the way of feeling or acting', that is, in general symptoms or general behaviour. While, in the beginning, Hahnemann used mainly mother tinctures and low potencies for homeopathic provings, he later switched to centesimal dilutions (30c), and many of his followers did the same. Most recent provings have been conducted with ultramolecular dilutions (>12c). It is highly unlikely that any original molecule is present in such medicines (Weingärtner, 2002). This raises the question whether the symptoms experienced by volunteers in homeopathic provings are mere placebo background noise (i.e. responses associated with placebo intake, such as expectation), or if they are different from placebo; this in turn raises the question of the possible mechanism producing specific symptoms (Walach et al., 2004). The authors concluded that homeopathic proving symptoms appear to be specific to the medicine and do not seem to be due to a local process. However, since this was a pilot study using only a small number of provers, the work needs to be replicated. According to Walach (2000), Weingärtner (2002) and Milgrom (2004) the action of homeopathic medicines has to be sought in something more general and cannot be experimentally isolated and pinned down to the consequence of the medicine alone. This could be the whole context of homeopathic treatment, including the patient, the practitioner and the remedy, with the remedy alone having a clear-cut effect only in this context, as proposed by Milgrom (2004), or it could be the remedy and the whole of its preparation history, together with the homeopathic experience that contains and produces the effect, and not only the remedy as such, as proposed by Walach (2000) and Weingärtner (2002).
- *Clinical toxological effects*: these may be acute, chronic, voluntary or accidental. Given the high doses involved they usually produce organic lesions.
- *Clinical therapeutic observation*: this observation has caused the pathological symptoms regularly cured by the remedy to be included in the drug picture. Some of these symptoms may have already been noticed during experimental provings and some may not. This is the source of many seemingly strange rubrics that one notices in some of the drug pictures.

In some instances the whole drug picture may be derived from toxicological or clinical observations and not from a true proving. For example, the drug picture of an organophosphate is based on the symptom picture resulting from accidental exposure of seven people to two such chemicals (Edwards et al., 1994). The drug pictures are collected together in weighty books known as materia medica, many of which have been computerised. These are usually consulted when an appropriate remedy is being chosen to treat a patient, as we shall see in Chapter 8. Until now, the most important method of studying homeopathic remedies has been to look at individual drug pictures in isolation. Another method, described by Scholten (1993), considers groups of mineral remedies (e.g. Natrum mur, Natrum phos and Natrum sulph), extracting that which is common to the drug pictures. These symptoms are then used in the various remedies that contain that chemical element. Blackie adopted a similar approach when describing the Natrum salts (Blackie, 1986).

A protocol for provings has been developed by the US based David Riley (Riley, 1995) and a number of remedies investigated in the USA (Riley and Zagon, 2005) and elsewhere. Sherr (1994) has also written a book on the methodology of homeopathic provings.

Fayeton and Van Wassenhoven (2001) have identified a need to clinically verify the symptoms from homeopathic proving and collect clinical symptoms not derived from homeopathic provings. This work has been started by Van Wassenhoven (2004) who carried out a clinical verification of Veratrum album within the framework of a specific homeopathic methodology. He verified the outcomes of patients prescribed Veratrum album by correlation against rubrics. The data from 24 patients were analysed and a good correlation in the results found. It is hoped that an evidence based repertory will be available in 2008.

Minimal dose

It is in this area that many people have extreme difficulty in accepting that homeopathic remedies can possibly work. When Hahnemann did his original work he gave substantial doses of medicine to his patients, in keeping with current practice, sometimes causing aggravations that, in some cases, amounted to dangerous toxic reactions. He experimented by diluting out his remedies in the hope of increasing safety. The advantages of simple dilution were clearly limited, for the medicine quickly became too weak to be effective. Hahnemann then submitted each dilution to a series of vigorous shakes or successions and discovered that progressive dilutions were then not only less toxic but also more potent. It is not known exactly how Hahnemann came upon the procedure; most likely it arose from his knowledge of chemistry and alchemy.

Tyler (1980) quotes Hahnemann in regard to common salt:

> If it be true that substances which are capable of curing disease are on the other hand capable of producing diseases in healthy organisms it is difficult to comprehend how all nations, even savages and barbarians, should have used salt in large quantities without experiencing any deleterious effects from that mineral. Considering that salt, when ordinarily used has no pernicious effect upon the organism, we ought not to expect any curative influence from that substance. Nevertheless salt contains the most marvellous curative powers in a latent state.

A teaspoonful of salt is unpleasant to take, and has little effect other than to make a patient very thirsty. However, when the remedy is serially diluted down to one part in a million it becomes extremely active in the treatment of many conditions, including violent and prolonged sneezing. Similarly gold, silver, charcoal and silica take on medicinal properties when they are diluted according to homeopathic procedures. Modern pharmacists are not alone in wondering how this could possibly happen. Even Hahnemann was surprised.

Potentisation

In the preamble to volume 4 of his *Materia Medica Pura*, Hahnemann asks: 'How can small doses of such very attenuated medicine as homeopathy employs still possess great power?' He then suggests that one can attribute this effect to the way in which the medicine is prepared. The preparation procedure (described in detail in Ch. 4) is very specialised, involving shaking or succussion at each dilution level. Because the remedy becomes stronger acting – that is, more potent – the process is known as potentisation. For very acute conditions one might well use centesimal potencies of 30c or more, that is, remedies diluted serially in steps of one part in 100 down to one part in 10^{60} (see p. 92). In this area it is extremely difficult to explain how the remedy works – indeed it is difficult to explain how homeopathy works at almost any level! Sceptics make much of the huge dilutions that are involved in some homeopathic treatments, many, it is claimed, that result in potencies that exceed Avogadro's number. Amedeo Avogadro (1776–1856) demonstrated that the number of molecules in one mole of any substance is 6.02554×10^{23}. (The value seems to vary in the literature amongst the lower decimal places.) Depending on the material involved, once it has been diluted beyond 12c (mathematically equivalent to 24x on the decimal scale) the Avogadro number has been exceeded and no molecules of medicine are theoretically left in solution. This idea has led James Randi (of whom we shall hear more in Ch. 11) to comment on his website that 'Dr. Steven Kayne, yet another homeopathic pharmacist . . . is . . . a person who prepares nothing, though with great scientific expertise' (Randi, 2001).

However, homeopathy is not only about such huge dilutions. Potencies such as 6c (see Ch. 4) are used frequently, and at this level there are still molecules left in the solution. In practice there is a cut-off point as the Avogadro limit is approached above which molecules, though theoretically still present, cannot be detected with present methods. Some homeopaths claim that this limitation of present techniques of measurement may provide an explanation for the apparent lack of active material in the very high dilutions too – that is, molecules are present, but simply cannot be found. However, with some potencies, for example 6x (10^{-6}), quantities of drug present are of the same order as normally prescribed amounts of thyroxine or digitalis.

Arndt Schulz Law

A hypothesis known as the Arndt Schulz Law has been used rather simplistically to help explain the phenomenon of potentisation. In the 1880s Dr H. R. Arndt and Professor H. Schulz of the University of Greifswald in Germany were interested in homeopathic actions. They formulated a law based on the following observations (the allopathic interpretations are given in parentheses):

- small stimuli encourage living systems (e.g. immunisation)
- medium stimuli impede living systems (e.g. interfere with biochemical pathways)
- strong stimuli destroy living systems (e.g. chemotherapy agents).

Thus, as solutions of homeopathic remedies become weaker, they should be expected to encourage the healing process. However, this does not explain the position when Avogadro's number has been exceeded.

Law of Cure

There is a homeopathic Law of Cure associated with minute dose levels. It states:

> *The quantity of action necessary to effect a change in nature is the least possible, and the decisive amount is always the minimum.*

The minute dose was an empirical discovery, and the 'law' is deliberately ambiguous. It is taken to mean that not only should a minute dose be administered, but that the dose should not be repeated at too frequent intervals.

Single remedy

Although Hahnemann experimented with the idea of multiple prescribing, his final principle was that of using a single remedy to treat patients' ills, because he believed that patients could not suffer from more than one disease at a time; symptoms, however diverse, were therefore all linked to a single cause. 'In no case under treatment is it necessary to, and therefore not permissible to, administer to a patient more than one single, simple medicinal substance at one time,' he wrote in the *Organon*. Classical homeopaths observe this rule carefully. All the drug pictures in the materia medica have been determined on this basis. Provings have not been carried out on mixtures of remedies and it is not known how – or if – remedies interact. Many health professionals would welcome this approach in modern orthodox medicine and be pleased to see the demise of polypharmacy. The combination of competing ingredients (e.g. expectorants and linctuses) in some OTC cough mixtures certainly appears to defy logic!

Having said this, it has become the practice among some practitioners, especially in France and Germany, to augment the classical approach by the use of remedy mixtures with specific indications. Many appear to be effective in treating the symptoms of a range of common complaints.

The above three principles of practice, together with a holistic approach to treatment, form the basis of homeopathy.

A summary of Hahnemann's life and main publications is provided in Box 2.1.

> **Box 2.1 Summary of Hahnemann's life and main publications**
>
> 1755 Born at Meissen
> 1779 Qualifies in medicine at Erlangen
> 1782 First marriage
> 1782–1805 Years of wandering
> 1790 Cinchona experiment
> 1810 Publishes first edition of the *Organon*
> 1811 Leipzig. Provings which result in publication of the *Materia Medica Pura*
> 1821 Köthen. Period of semi-retirement. Publication of *The Chronic Diseases*
> 1830 Death of first wife
> 1835 Marriage to Melanie. Moves to Paris
> 1843 Death in Paris

REFERENCES

Anon. (1987) *Health Physics*. May: 531–537.

Belon, P (1995) Provings: concept and methodology. *Br Homeopath J*, 84: 213–217.

Black, F (1843) On the preservative properties of belladonna in scarlet fever. *Br J Homeopathy*, 1: 129–141.

Blackie, MG (1976) *The Patient not the Cure*. MacDonald and Janes, London.

Blackie, MG (1986) *Classical Homeopathy* – repertory edition. Blackie Foundation Trust, London, pp 102–113.

Bradford, TL (1895) *The Life and Letters of Dr Samuel Hahnemann*. Boericke and Tafel, Philadelphia, pp 36–37.

Cook, TM (1981) *Samuel Hahnemann*. Thorson's, Wellingborough.

Coulter, HL (1994) *Divided Legacy. A History of the Schism in Medical Thought*. Vol 4. Twentieth century medicine: the bacteriological era. North Atlantic Books, Berkeley, pp 256–257.

Danciger, E (1987) *The Emergence of Homeopathy*. Century, London, p 12.

Edwards, DA, Ibarra-Ilarina, C and Ibarra, M (1994) Report on homeopathic proving based on organophosphate exposure in seven subjects. *Biol Ther*, 12: 257–260.

Fayeton, S and van Wassenhoven, M (2001) Working Group 'Clinical Verification of Symptoms', European Committee for Homeopathy. Clinical verification of symptom pictures of homeopathic medicines. *Br Homeopath J*, 90: 29–32.

Haehl, R (1922) *Samuel Hahnemann, His Life and Work*. Homeopathic Publishing Co., London, p 10.

Hahnemann, S (1786) *On Poisoning by Arsenic: its Treatment and Forensic Detection*. Lebrecht Crusius, Leipzig.

Hahnemann, S (1793) *Apotheker Lexicon* ('Apothecaries' lexicon'). Lebrecht Crusius, Leipzig.

Hahnemann, S (1796) Essay on a new principle for ascertaining the curative powers of drugs and some examinations of the previous principles. *Hufeland's Journal*, 2: 3–4.

Hahnemann, S (1805) *Aesculapius in the Balance*. Steinacker, Leipzig.

Hahnemann, S (1810) *Organon of the Rational Art of Healing*. Arnold, Dresden.

Hahnemann, S (1818) *Materia Medica Pura*. Arnold, Dresden, vol 4.

Hahnemann, S (1828) *Chronic Diseases, their Nature and Homeopathic Treatment*. Arnold, Dresden.

Hahnemann, S (1842) *Organon of Medicine*, 5th edn, trans Boericke. Available online at http://www.homeopathyhome.com/reference/organon/organon.html

Hobhouse, RW (1933) *Life of Christian Samuel Hahnemann*. CW Daniel, London.

Hunt, S (1993) Melanie Hahnemann. *Homeopathy*, 43(2): 25–30.

Medhurst, R (1995) A rational approach to homeopathy. *Aust J Pharm*, 76: 924–926.

Milgrom, LR (2004) Patient-practitioner-remedy (PPR) entanglement. Part 4: Towards classification and unification of the different quantum models for homeopathy. *Homeopathy*, 93: 34–42.

Mitchell, GR (1975) *Homoeopathy*. WH Allen, London, p 24.

O'Reilly, WB (ed) (1996) *Organon of the Medical Art*. Birdcage Books, Redmond, WA.

Randi, J (2001) James Randi Educational Foundation Commentary, 29 June. http://www.randi.org/jr/06-29-01.html. (Accessed 20 January 2005.)

Riley, D (1995) Proving report – Veronica officinalis. *Br Homeopath J*, 84: 144–148.

Riley, D and Zagon, A (2005) Clinical homeopathic use of RNA: evidence from two provings. *Homeopathy*, 94: 33–36.

Scholten, J (1993) *Homeopathy and Minerals*. CIP-data, Koninkliake Bibliothek, Den Haag.

Sherr, J (1994) *Dynamics and Methodology of Homeopathic Provings*. Dynamis Books, Malvern.

Singer, SP and Oberbaum, M (2004) The structure of the *Organon*. *Homeopathy*, 93: 151–153.

Townsend, W and Luckey, P (1960) Hormoligosis in pharmacology. *JAMA*, 173(1): 44–48.

Tyler, ML (1980) *Homeopathic Drug Pictures*. Jain Publishing Company, New Delhi, pp 567–568.

Van Wassenhoven, M (2004) Towards an evidence-based repertory: clinical evaluation of Veratrum album. *Homeopathy*, 93: 71–77.

Walach, H (2000) Magic of signs: a non-local interpretation of homeopathy. *Br Homeopath J*, 89: 127–140.

Walach, H, Sherr, J, Schneider, R, Shabi, R, Bond, A and Rieberer, G (2004) Homeopathic proving symptoms: result of a local, non-local, or placebo process? A blinded, placebo-controlled pilot study. *Homeopathy*, 93: 179–185.

Weingärtner, O (2002) Über die wissenschaftliche Bearbeitbarkeit der Identifikation eines 'arzneilichen Gehalts' von Hochpotenzen. *Forsch Komplementärmed Klass Nat*, 9: 229–233.

Chapter **3**

The development of homeopathy around the world

CHAPTER CONTENTS

Homeopathy in the UK	59	Homeopathy in Asia	70
Pharmacy	61	Homeopathy in Australasia	71
The main British organisations	62	Homeopathy in Europe	72
The British homeopathic hospitals	63	Homeopathy in Latin America	73
London	63	Homeopathy in the USA	74
Glasgow	66	History	74
Tunbridge Wells	67	The National Center for Complementary	
Bristol	68	and Alternative Medicine (NCCAM)	76
Other hospitals	68	Samuel Hahnemann Memorial,	
Homeopathy in Africa	68	Washington DC	77

Homeopathy is found in many countries worldwide, and outside Europe each has its own particular way of dealing with the therapy. The following account is not meant to be comprehensive; rather, it represents some of the countries with which I have had contact and is meant to indicate how widely homeopathy is practised.

HOMEOPATHY IN THE UK

Although preceded by a Dr Belluomini, the first British homeopath is generally considered to have been Dr Frederick Hervey Foster Quin (Hamilton, 1882; Jenkins, 1989; Leary, 1994a). Quin was born in London in February 1799. Despite a lack of firm evidence, it is widely stated in the literature that he was the illegitimate son of the Duchess of Devonshire whose maiden surname, Hervey, was included in his own. In 1817 he entered Edinburgh University, the first British university to offer a formal medical training. He graduated as Doctor of Medicine 3 years later at the tender age of 20 years, having presented a thesis on arsenic. On his return to London, and with the Duchess of Devonshire's influence, Dr Quin, known as the 'Cheery Doctor' because of his happy disposition, was appointed physician to the exiled Napoleon I, who had just discharged his Irish doctor. Unfortunately the Emperor died before Quin could take up the position on St Helena.

Dr Quin met Dr Necker, a disciple of Hahnemann's, in Naples and this prompted him to go to Leipzig to meet the founder in 1826, and find out more about the new system of medicine. Unfortunately the visit was not wholly successful from a medical standpoint, although the men became good friends.

During the great European cholera epidemic, Dr Quin went to Moravia to study the disease, and as a result of a deeper insight into the effective workings of Hahnemann's method his doubts began to evaporate. On his return he practised homeopathy in London, first in King Street, St James's and then at 13 Stratford Place, despite being forbidden to do so by the College of Physicians. Now fully convinced as to the worth of homeopathy, Dr Quin went to visit Samuel Hahnemann again, this time in Paris, where he studied with his mentor for several months.

A contaminated water pump in St James's, London, was suspected as the source of the cholera epidemic that reached Britain in 1853. The facilities of the London Homeopathic Hospital, founded by Quin in 1850, were turned over completely to the treatment of cholera victims. The outbreak occurred just as the General Board of Health came into being under the first Public Health Act. This meant that for the first time accurate statistics on health were available. In 1854 a report to the House of Commons gave the figures of death from cholera under orthodox treatment as 59.2% and under homeopathic treatment as 16.4% (10 out of 61 cases). In all 54 000 people died. These figures have to be viewed with care for at this time in many instances there was more risk from the treatments than from the disease being treated. It has been suggested that it may have been the withdrawal of dangerous treatments rather than the application of homeopathy that led to an apparent success for Hahnemann's methods. For example, every patient admitted to the Middlesex Hospital received a hot bath at 104°C followed by an emetic of mustard and salt, repeated once or more if the vomiting that ensued was not substantial. Hot fomentations and turpentine applications were applied and the whole chest was covered by a mustard plaster. Typically these procedures were then followed by the use of calomel, cod liver oil or lead acetate (Leary, 1994b). Dr Bernard Leary has pointed out that the expected mortality rate for patients not treated for cholera at all is stated as being around 50% in modern textbooks. However, given that the mortality rate claimed by the London Homeopathic Hospital in this epidemic was a mere 20%, it seems that a lack of debilitating procedures could not have been the only contributory factor to this relative success. It is likely that homeopathy played some active part in the recovery process, otherwise the death rate would have been much higher. Success in treating cholera and yellow fever was reported in the USA (see below).

A pilot study of the homeopathic treatment of cholera in Peru by Gaucher et al. (1993) appeared to show that it was effective, but a subsequent double-blind study found no difference between active and placebo treatments (Gaucher et al., 1994). Dr Gaucher has also considered the role of homeopathy in the treatment of tetanus and concluded here that homeopathy is effective in combination with orthodox treatment, but not on its own (Gaucher, 1995). The efficacy of such treatments is thus still to be resolved.

As a result of the apparent historic 'success' in treating cholera, a clause was added to the 1858 Medical Act during its passage through Parliament to ensure that properly qualified physicians could not be denied admission to the medical registrar merely because of an interest in homeopathy.

Dr Quin suffered from ill health throughout his life; latterly he was troubled with arthritis. His last illness was very brief, a sudden chill brought on a severe attack of bronchitis which his feeble constitution was unable to withstand, and he died on 18 November 1878.

Other outstanding British homeopaths were Drysdale, Hughes, Russell and Dudgeon. Of these, Dudgeon practised in Liverpool and made many contributions to the homeopathic literature but is probably more widely known for constructing the original sphygmomanometer.

In modern times, Dr John Weir of Glasgow was a great influence on the practice of homeopathy, restoring the classical nature of prescribing in Britain. He did much to establish the credibility of homeopathy and succeeded in breaking down many of his colleagues' prejudices. He was the instigator of the first educational meetings for doctors. His contribution was immense and on his death in 1971 it was a heavy responsibility that fell on the shoulders of the Dean of the Faculty of Homeopathy, Dr Margery Blackie. Dr Blackie was responsible for a rapid renewal of interest in homeopathy amongst British allopathic doctors. She was responsible for setting up courses and expanding the Faculty membership. Like John Weir (later Sir John), Dr Blackie was appointed Royal Physician, the first woman to hold this honour. I was privileged to work with Dr Blackie during the 1970s at Thurloe Place, London. Her rooms provided an excellent venue for a series of highly memorable parties that served to release the tensions of the long courses that took place at the Royal London Homeopathic Hospital (RLHH).

Scotland has always enjoyed an important homeopathic tradition. Dr Hamish Boyd was largely responsible for nurturing a resurgence of interest both in that country and further afield. Since the 1970s, there has been a substantial rise in the amount and quality of homeopathic research by physicians, veterinary surgeons, pharmacists and podiatrists.

Pharmacy

Own label homeopathic remedies were widely available from branches of Boots (priced at 6d. each) during the 1930s but with the development of the OTC market they fell out of favour until reintroduced in 1992. The pros and cons of homeopathy were discussed in papers in the pharmaceutical press in 1981 (Steinbach, 1981) and again 10 years later (Kayne, 1991). A debate at the British Pharmaceutical Conference in Birmingham 1992 supported a growing interest in the discipline by backing the supply of homeopathic remedies in pharmacies (Anon., 1992). Exposure to homeopathy and other complementary disciplines crept into the undergraduate (and postgraduate) training programmes during the 1990s and articles now appear regularly in the journals.

Within the discipline of homeopathic pharmacy in Britain, John Ainsworth, FRPharmS, deserves particular mention. In a distinguished career spanning well over 40 years, John was responsible for raising the profile of homeopathic pharmacy and developing important links with colleagues in Europe. Both John and the late Mervyn Madge, FRPharmS, a past member of the Council of the Royal Pharmaceutical Society of Great Britain, served as Chair of the British Homeopathic Association.

The main British organisations

After an abortive attempt in 1837 to found the British Homeopathic Society with five colleagues, Dr Quin eventually achieved his aim in 1844 at a dinner party held in his house to commemorate the death of Hahnemann a year earlier. Among the laws and regulations of the new Society were the following:

1. membership is open to medical practitioners and medical students only
2. new members are expected to prepare a Dissertation or paper before the Society
3. members who reside in London or within five miles of the Society's rooms (or who reside outwith London but happen to be in the Capital on the date of a meeting) shall be subject to a fine of 1s. for being absent from any ordinary meeting at which a quorum is not formed.

It was not until 1860 that the British Homeopathic Society began to issue a record of its proceedings. The first publication was called the *Annals and Transactions of the British Homeopathic Society and the London Homeopathic Hospital*. Subsequently it was known as the *Journal of the British Homeopathic Society* (1893) until 1913, when the Society took over the running of the *British Homeopathic Journal*, a monthly periodical launched 2 years previously. The journal became quarterly in 1920 and has remained the official organ of British homeopathy ever since. It has now been renamed simply *Homeopathy*.

In 1943 the British Homeopathic Society became the Faculty of Homeopathy and was incorporated under the Companies Act 1929 as a company limited by guarantee without share capital. It was then thought expedient that members of the existing Faculty should be incorporated and have powers conferred upon them by an Act of Parliament, and the Faculty of Homeopathy Act 1950 was passed. Under this Act, the Faculty has responsibilities to advance the principles and practice of homeopathy. Traditionally it was medically orientated, with only physicians and veterinary surgeons able to achieve membership. In recent years other professions including dentistry, midwifery, nursing and pharmacy have secured equal status.

In 1995 the Faculty relinquished its training duties and assumed an accreditation role for postgraduate courses offered in the UK by the Academic Department of Homeopathic Medicine in London and Glasgow and other educational groups in Oxford and Bristol as well as overseas. The Faculty also maintains a list of its Members, Diplomates and Associates.

In 1902 the British Homeopathic Association (BHA) was formed. Although it has always attracted a number of representatives from the medical professions, it exists primarily to spread the use of homeopathy among the general public. The Association ran seminars, training sessions and 'road shows' throughout the UK and had an impressive stock of books and self-help pamphlets at its London headquarters in Devonshire Street. It published a quarterly journal called *Homeopathy* for many years (not to be confused with the renamed *British Homeopathic Journal* currently published by the Faculty of Homeopathy). This was discontinued and replaced by the title *Health and Homeopathy* following the merger with the Homeopathic Society (see below). Although the BHA merged with the Faculty of Homeopathy in 2001 it has managed to maintain its own identity. The Queen Mother was patron of the BHA until her death in 2002.

The Homeopathic Trust (Patron HRH The Duke of Gloucester) was a registered charity that supported the training in homeopathy of statutorily registered health professionals, and funded research and educational activities. The Trust worked to advance homeopathy and secure its general availability and supported the Faculty of Homeopathy financially. The Scottish Homeopathic Research and Educational Trust (SHRET) has similar aims.

The Homeopathic Trust (HT) merged with the British Homeopathic Association in September 2000 and no longer exists as a separate entity. All the HT's funds were transferred to the BHA, and the HT's work is now part of the BHA's efforts.

The Blackie Foundation Trust was formed by Dr Margery Blackie to promote education and research into the science of homeopathy. During the 1980s and 90s it actively supported an annual Blackie Memorial Lecture and organised symposia, the proceedings of which are published on an occasional basis. The Trust also funded research projects and offered help and advice to researchers through the British Homeopathic Research Group. The Foundation is largely quiescent at the time of writing.

The Homeopathic Society was the public membership division of the charity the Homeopathic Trust, with which it merged in 1990 to further their mutual aim of securing the general availability of homeopathy in primary care. Founded in 1958 as the Hahnemann Society, it published a quarterly magazine entitled *Health and Homeopathy* but in 1999 the Society was completely subsumed by the BHA.

The Society of Homeopaths is the largest organisation registering homeopaths in the UK. The Society was founded in 1978 to forward the development of the profession. Its aim is high-quality homeopathic health care for all. Registered members (RSHom) complete 3 years full-time or 4 years part-time training and then undergo a further period of clinical supervision before becoming eligible for registration. The Society publishes a register of homeopaths with proven ability who have satisfied the registration criteria set out in the Society's Registration Standards and Procedures. These practitioners (often called professional homeopaths or non-medically qualified practitioners) have agreed to abide by the Society's Code of Ethics and Practice, and are subject to complaints and disciplinary procedures.

The British homeopathic hospitals

London

The Royal London Homeopathic Hospital has its origins in premises secured by Dr Quin at 32 Golden Square. The British Homeopathic Society opened a hospital there with 25 beds on 10 April 1850 (the anniversary of Hahnemann's birthday). The cost of fitting out the premises was given as £493 12*s*. 6*d*. By 1859 the hospital was proving to be too small, and Dr Quin then bought three houses in Great Ormond Street, including one that was the headquarters of the antislavery struggle, for conversion at a cost of nearly £15 000. This building was in use for 36 years, during which time the cumulative numbers of patients increased to over a quarter of a million.

Many of the great names in British homeopathy – including Robert Cooper, Richard Hughes, James Compton Burnett, John Henry Clarke, Edward Bach, Charles Wheeler, Donald Foubister and many others – have been associated with the hospital. Robert Dudgeon was a stalwart of the hospital in the late 19th century, and something of a polymath. Apart from translating virtually all of Hahnemann's voluminous writings into English, he invented the sphygmograph, a device for recording the pulse, a marvel of Victorian miniature engineering, as well as spectacles for use underwater.

A cache of 300 volumes containing the case notes of 1426 patients treated at the hospital between 1889 and 1923 was discovered in the vaults in 1992. Most patients appeared to be manual workers including lacquerers, fancy box makers, ostrich feather workers, fancy stationers, and other long-vanished occupations. Phthisis and consumption (both forms of TB), bronchitis, rheumatism, gastric ulcer and female health problems were among the most common diagnoses. Outcomes of treatment varied from specialty to specialty: for diseases of women, for example, 74% were reported cured, 19% improved, 5% were unchanged and 2% died; for respiratory problems 62% were cured, 21% improved, 4% unchanged and 13% died. Duration of admission averaged over a month.

The case notes show the so-called 'new wind from Chicago' blowing through the hospital. The 'new wind' was the high potency, repertory-based homeopathy of Dr James T. Kent of Chicago. It arrived with a paper read by Dr Octavia Lewin in 1903, and within a decade had revolutionised practice at the hospital, which was to remain a bastion of Kentian homeopathy for many years to come. Dr Lewin herself was the first in a line of distinguished women homeopathic physicians on the staff of the RLHH, although her successors Drs Margaret Tyler and Margery Blackie are better known.

The RLHH suffered severe bomb damage during the Second World War. The gallantry of the staff during the raids was recognised by the award of four George Medals. During this period refugees from Nazi persecution, notably Drs Otto Leeser and Erich Ledermann, joined the staff.

Various extensions and modifications were carried out to the London Homeopathic Hospital in the ensuing years (Fig. 3.1). In September 1948, in time for its centenary celebrations the following year, King George VI conferred the title 'Royal' on the hospital. During the 1950s and 60s the RLHH's influence spread internationally through young overseas doctors who attended the hospital for clinical attachments. These include Dr Diwan Harish Chand, homeopathic physician to the President of India and the influential Argentine homeopath Dr Francisco Eizyaga.

The Royal London Hospital reached its peak in the early 1970s when it had 170 beds, over 20 000 outpatients and 152 nursing staff. Since then facil-

Figure 3.1 A plaque commemorating the 1909 extension at the Royal London Homeopathic Hospital

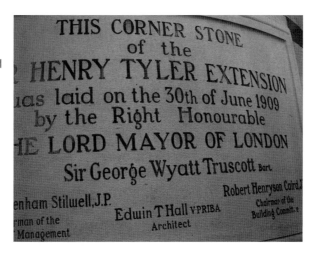

ities have declined as a result of National Health Service rationalisations. On 18 June 1972 the RLHH suffered a devastating blow when a Trident airliner crashed at Staines, close to Heathrow airport. Sixteen doctors and colleagues, including Dr John Raeside, who had been on their way to the International Homeopathic League Congress in Brussels, were killed. This marked the beginning of a period of sharp decline. NHS reorganisation resulted in loss of independence and a series of closures. The operating theatres and surgical, children's and geriatric wards were closed, and the number of beds fell to 45.

The RLHH responded actively to these changes, developing and diversifying its complementary medicine services. Dr Ralph Twentyman pioneered complementary cancer care, Dr Anthony Campbell established an acupuncture clinic and Dr Michael Jenkins developed environmental medicine. The RLHH also introduced manual medicine and autogenic training. All of these were the first, or among the first, services of their kind in the NHS.

Nevertheless, by the early 1990s many perceived closure of the hospital as inevitable. This was averted by a bid to become an autonomous NHS Trust. The success of the bid owed much to the Trust's first Chairman, Dr J. Dickson Mabon, who, apart from being a homeopathic doctor, had been an MP and Government Minister for many years. The public consultation on the RLHH's Trust bid attracted one of the largest postbags for any such application, letters from the public were overwhelmingly supportive, and the RLHH became a Trust on 1 April 1993 (Fig. 3.2).

The Trust made a number of major changes, including the establishment of the NHS's first musculoskeletal service and an academic centre with directors of education and research. A range of multidisciplinary packages of care, including complementary cancer care, were set up. But eventually the financial burden of maintaining a Board and the associated management structure proved too great and in April 1999 the RLHH Trust merged with Parkside Health NHS Community Trust. This arrangement was shortlived because in April 2002 Parkside, along with all other Community Trusts, was abolished. However, this period resulted in an enduring achievement: the acceptance by the NHS of an ambitious plan to completely redevelop the

Figure 3.2 Royal London Homeopathic Hospital in 2005

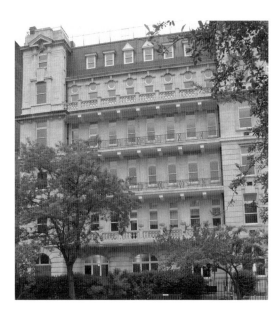

hospital's building, at a cost of £18.5 million. Work began in summer 2002 and was completed in 2005.

Following the demise of Parkside, the RLHH joined University College London Hospitals NHS Foundation Trust (UCLH), as apart of its Specialist Hospitals Board, alongside other famous names such as the National Hospital for Neurology and Neurosurgery, Queen Square and the Elizabeth Garrett Anderson women's hospital. UCLH is a large NHS Trust with strong academic links. There is widespread enthusiasm among its clinicians to integrate homeopathy and other forms of complementary and alternative medicine in their work.

Joining UCLH, combined with the redevelopment of the building, completes a dramatic revival in the fortunes of the RLHH. It now stands well placed to become a 21st century centre of excellence for homeopathy and other forms of complementary and alternative medicine.

Glasgow

A homeopathic dispensary was opened in Glasgow in about 1880 by a group of doctors but after a few years of good work closed down through lack of funds. Subsequently a consulting room was set up in 1909 by Dr R. G. Miller, following his return from tutelage under Dr Kent in Chicago, but this also closed because it could not cope with the demand. Some 5 years later a house on Lynedoch Crescent (having been purchased with a legacy from Miss Houldsworth of Ayr) opened as the Houldsworth Homeopathic Hospital, with 12 beds and four cots. A further legacy from the Houldsworth family enabled the inauguration of a much larger facility in Great Western Road in 1931, then known as the Glasgow Homeopathic Hospital. Despite plans in 1938 for a substantial new hospital with 200 beds being interrupted by the Second World War, it was not until 1999 that a new facility became available.

Figure 3.3 Glasgow Homeopathic Hospital

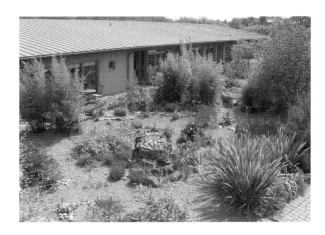

In 1921 Mr and Mrs Fyfe gifted the Homeopathic Children's Hospital on the east side of the city; this closed in 1981, ostensibly because of falling demand, and an outpatients' clinic was set up at a health centre in nearby Baillieston. When the hospital vacated the Houldsworth premises in Lyne-doch Crescent the building was converted into a busy outpatients' clinic which functioned until it was transferred to Great Western Road in 1987. At the same time the bed capacity at the hospital was reduced from 31 to 20. Following rationalisation of homeopathic services in the Glasgow area in 1995, all outpatient facilities were then transferred to Great Western Road. These premises were sold in 1999 and the first phase of a new purpose built hospital opened in the grounds of the Royal Gartnavel Hospital in Glasgow.

The hospital was designed by Maclachlan Monaghan Architects, who were selected for the job after winning a national competition. The aim was to create a building in keeping with homeopathic ideology linking harmony with healing. The architects achieved a look which is both contemporary and welcoming with lots of light and space. Inside the colours are soft and clear and Jane Kelly the artist has worked closely with the architects to create a very attractive interior with lots of natural materials, comfortable seating and beautiful plants (Fig. 3.3).

The hospital is the base for the Scottish branch of the Faculty of Homeopathy who are extremely active in promoting homeopathic education and research among health professionals. After securing an earlier reprieve, the Baillieston Clinic was unfortunately closed during 1996.

A more detailed history of homeopathy in Glasgow may be accessed at http://www.homeoint.org/morrell/glasgow/preface.htm.

Tunbridge Wells

The Tunbridge Wells Hospital (Leary, 1993) developed from a dispensary that opened in the Pantiles in 1863 and moved to Hannover Road in 1886. The following year two houses were purchased in Upper Grosvenor Road and a hospital was opened in them in 1890. By 1902 this hospital had doubled in size. The following year the present hospital was opened in Church Street, the freehold having been purchased by Dr Francis Smart. A new wing was added in 1921 and named as a memorial to him. There were further extensions in 1930. The hospital has 10 beds reserved for homeopathy and a further 20 for surgery and rheumatology.

Bristol

The history of homeopathy in Bristol began in 1852 with the establishment of a dispensary in Queen Square. The Cotham House and grounds were purchased by Mr and Mrs Melville Wills of the cigarette firm W. D. & H. O. Wills in 1917, and donated to the hospital in memory of their son who was killed while trying to rescue a wounded brother in the First World War. The foundation stone of the present hospital was laid in the grounds of Cotham House by the then Prince of Wales (later Duke of Windsor) in 1921, and the new building opened by Princess Helena Victoria in 1925. The Bristol Homeopathic Hospital continued to provide a full range of services until 1986 when the inpatient facilities were transferred to the Bristol Eye Hospital, where they continue to be provided, and outpatient services were moved to the ground floor of the Cotham Hill site. In 1994, following the sale of the main building to the University by the Bristol and District Health Authority, a new purpose-built Department has been provided in the Annexe buildings adjoining the original Cotham House. The Bristol hospital is active in research and education (Fig. 3.4).

The above hospitals all provide treatment under the UK National Health Service. There is also a privately run homeopathic clinic in Manchester.

Other hospitals

In the early days of British homeopathy the Liverpool branch of the British Homeopathic Society was particularly active. A hospital was built and equipped in the city by Sir Henry Tate of Tate & Lyle, the sugar refiners, in 1837 and served the community for many years before its eventual demise in the 1970s. An outpatient clinic still exists.

Around the start of the 20th century there were homeopathic hospitals in Bath, Birmingham, Bournemouth (Hahnemann Convalescent Home), Bromley (Phillips Memorial Homeopathic Hospital), Eastbourne, Leicester, Liverpool, Plymouth (Devon and Cornwall Homeopathic Hospital), St Leonards (Buchanan Hospital) and Southport.

HOMEOPATHY IN AFRICA

South Africa provides an environment in which homeopathy can make considerable progress. The ongoing 'war' between medically qualified doctors and dentists and non-medically qualified homeopaths has been resolved. The two codes are now working side by side. Homeopaths are able to request medical tests, receive referrals from other health professionals, hospitalise patients when necessary and visit hospitals as part of their training programme. A comprehensive training course is offered by institutions in Durban and Johannesburg. This was set up in association with the statutory

Figure 3.4 Bristol Homeopathic Hospital

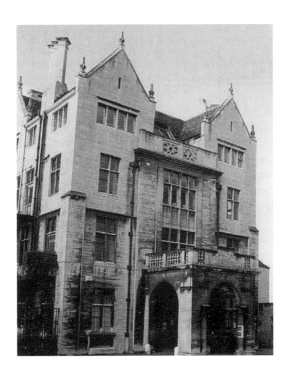

body with whom all homeopaths must register. On a recent visit I was impressed by the training facilities available and the intensity of the 6 year curriculum. There are approximately 450 registered homeopaths in South Africa.

Training for health professionals (physicians, dentists and pharmacists) has been provided by the British Faculty of Homeopathy with local assistance. Students have sat both the Primary Care Certificate and the more advanced MFHom examinations. However, veterinary homeopathy is in its infancy. A number of South African medical homeopaths have settled in the UK where their contribution to homeopathic practice and education has been greatly appreciated.

Homeopathy has been practised in Nigeria for at least 40 years, with the first formal organisation, the All Nigeria Homeopathic Medical Association, being founded in 1961, shortly after the country gained independence from Britain. Dr Peter Fisher visited Nigeria in 1989 and found it difficult to identify the number of homeopaths practising, partly because of the problem of defining exactly what constituted a homeopath (Fisher, 1989). There were about 50–100 homeopaths with an 'acceptable' level of training at that time. Generally speaking the standards of training were below what would be expected in developed countries. Dr Fisher said that there were a number of homeopaths in and around the federal capital Lagos and in the east of the country, particularly in Imo and Anambra states. By 1991 some progress had been made, with acceptance of the medical and dental professions having been secured (Okpokpor, 1991). Further advances have been hampered by political pressures.

HOMEOPATHY IN ASIA

Dr Mitchell gives a good account of homeopathy in India (Mitchell, 1975). He claims that homeopathy can be traced in India to as early as 1810, having been introduced by a German geologist working in the country on a survey. Remedies were distributed to servants and poor Bengalis. At some later time (no date is available) an Englishman called Mullins arrived in Calcutta, at that time the capital of India, and administered homeopathy to the poor.

The third important character in Indian homeopathy was Julian Martin Hoenigsberger, who was described as an 'adventurer'. He had spent 35 years travelling throughout the East and set off to study homeopathy under Hahnemann in the 1830s. On his way back to India in 1839 he contracted cholera in Vienna and is reported to have cured himself within 6 hours with homeopathic Ipecacuanha. Hoenigsberger was appointed physician to the Court of Lahore. He won fame by treating the Maharajah of Punjab successfully, but incurred the hostility of Indian doctors. The Civil Service and the military provided some notable amateur homeopaths.

Calcutta became the centre of homeopathy in India, the discipline growing through the agency of physicians and lay homeopaths. Because of its huge geographical area and population, India has always had a shortage of medically qualified practitioners; lay practitioners therefore perform an important role in supporting medical services. In 1861 Babu Razan Dutta, a man who had acquired a sound knowledge, took over a homeopathic practice from a French doctor whom he had sponsored but who had proved inadequate. About 6 years later, the Indian physician Mahedra Lal Sircar popularised homeopathy and the discipline has flourished ever since.

Homeopathy is recognised and actively encouraged by the central Government, with sponsorship of homeopathic clinics, dispensaries and hospitals throughout the country. India has many homeopathic journals and publishes a large range of the classical homeopathic books, many of which are exported. The name of B. Jain, publishers, of Delhi is well known throughout the world.

Dr P. Sankaran (1922–1979), the father of the well-known Indian homeopath Rajan Sankaran, was one of the greatest homeopathic teachers and practitioners in India. P. Sankaran's writings were based on his clinical experiences in his busy practice. He was a convert to homeopathy, having been cured by it after allopathy and Ayurvedic medicine had failed. He took up the study and practice of homeopathy with intensity and passion, studying in London under the guidance of Dr Blackie and other revered names in British homeopathy. His son Rajan graduated from the Bombay (Mumbai) Homeopathic Medical College (now known as Smt. Chandaben Mohanbhai Patel Homeopathic Medical College). He is well known for teaching psychology and philosophy and a concept known as the 'soul of remedies'.

The regulatory situation in Israel is rather confusing. The influx of Jewish refugees from countries of the former Soviet Union has caused a substantial increase in demand for homeopathy. A large number of the immigrant practitioners are preparing their own remedies (as indeed Hahnemann and his followers did) but without any standards being enforced. Contact with Europe (mainly through visiting lecturers from France, Germany and the UK) has helped to establish trained practitioners, and at the time of writing discussions are in progress to regulate homeopathic practice and manufacture (A. Moschner, homeopathic pharmacist, Tel-Aviv, personal communication, October 1999). The Israel Association of Classical Homeopathy is active in promoting homeopathic practice and maintains contact with the Israeli authorities.

Malaysia received its introduction to homeopathy during the Second World War through Indian soldiers who were fighting with the British Army and influence from the subcontinent is still strong. Teaching began in 1979 under the auspices of the Faculty of Homeopathy Malayasia. There were four homeopathic medical centres in the country in 1988 (Nasir and Zain, 1988). Enquiries have established that although the Government allows complementary medicine there are no formal registration procedures for practitioners. An organisation called the Registered Malaysian Homeopathic Medical Practitioners Association was established in 1985 to unite all qualified homeopathic practitioners. Without standards it is uncertain as to exactly what constitutes qualification. The group has about 500 members.

Singapore recognises homeopathy but there is no legislative framework to control its practice. Few, if any, practitioners are medically qualified.

HOMEOPATHY IN AUSTRALASIA

Some time in the 1840s Dr Albert Scholz, a military surgeon, migrated from Silesia to southern Australia and brought with him the practice of homeopathy, importing his remedies from Germany. After 20 years in the Barossa Valley he moved to Jindera, near Albury. By the 1850s a small number of British homeopaths were practising in Sydney and Melbourne, where a 60 bed hospital opened in 1869. The holistic nature of homeopathy and herbalism appealed to the population, much to the chagrin of the orthodox medical profession, especially as there was no legislation to guarantee their monopoly at this time. However, subsequently the medical profession established the authority to limit the practice of medicine to those considered 'suitably qualified' and homeopathy began to decline. In the 1920s doctors moved to limit the numbers of their own members for whom homeopathy was an approved therapy as well. The situation is considerably improved now and pharmacies throughout Australia are seeing an increase in the demand for homeopathic medicines. At present there is no requirement for non-medically qualified homeopathic practitioners to be registered in Australia (de Brenni, personal communication, December 1994). There have been calls for an expansion of research in Australia over the next 5–10 years and Bensoussan and Lewith (2004) have proposed a funding model based on a proportion of the GST (VAT) collected on CAM sales and services.

The origin of homeopathy in New Zealand is linked with the name of Dr William Purdie, a graduate of Glasgow Medical School, who arrived at Port Chalmers in South Island from Port Glasgow in 1849. Subsequently most homeopathic development took place in the north (McDermott, 1991). A Homeopathic Association was established in 1857 and a hospital and dispensary opened in Auckland a year later, only to close after 5 years when the Government appropriated the buildings for official offices. Homeopathy was recognised in the Pharmacy Act of 1880 as a valid system of medicine,

Figure 3.5   Postage stamps

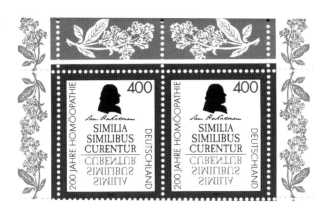

but prescribing declined during the next 80 or so years as modern high-powered drugs became available, until the incorporation of the New Zealand Homeopathic Society signalled a revival in 1962. Today the Society, based in Auckland, has a library of books and tape-recorded lectures. It is estimated that 80% of New Zealand pharmacies now keep homeopathic remedies. Training courses for pharmacists and non-medically qualified homeopaths are readily available through several colleges of homeopathy. The schools of pharmacy in Auckland and Otago give exposure to complementary medicine to undergraduate pharmacy students.

Training opportunities for doctors are at their own expense.

HOMEOPATHY IN EUROPE

A detailed history of homeopathy in Germany may be found at http://www.hpathy.com/Status/homeopathyGermany.asp. From its birthplace, homeopathy spread throughout Europe and beyond (Gaier, 1991). The first phase, in the 1810–1835 period, included Austria, Belgium (1829), France (1830), Hungary, Italy, the Netherlands (1827), Poland (1820s), Russia and Switzerland (1832), followed in 1820–1850 by Greece, Ireland, Portugal (1838), Scandinavia and Spain (1833).

Commemorative sites honouring Hahnemann in Germany are few and far between (see Ch. 2) but the German Post Office did issue a special stamp in 1996 (Fig. 3.5).

Of particular note in the Netherlands is Jan Scholten. Scholten is known for working with remedy groupings, particularly mineral salts. His books *Homeopathy and the Minerals* and *Homeopathy and the Elements* are now considered fundamental texts for understanding and utilising mineral remedies in the periodic table. The concept of the whole new perspective of the periodic table is now being applied to the plant families and other areas of homeopathic materia medica.

Although only officially allowed in Russia since 1992, homeopathy was unofficially widely available in the former Soviet Union, many practitioners preparing their own remedies. Homeopathy is taught in medical schools and minimal standards have been introduced to try and standardise remedies, many of which are now being prepared by pharmacies. International congresses are held by the Russian Homeopathic Association on an irregular basis (http://www.homeoint.org/books4/kotok/).

Homeopathy is currently available in Bulgaria, Hungary, Poland and Romania. It is generally restricted to medical doctors but in some cases pharmacists are also involved. Small active communities are working hard to establish its popularity.

HOMEOPATHY IN LATIN AMERICA

Homeopathy is practised in Argentina, Brazil and Mexico. Of the three, Mexico is the best organized (P. Guajardo of the Instituto de Investigaciones en Ciencias Veterinarias, University de Baja California, Mexico, personal communication, October 1999), with training to become a medical doctor and homeopath available from two facilities in Mexico City. Three other institutions offer postgraduate training. In 1996 the National School of Medicine and Homeopathy (Escuela Nacional de Medicina y Homeopatía) celebrated its 100th anniversary. In fact, homeopathy in Mexico dates back to 1850, when migrating physicians from Spain taught local physicians (J. A. Oceguera, Sección de Estudios de Posgrado e Investigación, Escuela Nacional de Medicina y Homeopatía, Mexico DF, personal communication, translated by Germán Guajardo-Bernal, October 1999). One of the first successes was attributed to a Dr Carbo who in 1854 treated 45 patients during a yellow fever epidemic on the island prison of San Juan de Ulúa. His success was rewarded by President Antonio López de Santana who granted Dr Carbo a certificate to practice medicine in Mexico. In 1867, the first homeopathic pharmacy was founded and this was followed by the first homeopathic hospital at San Miguel de Allende Guanajuato 4 years later.

Many pharmacies now keep remedies and several others manufacture. Although only medical practitioners are supposed to practise homeopathy there are many other non-medically qualified practitioners operating. One state in Mexico even allows training for these practitioners. Dr Sanchez Ortega is a Mexican homeopath known throughout the world for his writings on miasms (see Ch. 7).

In Brazil, homeopathy as a therapeutic option to the services provided by traditional medicine only became a politically viable possibility in the 1980s in spite of the existence of homeopathic medicine in the country since 1840 (Luz, 1992). There are problems overcoming resistance from academic and clinical sources. Only medical doctors, dental surgeons and veterinarians are legally able to prescribe homeopathic remedies. However, supplies are also possible from pharmacies and *Drogeries* whose exact status I found difficult to identify while attending a convention in early 1999. They appeared to sell most of the items found in pharmacies but without a qualified pharmacist on the premises. There is a small but active group of homeopaths in the country, using different approaches to prescribing.

Argentina also has a small number of homeopaths (around 1500) but relatively little is known about the methods being used to treat patients or the distribution of the services on offer. Dr Eugenio Candegabe is known as a leading South American homeopath who was a founding member of the Argentine School of Homeopathic Medicine in Buenos Aires.

His interest in homeopathy began as a result of successful homeopathic treatment of members of his family, and in 1954 he went on to study the subject under his great mentor, Dr Tomás Pablo Paschero, with whom he subsequently worked closely. Dr E. Candegabe served as Professor of Materia Medica from 1971 until 1986, when he was nominated Emeritus Professor.

Homeopathy is popular in Costa Rica with over half the population using the therapy regularly. Training is available for both medical doctors and non-medically qualified practitioners.

During 1999 I visited Cuba and was delighted to find that the discipline was well organised in this republic of 20 million people. Some Mexican doctors helped reintroduce homeopathic practice to Cuba 1992 when it was incorporated into the National Health Service. A year later some Brazilian homeopaths offered the first formal medical training. Other health professions – pharmacy, dentistry and veterinary surgery – followed shortly after. There are now a total of 922 homeopaths in Cuba including 320 physicians, 220 veterinary surgeons, 161 pharmacists and 141 dentists. Teaching uses a national homeopathic curriculum and leads to the award of a diploma after 1 year of study. Unfortunately, further development is being hampered by a shortage of literature and remedies, particularly in the hospital environment.

All the municipalities around Havana and many elsewhere in the island offer homeopathic facilities through family doctors and clinics. Many pharmacies, including a magnificent new homeopathic pharmacy in Havana, dispense homeopathic prescriptions. They are all state owned. The 48 homeopathic dentists in the capital have performed 667 extractions collectively with the aid of 'homeopathic anaesthesia' achieved with the remedy Hypericum 200c given by mouth. Gathering statistics about consultations is a little difficult because homeopathy is officially included with other therapies under the heading 'Traditional Medicine' by the health authorities but it is known that there is considerable sympathy for the discipline at high levels within the Government. I was privileged to meet with the Minister of Health who reiterated a commitment to providing homeopathic facilities. Homeopathy is used by the medical facilities at Havana International Airport. Almost all the 200 patients who attended last year improved within 20 minutes of receiving their medicines; some 49 different remedies were used, the most popular being Baryta carb and Nux vom.

A considerable amount of homeopathic research is being carried out, particularly with animals. For example, homeopathic veterinary surgeons have reported that homeopathy can be used as a growth promoter for animals in the food chain, especially cows, pigs and chickens, and also to treat mastitis.

HOMEOPATHY IN THE USA

History

Homeopathy was brought to the USA in 1825 by Hans Burch Gram (1786–1840), a doctor born of Danish parents in Boston. He was trained in

Copenhagen by Dr Lund, a pupil of Hahnemann's (Winston, personal communication, January 1995). Within a few years of his return to New York, Dr Gram converted several orthodox practitioners in the New York City area and one, Vanderburgh, was responsible for teaching homeopathy to several other physicians who in turn spread it to other states in New England and the Mid-West. At this time there were many practitioners of botanical medicine, some of whom had learnt from Native American herbalists. At a time when regular medical training consisted of 6 months of lectures and 2 years of supervised practice, the care offered by the herbalists was often better than the bleeding, purging and taking of chemicals prescribed by the orthodox physicians.

At about the same time that Gram settled in New York, William Wesselhoeft and Henry Detwiller, two German physician émigrés who were living near Bethlehem, Pennsylvania, began studying Hahnemann's *Organon* and *Materia Medica*. When Detwiller cured a patient with a dose of Pulsatilla in 1828, the two became homeopaths. By 1833, when Dr Constantine Hering arrived in the US, the practice of homeopathy was well under way in the German communities in the area around Philadelphia. Hering was born at Oschatz, Germany, in 1800, and first studied homeopathy with the intention of writing an essay refuting Hahnemann's teachings, but instead was converted to them (Fie, 1990). Hering emigrated to America and became the guiding force behind American homeopathy, founding in 1835, together with several other physicians, the first medical school in the world to teach homeopathy. Although the Allentown Academy, as it was called, lasted for only 2 years before its funds ran out, it became the training ground for some of the finest homeopathic doctors of the next generation. In 1844, 3 years before the American Medical Association was formed, Hering, with a group of doctors from New York and Boston, founded the American Institute of Homeopathy, and this body is still in existence. Four years later Hering, Williamson and Jeanes founded the Homeopathic Medical College of Pennsylvania, later to become the Hahnemann Medical College.

By the 1880s there were over 20 homeopathic medical colleges in the USA and every state had a homeopathic medical society. As the century drew to a close, however, most of the homeopathic schools began to teach what might be called a symptomatic or 'this for that' approach to homeopathy and ignored the holistic teachings of Hahnemann. In 1880, shortly before the death of Hering, a group of physicians, headed by Adolph Lippe and H. C. Allen, established the International Hahnemannian Association (IHA). The IHA decried the move away from Hahnemannian teaching and began to establish its own educational institutions.

At the same time, James Tyler Kent began his study of homeopathy in St Louis, and emerged as one of the prominent homeopathic practitioners and educators for the next 30 years. It was Kent who restored the classic features of homeopathic practice. He left a lasting memorial in the form of his huge text *Repertory of the Homeopathic Materia Medica*.

A little known fact of history is that homeopathic medicine developed its popularity in the USA (as well as in Europe – see above) because of its successes in treating the infectious epidemics that raged during the 19th century

(Ullman, 1991). In 1849 the homeopaths of Cincinnati claimed that in over 1000 cases of cholera only 3% of the patients died. To substantiate their results they even printed the names and addresses of patients who died or who survived in a newspaper (Bradford, 1900). The death rate of patients with cholera who used conventional medicines generally ranged from 40 to 70%.

The success of treating yellow fever with homeopathy was so impressive that a report from the US Government's board of experts included several homeopathic medicines, despite the fact that the board was primarily composed of conventional physicians who despised homeopathy (Coulter, 1979).

In 1910, an evaluation of medical education in the USA led to the closing of many medical schools, among them most of the homeopathic schools. In 1916, Kent died, and it was his pupils who in large part helped to keep homeopathy in the USA alive during a time when it was seen as unscientific and old-fashioned.

In an 1890 issue of *Harpers Magazine* Mark Twain acknowledged the special value of homeopathy, noting, 'The introduction of homeopathy forced the old school doctor to stir around and learn something of a rational nature about his business' (Twain, 1890). Twain also asserted: 'You may honestly feel grateful that homeopathy survived the attempts of the allopathists [orthodox physicians] to destroy it.'

In 1922, Julia M. Green, MD, founded the American Foundation for Homeopathy, in an effort to continue training physicians in homeopathy. When Hahnemann College in Philadelphia stopped teaching even its elective course in homeopathy in 1959, it looked as if the discipline was all but dead. The resurgence in the rise of natural therapies led to the development of the two naturopathic colleges on the west coast, and the emergence of a new crop of well-trained homeopaths.

The roots of the homeopathic pharmaceutical industry in the USA stem from a handful of companies founded between 1840 and 1910. Of the active companies remaining, only Standard Homeopathic (1903) and Luyties Pharmacal (1853) are still American owned. The rest are now owned by European interests. Boericke and Tafel (1843) is Dutch owned and Borneman (1910) is French owned. In addition, numerous new companies have established themselves, including Natra-Bio, Dolisos and HomeoLab. An increasing trend is the development of marketing companies who do not produce their own products but sell their own brands made under contract (Sunsource, Pharmavite, NaturaLife, Lake Pharmaceutical and Schmid Laboratories). The trend for non-pharmaceutical companies to enter the field continues with an increased number of allopathic marketers exploring the field (Borneman, personal communication, November 2004).

The National Center for Complementary and Alternative Medicine (NCCAM)

In October 1991, the US Congress passed legislation (P.L.102-170) that provided $2 million in funding for fiscal year 1992 to establish within the National Institutes of Health (NIH) a centre to investigate and evaluate promising unconventional medical practices. The NIH is one of eight agencies under the Public Health Service (PHS) in the Department of Health and Human Services (DHHS).

The NCCAM is dedicated to exploring complementary and alternative healing practices in the context of rigorous science, training CAM researchers and disseminating authoritative information to the public and professional communities.

The four primary areas of focus are:

- the support of clinical and basic science research projects
- provision of research training and career development
- sponsoring of conferences and educational exhibits
- the integration of scientifically proven CAM practices into conventional medicine.

The NCCAM Strategic Plan (2005–2009) presents a series of goals and objectives to guide NCCAM in managing its portfolio in the future. This action is in order to concentrate on efforts likely to yield the greatest impact on the health and well-being of people at every stage of life, using the following set of master health goals as important, but not exclusive, selection criteria:

- Enhance physical and mental health and wellness
- Manage pain and other symptoms, disabilities, and functional impairment
- Have a significant impact on a specific disease or disorder
- Prevent disease and empower individuals to take responsibility for their health
- Reduce selected health problems of specific populations.

The document is based on extensive public input, the advice of NCCAM staff, and the recommendations of a distinguished group of outside experts. In this document, NCCAM's first 5 years are reviewed. Goals for four strategic areas have been specified:

- Investing in research
- Training CAM researchers
- Expanding outreach
- Advancing the organisation.

The document can be viewed and/or downloaded at http://nccam.nih.gov/about/plans/2005/index.htm. A more detailed history of homeopathy in the USA may be accessed at http://www.homeopathic.com/articles/intro/history.php.

Samuel Hahnemann Memorial, Washington DC

An impressive memorial to Samuel Hahnemann stands to the east of the Scott Circle, near the cross-section of Massachusetts and Rhode Island Avenues, Washington DC. The idea of a monument to Hahnemann was proposed in 1881 by J. H. McClelland, but a further 19 years was to pass until it was authorised by Congress in January 1900. The sculptor was Charles Henry Niehaus, a resident of Cincinnati, who used as his model a bust of Hahnemann aged 82, given by Melanie Hahnemann, the Founder's colourful second wife. The architect was J. Harder of the firm Israel and Harder,

New York. The monument was the gift of the American Institute of Homeopathy and was unveiled the following June. The bronze statue shows Hahnemann seated on a pedestal centered in front of a curving wall of New Hampshire granite. The pedestal bears the well-known principle of homeopathy, expressed in the Latin phrase *Similia similibus curantur*. Four large bronze bas-relief panels on the wall depict Hahnemann as a student surrounded by books, a chemist in the laboratory, a teacher in the lecture room, and a physician at the bedside. In June 2000 a ceremony was held in the presence of an international audience to rededicate the memorial. As in 1900 a marine band played and a colour party from the US Forces added formality to the rededication ceremony. The US President was not present on this occasion, but he did send a letter of congratulation.

REFERENCES

Anon. (1992) Conference backs homeopathy. *Pharm J*, 249: 343–344.

Bensoussan, A and Lewith, GT (2004) Complementary medicine research in Australia: a strategy for the future. *Med J Aust*, 181: 331–333.

Bradford, TL (1900) *The Logic of Figures or Comparative Results of Homoeopathic and Other Treatments*. Boericke and Tafel, Philadelphia.

Coulter, HL (1979) *Divided Legacy: The Conflict Between Homoeopathy and the American Medical Association*. North Atlantic Books, Berkeley, CA.

Fie, WB (1990) Vasodilator theory for angina pectoris: the intersection of homeopathy and scientific medicine. *J Hist Med*, 45: 317–340.

Fisher, P (1989) Homeopathy in Nigeria. *Br Homeopath J*, 78: 171–173.

Gaier, H (1991) *Encyclopaedic Dictionary of Homeopathy*. Thorsons, London.

Gaucher, C (1995) The role of homeopathy in the treatment of tetanus. *Br Homeopath J*, 84: 149–155.

Gaucher, C, Jeulin, D, Peycru, P, Pla, A and Amengual, C (1993) Cholera and homeopathic medicine: the Peruvian experience. *Br Homeopath J*, 82: 155–163.

Gaucher, C, Jeulin, D, Peycru, P and Amengual, C (1994) A double blind randomised placebo controlled study of cholera treatment with highly diluted and succussed solution. *Br Homeopath J*, 83: 132–134.

Hamilton, E (1882) A memoir of FHF Quin. *Ann Trans Br Homeopath Soc*, 9: 1–112.

Jenkins, H (1989) The history of the Royal London Homeopathic Hospital. *Br Homeopath J*, 78: 198–202.

Kayne, SB (1991) Homeopathy – demand and scepticism. *Pharm J*, 247: 602–604.

Kent, JT (1969) *Repertory of the Homeopathy Materia Medica*. S. Dey, Calcutta.

Leary, B (1993) The smaller homeopathic hospitals. *Homeopathy*, 43(6): 127–130.

Leary, B (1994a) The foundations of the British Homeopathic Society. *Br Homeopath J*, 83: 185–186.

Leary, B (1994b) Cholera 1854: update. *Br Homeopath J*, 83: 117–121.

Luz, MT (1992) The incorporation of homeopathy into public health. *Br Homeopath J*, 81: 55–58.

McDermott, L (1991) Homeopathy and its development in New Zealand. BSc Degree Project, University of Otago, Dunedin.

Mitchell, G (1975) *Homeopathy*. WH Allen, London, p 24.

Nasir, N and Zain, M (1988) A brief history of homeopathy in Malaysia. *J OMHI*, 1: 26.

Okpokpor, SO (1991) Homeopathy – Nigerian update. *Homeopathy*, 41: 140.

Quin, FH (1862) Address of the President. *Homeopathic Annals and Transactions*, 1: 3–13.

Steinbach, D (1981) The pros and cons of homeopathy. *Pharm J*, 227: 384–387.

Twain, M (1890) A majestic literary fossil. *Harpers Magazine*, February: 444. (Cited by Ullman, D (1991) *A Condensed History of Homeopathy* (from *Discovering Homeopathy: Medicine for the 21st Century*, North Atlantic Books Berkeley CA). Available online http://www.homeopathic.com/articles/intro/history.php. (Accessed January 2005.)

Ullman, D (1991) *A Homeopathic Perspective on Infectious Disease: Effective Alternatives to Antibiotics*. Homeopathic Educational Services. Available online http://homeopathic.com/articles/using_h/inf_disease.php. (Accessed January 2005.)

PART 2

Procedures

PART CONTENTS

4. Preparing the remedy   81

5. Supply of a named remedy   121

6. The provision of homeopathic
   treatment   137

Chapter **4**

Preparing the remedy

CHAPTER CONTENTS

The Homeopathic Pharmacopoeia	81	Other methods of potentisation	97
Sources of raw materials	83	Pharmaceutical presentations available	100
Plant material	83	Oral dose forms	100
Animal and insect material	85	Solid dose forms	101
Biological material	85	The medicating process for solid dose	
Chemical material	87	forms	103
Miscellaneous source material	87	Topical preparations	105
New sources of remedies	88	Other dose forms	105
Preparation of remedies	89	Quality control	107
Extraction	90	Packaging and storage	109
Potentisation	92	Nomenclature	110
Dilution	92	Legal status of homeopathic remedies	113
Succussion	93	Further information for pharmacists	117
Terminology – centesimal and decimal			
scales	95		

THE HOMEOPATHIC PHARMACOPOEIA

In the very simplest terms homeopathic remedies may be defined as being 'medicines used according to the principles of Samuel Hahnemann'. This is not entirely true, however, for several 'new' ways of using homeopathy have emerged since Hahnemann's time, for example drainage therapy (see Ch. 8). Complex remedies have never been subject to provings (although their constituents may have been proven individually) so they cannot be administered according to the similimum. Mother tinctures are generally considered to be homeopathic, but many have not been proven either and are used more in a herbal manner than homeopathically. Modern definitions tend to focus on what remedies *are* rather than how they are used. The wide-ranging definition given in both the EU Directive for Medicinal Products (1992) and UK Statutory Instrument (SI 1995/308) is as follows:

> *Homeopathic medicinal product means a medicinal product (which may contain a number of principles) prepared from products, substances or compositions called homeopathic stocks in accordance with a homeopathic manufacturing procedure described by the European Pharmacopoeia or, in the absence thereof, by any pharmacopoeia used officially in an (EU) member state.*

The UK Medicines and Healthcare Products Regulation Authority (MHRA) and other European regulatory bodies uses the term *stocks* for the starting solutions, usually *mother tinctures*, from which homeopathic potencies are prepared.

For many years, British manufacturers relied on a selection of foreign reference works for most of their information, particularly with regard to the analysis of starting materials. They used principally the *German Homeopathic Pharmacopoeia (Homëopathisches Arzneibuch or HAB)*, with its various supplements, together with the French and the *Homeopathic Pharmacopoeia* of the USA (*HPUS*), the first of which was produced by the American Institute in 1897 with the help of Otis Clap and Sons. This became the official text in 1938. The *German Homeopathic Pharmacopoeia*, usually abbreviated to *HAB* or *GHP*, was first published in 1825 by Dr Caspari of Leipzig and then again by Schwabe in 1872, and was translated into English by the British Homeopathic Association in 1990. The English version is now available from ECHAMP, the European Coalition on Homeopathic and Anthroposophic Medicinal Products, at the following website: http://www.echamp.org/home.php.

There is also an *Indian Homeopathic Pharmacopoeia* in four volumes produced with the help of the Indian Homeopathic Pharmacopoeia Committee appointed in 1962 (Banerjee, 1991).

The first edition of the *British Homeopathic Pharmacopoeia* was published by the British Homeopathic Society in 1870 with later editions in 1876 and 1882 by E. Gould and Son of London. It then went out of print for over a century. New editions of the *BHomP* were published by the British Association of Homeopathic Manufacturers (BAHM) in 1993 and 1999. The book is in a clear loose-leaf format and reflects many of the current practices developed by British manufacturers by adapting German methods. It is designed to be used in conjunction with the *HAB*. The *British Homeopathic Pharmacopoeia (BHomP)* has no official status, having not been adopted as a national standard by the MHRA. The first section of the book contains background information to the manufacture of homeopathic preparations, including abbreviations, analytical methods, reagents and general regulations for the manufacture of homeopathic medicines. Cross-reference is made to the *HAB* and other pharmacopoeias. At the start of the section on manufacturing methods there is an index to all the methods of preparation, referencing the source of the method concerned. The monographs are set out in the second part. The development work for the British methods and monographs took place in the laboratories of BAHM members.

Unfortunately some of the standard methods of manufacture are not as specific as they could be, especially with regard to diluents. Another important omission is the lack of standardisation for unit dose forms. The inclusion of Bach flower remedies in the book causes concern to many homeopathic pharmacists, for the reasons outlined in Chapter 10.

Following many years' work by the Scientific Committee of the International Committee of Homeopathic Pharmacists (CIPH), the German Health Ministry took the initiative in 1988 to invite member countries to an informal meeting to discuss the feasibility of establishing standards for homeopathic medicines. Later that year, in November, an international meeting convened in London by the Faculty of Homeopathy adopted a proposal to establish a European Homeopathic Pharmacopoeia Commission comprising representatives from the then 12 members of the European Community. In May 1989 the Chairman of the European Pharmacopoeia Commission invited representatives of the main homeopathic manufacturers, pharmacists and representatives of several European Health Ministries to a meeting in Strasbourg. It was greed that a European Homeopathic Pharmacopoeia should be produced for use in the EU and EFTA countries. Subsequently it was agreed that the European Pharmacopoeia should include homeopathic monographs and the first appeared in 2002.

SOURCES OF RAW MATERIALS

In many instances it is not possible to be specific about the exact source of material and to equate it exactly with the material used by Hahnemann and others in early provings. For example, we do know that the drug picture of Apis mellifica, the bee, was derived originally from provings of bee venom, whereas now the whole insect is used. The controversy over this particular remedy has raged for a long time. In his book *Guiding Symptoms* (1879) Constantine Hering wrote:

> It is foolish to take the whole bee with all the foreign matter and impurities. There is but one kind. It is the pure poison, which is obtained by grasping the bee with small forceps and catching the minute drop of virus suspended from the point of the sting.

It is claimed that some manufacturers do not adhere to the standardised practices set down by Hahnemann (Barthel, 1993). Among more modern remedies becoming available there is considerable discussion as to the source for RNA and DNA remedies.

Despite these potential problems, homeopathic pharmacy routinely produces over 3000 remedies, of which about 1250 are in common use, in a variety of potencies (Ainsworth, 1991).

For details on how remedies prepared from the following sources are used in homeopathic practice, see Chapter 8.

Plant material

About 65% of all remedies are prepared from extracts of plant materials, and because of this homeopathy is often confused with herbalism by many people. The manner of producing the two types of medicine is quite different, however. Herbal products are generally the result of an aqueous or alcoholic extraction alone, whereas in homeopathy an additional dilution process is involved. Either the whole plant may be used or only the leaves, flowers, stems or roots as specified in the pharmacopoeia monographs. The species of plant, the parts taken, the time of collection and the extraction procedures may well differ according to the particular pharmacopoeia monograph being consulted (Belgian Pharmaceutical Society, 1995). For Calendula, for instance, the *HPUS* specifies flower tips, the *French Pharmacopoeia* specifies fresh leaf tips, and the *HAB* the whole aerial flowering parts. Depending on where the plant material is grown, harvesting may extend over several months, and the active ingredients vary in both quality and quantity. Patients' delight at being offered familiar remedies abroad should be tempered by the strong possibility that these remedies are likely to differ in therapeutic strength from those obtained at home. It is important that incoming foreign travellers are also made aware of this fact. Figure 4.1 represents high-performance liquid chromatography (HPLC) traces of Urtica mother tincture derived from two different species of the plant. A clear difference in the peak patterns and therefore the constituents can be seen.

Work carried out by a homeopathic Master's student at Durban Institute of Technology using NMR spectroscopy has demonstrated differences in the traces associated with remedies obtained by different methods of production (Hofmeyr, 2004).

The specimens are usually collected in dry, sunny weather and cleaned by careful shaking, brushing and rinsing with distilled water. They are then

Figure 4.1 HPLC traces of Urtica from different sources. A: Tincture of the whole fresh plant of *Urtica dioica*. B: Tincture of the whole fresh plant of *Urtica urens*. (Courtesy of Weleda, UK Ltd.)

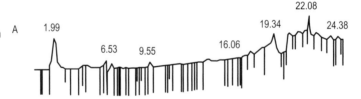

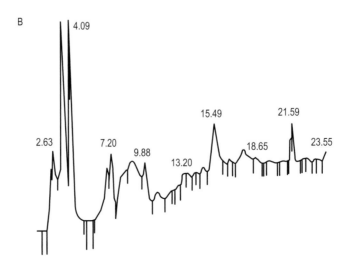

examined to ensure the absence of moulds and other imperfections. Berries, fruits and seeds are generally gathered when ripe and must be perfect. Non-resinous barks are harvested from young trees late in the autumn or, depending on the species and if resinous, at the development of blossom. Woods are collected from young trees and shrubs before the sap rises. A record is kept of all growing conditions and time of collection. Fresh plant material is really desirable, but for a variety of reasons dried specimens are sometimes used. Arnica, for example, grows best above 3000 m and is often subject to conservation orders at certain times of the year, while Nux vomica is readily available by the sack-load, but difficult to obtain in the very small quantities required by pharmacists. Soil differences may mean that the easily accessible plants are not the most suitable. Crataegus, the hawthorn, varies in quality from country to country, while Hydrastis from Canada is preferable to samples from USA. These difficulties may be appreciated if one considers the analogy of wines: grapes grown in different soil and climatic conditions, even if adjacent to each other, can produce wines with totally different characteristics.

Animal and insect material

This material must be obtained from healthy specimens. Lactrodectus is a spider whose venom is sometimes used in the treatment of angina. The bee yields Apis, a remedy used to treat peripheral oedematous conditions and the effects of stings. Apis is a good example of the origins of homeopathy in folk medicine. The remedy was introduced by a Dr Frederick Humphries following the intervention of a Native American to help treat a young boy in Providence, Rhode Island, in 1847, although it had been used a few years earlier to treat horses by a German clergyman.

Jeremy Sherr proved a remedy derived from the scorpion in 1985. The insect has been known to be a medicine since the earliest times; specimens burnt alive have been used in the treatment of gall stones, and their ash used as a diuretic and for renal colic. Sherr killed his scorpions by injecting 95% alcohol into their rectums; he preserved them in a similar vehicle. They were then triturated for 3 hours with yet more 95% alcohol, using a pestle and mortar, and he eventually potentised the resulting solution in the normal way (Sherr, 1990).

The insect remedies are usually quick acting, and are especially useful in inflammatory and immune responses. Examples of remedies from some insect and marine sources are summarised in Table 4.1. There are also remedies made from snake, lizard and salamander venoms (Walker, 1995). Other sources are musk oil and the juice of the cuttlefish (Sepia).

It is important to be aware of any common remedies made from animal or insect material, as patients occasionally ask not to be treated with medicines derived from these sources.

Biological material

Material may be used from healthy animal or vegetable secretions or from bacterial cultures; the resulting remedy is then known as a *sarcode*. It may

Table 4.1 Examples of remedies made from animal/insect tissue

Remedy	Source	Main use
Apis mellifica	Honey bee: crushed	Oedema, inflammation
Astacus fluviatilis	Crawfish	Urticaria
Badiaga (Spongilla fluv)	Fresh water sponge	Soreness of muscles
Blatta orientalis	Indian cockroach	Asthma
Cantharis vesicator	Spanish fly	Burns, cystitis
Cimex lectularoius	Bedbug	Intermittent fever
Coccus cacti	Cochineal (insect)	Spasmodic/whooping cough
Formica rufa	Crushed live ants	Arthritic conditions
Helix tosta	Snail, toasted without shell	Haemorrhage, chest diseases
Homarus	Lobster digestive fluids	Dyspepsia, sore throat
Latrodectus mactans	Spider	Angina
Pulex irritans	Common flea	Prickly itching skin
Tarantula hispanica	Tarantula (spider)	Nervous hysteria

also be derived from diseased tissue, when the finished remedies are known as *nosodes*. For example, Pertussis is a sarcode produced from a culture, while Pertussin is a nosode prepared from infected sputum. A third variant, known as a *tautopathic* (see below), is made from the allopathic vaccine. This differentiation is important for it has implications for the way in which these remedies are used. Often, it is unclear from the label whether an old remedy is a nosode or a sarcode. This is due to the records of original source material being lost. Staplococcus is a remedy that falls into this category. Modern manufacture involves the fixing of infective material before extraction. The preservation of accurate records is an important development.

Sarcodes may be used according to the similimum or as a prophylactic. Examples of sarcode source material are:

- plant sarcodes: Terebintha, the oleic exudation from pine trees
- animal sarcodes: RNA and DNA; Cholesterinum, Folliculinum
- bacterial sarcodes: Penicillin derived from a culture.

Nosodes may be used to treat pathological conditions; some historical nosodes also have drug pictures. Examples of nosode source material are:

- plant nosodes: examples include remedies derived from Secale cornutum (ergot); Ustilago maydis (corn smut); Solanum tuberosum aegrotans (diseased potato). A drug picture of the latter, accredited to Benoit More (1809–1858), may be found in a fascinating book entitled *Homoeopathy in the Irish Potato Famine* (Treuherz, 1995). The isopathic use of this remedy is advocated by inoculation of healthy potatoes as a form of prophylaxis against the blight (Kennedy, 1997)

- animal nosodes derived from pathological secretions, for example: Ambra grisea (from sperm whale)
- microbial nosodes derived from pathological samples, for example: Syphilinum (Lueticum) spirochetes in syphilitic exudate; Variolinum from smallpox vesicle
- pathological autonosodes: made from patients' own body fluids, exudates and infected lesions (e.g. vesicles and pustules) can be useful in dealing with long-standing chronic infections, particularly those showing resistance to orthodox homeopathy. This treatment is not carried out routinely and the preparation of the remedies necessitates substantial precautions to prevent the spread of disease.

Treatment using remedies in this group is often termed isopathic and involves treating 'same with same', as opposed to classical homeopathy, when 'like is treated with like'.

Chemical material

About 30% of all source material is chemical in nature. Highly purified laboratory grade material is rarely used in the preparation of remedies. The original provings carried out by Hahnemann used naturally occurring chemicals together with their trace impurities, which are considered to contribute to the overall activity of the remedy in a symbiotic way. Thus Calc carb is obtained from the middle layers of mussel (or oyster) shells and is not prepared in the laboratory. Considering how far Hahnemann's home was from the nearest oyster beds it is perhaps surprising that he should have chosen this source when other forms of the mineral were far more accessible locally. Natrum mur is derived from sea salt and Sulphur is obtained from a naturally occurring source; neither is prepared pure in the laboratory. A remedy known by the delightful name of Skookum chuck comprises chemical salts obtained from the water of Medical Lake near Spokane, Washington. Sanicula is a similar remedy from the water of Sanicula Springs, Ottawa, Illinois. The springs have long since dried up, however, and there is barely enough remedy in circulation to satisfy requirements (Satti, 1997). Hecla lava is derived from the laval flow of Mount Hecla in Iceland. One synthetic success can be recorded, however. Petroleum was formerly obtained from the naturally occurring Rangoon rock oil but during the war years the source was inaccessible. In this case the chemically pure substitute was found to be as active as the original material.

Miscellaneous source material

This grouping covers a mixed bag of source materials including allergens such as pollens, flowers, cat and dog hair, feathers and various foods (coffee, chocolate, eggs, milk, etc.), known as **allergodes,** together with about 150 allopathic drugs and vaccines including aspirin, chloramphenicol and penicillin known collectively as **tautodes** or **tautopathic remedies**. Remedies made from industrial chemicals (e.g. solvents, paints, etc.), insecticides (e.g. organophosphates, sheepdips, etc.) and household fluids (e.g. disinfectants, washing-up liquids) are also said to be tautopathic. They are generally (but not exclusively) used for the isopathic treatment of allergies and chemical irritation.

Propolis is a brownish resinous material derived from the buds of trees. It is also called 'bee glue' for it is used by bees to seal cracks in the hive comb, or for covering foreign objects in the hive that cannot be removed.

The remedy Tela aranearum is prepared from the web of a fully grown cross or garden spider (Schober and Luckert, 1994). According to Hering:

> the insect is made to run along a hoop and then made to fall by shaking, so that it hangs by its own thread. The hoop is then rotated and as much thread as possible extracted . . . in order to extract one grain several hours of strenuous work (involving many spiders) are necessary.

The drug picture of Tela is rarely listed but doses of the remedy are reported to have engendered a peaceful happy mood and an undisturbed refreshing sleep. In today's stressful world it is surprising that it does not enjoy more exposure.

There are a few remedies in the materia medica, for example Electricity (electric current), Radium bromide (radiation), Sol (sunshine), X-ray and Mag pol Aust (magnetism), that are made by exposure to the agents indicated. Another example is Luna (moonlight). A proving for this remedy was carried out by King and Lawrence in England in 1993.

New sources of remedies

The list of remedies available has grown in recent times. Some of the newer remedies do have full drug pictures (Julian, 1979), and from time to time new provings are reported in the journals. Modern provings of Chocolate have revealed an extensive drug picture containing emotional applications such as 'excitement, difficulties in concentrating, and aversion to company' (Dynamis School, 1994a). The US Food and Drug Administration (FDA) has published a monograph for chocolate manufacturers that specifies that up to 4% by weight may contain cockroach 'parts' since it is impossible to prevent the insects from contaminating vats in which chocolate is manufactured. A homeopathic remedy manufactured from chocolate in the USA may therefore show different characteristics to a similar remedy manufactured in Northern Europe. One British producer offers a potency made from the Berlin Wall, and claims success in treating patients suffering from trembling associated with terror. Hydrogen has also been proved (Dynamis School, 1994b). At the Russian Homeopathic Congress in Moscow in 1992, a remedy called Aqua crystalisata (ice) was reported by a participant. The preparation was made by adding ice crystals to alcohol and potentising the resulting solution. It appeared to have a localised role and 'activated the liquid crystal protein in the body' according to the Lithuanian doctor who

Box 4.1   PC Computeris

Progress in producing new remedies is slow and laborious. A relatively recent addition to the materia medica known as 'PC Computeris' was first reported by Dr Barry Rose. The source material has been extensively used by him, and the provings are therefore statistically reliable. The drug used by Barry for this proving can be obtained from a specialized high street store or through the post. It comprises three separate parts: a central processing unit (CPU), a keyboard and a video display unit (VDU), none of which seem to be much use unless connected to the other two. An electrical source is essential. The drug apparently causes a form of insomnia during which the patient may be found tapping on the keyboard for several hours at a time. The symptoms seem to be worse between midnight and 3 a.m. Very often the patient becomes involved in a conversation with the screen, and this periodically degenerates into a one-sided swearing match. The screen for its part merely flashes its cursor repeatedly, inviting even more abuse. Experimental work carried out by the author has shown that the effects of the drug can be antidoted by the use of a mother tincture known as Maltus singlus major, an amber-coloured liquid originating from an aqueous cereal extract. Another liquid remedy, Vinium rubrum, is said to have a similar effect. Excessive amounts of either have been known to result in a dissociated type of reaction leading to confused entries on the VDU. The source of supply of these liquids is critical.

While promising to be an effective remedy, PC Computeris should not be overused, for such action inevitably results in the output of garbage. (I am obliged to Dr Barry Rose, former Dean at the Faculty of Homeopathy, for permission to adapt the above from an article of his that first appeared in the *British Homeopathic Journal* in June 1987.)

presented several case studies, including the treatment of obesity (Kayne, 1992). An attempt has been made to prove Sequoia sempervirens, the Californian redwood. Possible indications include ailments from grief and Lyme's disease (Birch and Rockwell, 1994). Bonnet, long associated with the toxicology of insects, has highlighted several new remedies including the venoms of the Laxosceles spider (Bonnet, 1996) and the Androctonus scorpion (Bonnet, 1997).

Homeopathic dilutions of RNA have also been used clinically (Riley and Zagon, 2005).

For a final new remedy, see Box 4.1.

PREPARATION OF REMEDIES

The following approach is not suggested, but may serve as an amusing interlude:

> Take a sparrow's leg, the drumstick merely,
> Place in a tub, filled with water nearly,
> Set it out doors, in a place that's shady;

Let it stand a week (three days for a lady);
Drop a good spoonful in a fine large kettle,
Which should be of tin (or any sim'lar metal);
Add one grain of salt; for thickening – one rice kernel.
To light the fire – use the *Homeopathic Journal*.
Fill the kettle up and set it a-boiling
Strain the mixture well, to stop it oiling;
Let the liquor stew for an hour – no longer,
(For a man, of course it'll need to be stronger.)
Should you now desire the soup to be 'flavoury',
Stir it well, once round, with a stick of savoury.
When the broth is made, nothing can excel it,
So three times a day, let the patient smell it.
If he chance to die, say 'T'was nature did it',
If he chance to live, give the soup the credit.

(Adapted from an anonymous poem published in the *British Homeopathic Journal* in April, 1994, with the Editor's permission.)

Extraction

Mother tinctures are the liquid preparations resulting from the extraction of suitable source material with alcohol/water mixtures which form the starting point for the production of most homeopathic medicines. Comminution followed by standard percolation, maceration and squeezing techniques are used on fresh plants (which yield around 350 ml of juice per kg) and succulents (which yield up to twice the plant harvest), while dried specimens are subjected mainly to percolation with alcohol on a column similar to those illustrated in Figure 4.2.

It has been shown that the concentration of alcohol used in the extraction process can affect the quality of the final product and that the best solvent is 70% w/v alcohol (Nandi, 2002).

The resulting solutions are strained and can contain one part drug to three parts mother tincture, although this strength can vary from 10 to 50% depending on the species and monograph being used. When the final tincture represents one-tenth of the concentration of original drug it is, in effect, a 1x dilution.

Methods of preparing mother tinctures differ between the *FrHomP* and *HAB*. In the former it states that the material is macerated for at least 3 weeks whereas the *HAB* specifies that it is left for at least 10 days at a temperature not exceeding 20°C.

In later life, around 1835, Hahnemann is reported to have stopped using the mother tincture method of preparing potencies for soluble source material, preferring to process crude plant drugs, expressed juices and fresh plants by trituration with lactose (Dellmour, 1994). Trituration is the grinding of powders in a mortar with a pestle. It is the primary mode of mixing used for the preparation of powdered dilutions in homeopathy. Initially this trituration process was taken to the 12c level, but subsequently he changed to the 3c, producing higher potencies in fluid form. Compared with medicines produced from mother tinctures and solutions, this offered advantages

Figure 4.2 Percolation columns

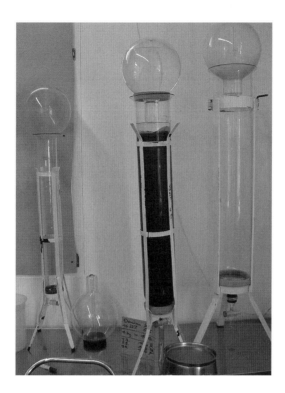

in more powerful action, longer shelf-life and retained constituents. Hahnemann processed a total of 54 mineral and plant remedies in this way. Although it would appear to be beneficial, the method is not generally used by modern producers other than for insoluble material.

Two other methods of extraction are available, although Hahnemann claimed that they produced remedies with different degrees of therapeutic activity.

Hahnemann knew of the medicinal use of powdered gold from his study of the early medical literature and in 1818 he triturated Aurum (as gold leaf) with lactose, finding the 1c potency to be effective in the treatment of suicidal depression. He triturated the remedy to produce higher potencies and subsequently suggested that the process should be adopted as a general method for making lower-potency remedies in homeopathic pharmacy.

With insoluble chemicals such as Aurum (gold), Plumbum (lead) or Sulphur (and many isopathic preparations) the solid material must be triturated and serially diluted with lactose powder using a pestle and mortar in a precise and documented manner. The process should be carried out in a warm dry atmosphere with perfectly clean equipment. According to the *HAB*, the lactose should be divided into three parts, and a third of the diluent is triturated with the starting material for 6 minutes and then scraped off the mortar and pestle with a spatula for 4 minutes. The process is repeated before adding the second and third aliquots in a similar manner. The length of time and physical effort required for the trituration can vary, depending on the material being processed. Hard substances (e.g. Zincum met) produce finer particles than do soft substances (e.g. Plumbum met).

When triturating Ferrum met, moisture must be removed by warming up the mortar from time to time.

The resulting triturate may be compressed directly into trituration tablets or administered as a powder if the remedy is required at potencies where it is still insoluble. More usually, however, trituration continues until the particle size has been reduced sufficiently to facilitate the preparation of a solution, usually achieved after three to six serial dilutions, depending on the scale being used. This solution is sometimes inaccurately called a mother tincture, but in fact could be a 6x or even 8x potency. From this point the standard potentisation procedure described in the following section can be followed. Some remedies are therefore not available as mother tinctures or very low potencies; for example, the first potency of Sulphur that can be made by surface inoculation of blank tablets is a 6x. (A supplier will be able to advise on this matter.)

In the case of soluble chemicals, solutions of known concentration in distilled water or alcohol can be initially prepared. Argent nit is prepared as a 10% solution (equivalent to 1x) while Merc cyan and Kali perman are both prepared as a 1% solution (equivalent to 2x or 1c). There is also an extraction process based on the use of equal weights of alcohol and glycerol on raw material of plant origin, for example buds, shoots or more rarely rootlets, seeds, or bark (Belgian Pharmaceutical Society, 1995).

Potentisation

With some remedies, for example Arnica or Calendula, the mother tincture may be applied directly to the skin, or it may be diluted and used as a gargle; Crataegus mother tincture is often administered as five drops in water.

Most other mother tinctures, however, are subjected to a very special two-stage process involving dilution and succussion. Because it increases the therapeutic strength, this process is known as potentisation. It is also called dynamisation. There are several methods of potentisation, of which the Hahnemannian method, devised by the Founder after a series of experiments, is the most common in the UK. Other methods are described below.

Dilution

The *Hahnemannian method* offers two scales of dilution, centesimal and decimal. In the former, one drop of mother tincture is added to 99 (or 9) drops of diluent in a new clean screw cap glass vial (Fig. 4.3).

In modern pharmaceutical practice it is common to use a triple distilled alcohol and water system, the strength of which varies from 20 to 60%, in the preparation of homeopathic dilutions. Hahnemann in 1827 recommended good brandy as a diluent. Brandy contains a lot of accompanying substances in addition to ethanol.

Lorenz et al. (2003) compared two dilution media to investigate the diluent's influence. Within the limitations of the test system the dilution media were as similar to good brandy as possible and like purified ethanol. Dilutions of histamine were prepared with both media. As test system they used modified basophil activation in an in vitro cell system. The results

Figure 4.3 The potentisation process

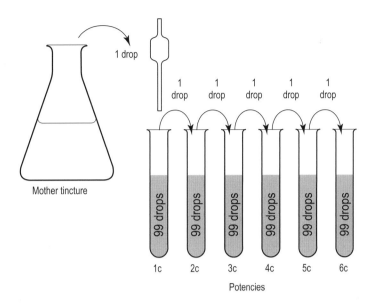

appeared to support the hypothesis that the dilution medium may influence the effects of high dilutions. This could be of importance for homeopathic pharmaceutical practice as well as for ultra-high dilution experiments.

Traditionally a single drop of mother tincture was obtained by tipping the container and carefully manipulating a cork stopper. This required a great deal of dexterity and often lead to minute traces of cork becoming incorporated into the potencies (R. Davey, personal communication, January 1995). To ensure no such contamination occurs, a disposable glass capillary or dropper bottle is now used for this transfer. For accuracy the 99 drops are usually measured with a special calibrated glass pipette.

Succussion

The solution resulting from admixture of the two liquids is subjected to the vigorous shaking with impact known as succussion. In Hahnemann's day the procedure was effected by striking the vial on a large leather-bound book, typically the family Bible. Nowadays, in a more secular environment, the same effect is usually obtained with a special mechanical shaker.

There are a few pharmacists who still succuss by hand, striking the vial on the heel of their palms. For quite some time Hahnemann could not decide on the number of succussions necessary. The extent to which the vials are shaken depends on the individual concerned and the pharmacopoeia being used – somewhere between 20 and 40 times is often quoted as being appropriate, although one British manufacturer claims to hand-succuss for 20 minutes and another machine-succusses for 10 seconds (Griffiths, 1993). The *French Homeopathic Pharmacopoeia* of 1965 (eighth edition) sets the number at 100.

Within each manufacturing process the number of succussions remains constant. A comparative study of the merits of hand-succussion and machine-succussion has been carried out (Jones and Jenkins, 1983). The study used the remedy Pulsatilla at 4c and 8c potencies, known to produce an increase in the growth of yeast, and found a gradual increase in the growth response rate of yeast cultures in the remedies that had been hand-succussed up to 60 times. Above this no further enhancement was observed. Unfortunately the workers were unable to formulate a result for the mechanical potencies and so a comparison could not be made. They suggested that a wait period of around 3 minutes between successive dilutions may be advantageous. We know from clinical observations that this agitation is vitally important to the therapeutic efficacy of the remedy; dilution alone is not sufficient to produce the phenomenon.

Vithoulkas (1980) has commented on the subject as follows:

> Succussion adds kinetic energy to the solution which is crucial. If one merely succusses a solution without diluting it further, a raise in level of only one potency occurs, regardless of how many times it is succussed; therefore both succussion and dilution are required. We also know that the more there is succussion and dilution, the more the therapeutic power is increased, even beyond the point of there being even one molecule of the original substance remaining.

It has been argued that succussion drives the homeopathic tincture undergoing potentisation to a turbulent regime where vortices continually form and disappear, ranging in size from the linear extent of the container to a minimum scale determined by viscosity and the rate of energy dissipation (Torres, 2002). Input of mechanical energy cascades down this population of eddies and becomes available at the microscopic level to perform work (chemical, electrical, etc.). A structure generated in the tincture would be interrupted by vortices smaller than it, and this sets definite limits on the strength of succussion so the power input leads to larger vortices than the structures one is trying to create and preserve through potentisation. This hypothesis has still to be tested experimentally although Torres has suggested a method.

If one merely succusses a solution without diluting it further, a raise in level of only one potency occurs, regardless of how many times it is succussed; therefore both succussion and dilution are required. We also know that the more there is succussion and dilution, the more the therapeutic power is increased, even beyond the point of there being even one molecule of the original substance remaining. The structure of solvent molecules may be electrochemically changed by succussion, enabling it to acquire an ability to 'memorise' an imprint of the original remedy. It is acknowledged that this concept is difficult for many highly trained personnel with scientific backgrounds to accept. Whether succussion imparts a certain energy or whether it merely facilitates complete mixing is, like much of homeopathy, still a topic for lively debate. We will look at some more theories on how the potentisation phenomenon is thought to work in Chapter 11.

Successive dilution and succussion may permanently alter the physico-chemical properties of the aqueous solvent (Elia et al., 2004). The modification of the solvent could provide an important support to the validity of homeopathic medicine which employs 'medicines without molecules'. The nature of the phenomena described by Elia et al. remains unexplained.

Figure 4.4 Skinner
potentising machine

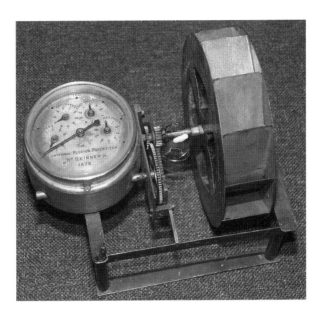

fluxion method, where a flow of tap water is run over 5 ml of potency contained at the bottom of a glass tube that is agitated. The original potency is progressively washed away to obtain the required potency. With this method it takes 75 hours and 180 litres of tap water to raise a 10M potency to a CM. There is no wonder that sceptics find it hard to believe that a medicine could possibly work at this dilution. How one works out the true final potency in Hahnemannian terms is also a matter for conjecture!

Quinquagintamillesimal potentisation method (LM). Some homeopaths use potencies based on serial dilutions of 1:50 000 at each level. These are called either 50 millesimal potencies (abbreviated to LM) or quinquagintamillesimal (thankfully abbreviated simply to Q) and became available commercially during the 1950s (Barker, 1997). This rather unusual method was suggested by Hahnemann towards the end of his life following a review of his earlier experiments with different degrees of dilution and succussion and is contained in paragraph 270 of the sixth edition of the *Organon*. They provided a method of lessening the aggravation caused by certain remedies. Remedies were first triturated to the 3c level with lactose, before being serially diluted on the new scale:

> *In order to best obtain this development of power, a small part of the substance to be dynamised (say one grain) is triturated for three hours with three time one hundred grains sugar of milk according to the method described below up to the one millionth part in powder form.*

A degree of dubiety exists as to whether some LM potencies are prepared exactly as Hahnemann instructed and also whether LM and Q potencies from different manufacturers are exactly interchangeable. A modern LM1 potency is sometimes understood to represent a dilution of 1:50 000 and a LM2 a dilution of 1:2500 000 000; that is, the potencies are made directly

Figure 4.5 Diagrammatic summary of the manufacturing process

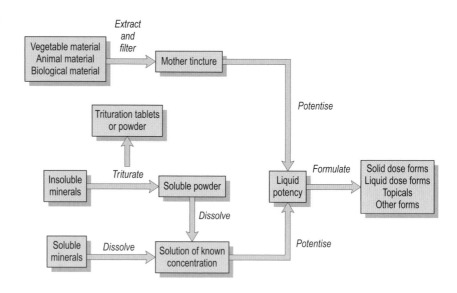

from mother tinctures without the intervention of a 3c stage. By convention the number signifying the level of millesimal dilution follows the scale letters, to distinguish it from centesimal potencies. Thus 50M (rather confusingly sometimes written as LM) is a 1:100 centesimal dilution carried out 50 000 times, while a LM1 potency is a 1:50 000 millesimal dilution carried out once. Remedies prepared in this way are claimed to be more gentle, more effective, and have a longer shelf-life.

A potency prepared by one of the methods described above in a high concentration alcohol vehicle may be used in the preparation of other dose forms (when it is known as a medicating potency) or the alcohol content may be adjusted to 20–30% and the potency administered orally (when it is known as a liquid potency). In most cases topical preparations are prepared by incorporating a mother tincture in a suitable vehicle, but occasionally a potency or a trituration powder may be used instead, for example Graphites or Sulphur.

The manufacturing process described above is summarised in Figure 4.5.

PHARMACEUTICAL PRESENTATIONS AVAILABLE

Oral dose forms

Linctus. A syrup preparation, usually containing honey or similar base in which may be dispersed one or more homeopathic mother tinctures (e.g. Bryonia) or 95% alcohol preparations of a homeopathic potency to the required concentration. Intended for oral use in the treatment of coughs and acute throat pain. Sometimes termed 'homeopathic elixir'.

Liquid potency. Liquid dosage form, typically composed of a 20–30% solution of alcohol in purified water combined with one or more homeopathic potencies. Intended for oral use, directly or in water via a dropper mechanism contained within the bottle. Also sometimes termed 'homeopathic drops'. Dispensed in amber glass bottles with non-absorbent dropper insert and screw cap.

NOTE

Homeopathic medicating potency. Liquid form of a remedy, typically composed of a 95% solution of alcohol in purified water. used to prepare homeopathic dosage forms by process of 'medicating'.

Not for administration as a medicine.

Mother tincture. Alcoholic primary plant extract, where applicable prepared to the standards of a national homeopathic pharmacopoeia. Forms the source material for the preparation of subsequent potencies of a homeopathic remedy. In some cases the mother tincture may be the medicine itself and may be diluted in water for direct oral administration or for use as a gargle/mouthwash. Dispensed in amber glass bottles, with non-absorbent dropper insert and screw cap if appropriate.

Oral solution. Liquid dosage form, typically composed of a 10% solution of alcohol in purified water combined with the 95% alcohol preparation of one or more homeopathic potencies intended for direct oral use. Dispensed in amber glass bottle with screw cap.

Solid dose forms

Solid dose forms are illustrated in Figure 4.6. They are shown in 14 g glass vials.

In allopathic medicine, tablets and capsules are made in different forms to control the speed at which the active ingredient is delivered. In homeopathy we are not faced with a necessity for sustained release or enteric coated preparations so the choice of carrier is governed by convenience rather than therapeutic efficiency. There is presently no standard for solid dose forms in the *BHomP*, so size and ingredients are likely to vary from one manufacturer to another.

Crystals. Solid preparations composed of sucrose, resembling granulated sugar and intended for oral or sublingual use. Coated ('medicated') with a 95% alcohol preparation of one or more homeopathic potencies and usually administered by measuring approximately 10–20 crystals per dose. Usually

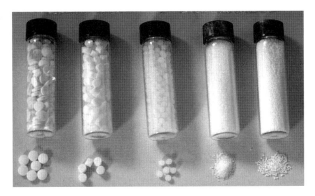

Figure 4.6 Solid dose forms (from left: tablets, soft tablets, pills, crystals and granules)

dispensed in clear or amber glass vials with screw cap or in a single dose sachet, similar to homeopathic powders.

Granules. These are also called 'non-pareils', 'globules' and 'globuli', causing some confusion with pills (see below). Very small solid spherical preparations composed of sucrose, and intended for oral or sublingual use. Coated ('medicated') with a 95% alcohol preparation of one or more homeopathic potencies and usually administered by measuring approximately 10–20 granules per dose. Usually dispensed in clear or amber glass vials with screw cap or in a single dose sachet, similar to homeopathic powders. Size and composition vary by manufacturer, but sucrose granules of approximately 0.8–1.0 mm diameter have been common in the UK although a much finer product is now also used (see Fig. 4.6).

Pills. These are also called 'pillules', 'granules' or 'globules' in some non-English-speaking countries, causing some confusion with granules (see above). Pills are solid spherical dose unit preparations composed of sucrose, lactose or a compound of the two intended for oral or sublingual use. Coated ('medicated') with a 95% alcohol preparation of one or more homeopathic potencies. Pillules are often found to be non-uniform in their size and shape, particularly if the manufacturers have obtained their stocks from food manufacturers rather than from specialist producers. In many cases the pills are built up by adding successive aliquots of liquid sucrose in a revolving drum, and it is rather difficult to control the dimensions of the finished product using this method. Continental European and South American suppliers offer pillules in different sizes and their product tends to be more uniform (weighing on average 0.0435 g) but naturally more expensive. Pillules of approximately 3–4 mm diameter are most common in the UK. Dispensed in clear or amber glass vials with screw cap.

Powders – individual. Made from lactose impregnated with liquid potency, individual powders are especially useful for combined medicated and placebo treatments or where one remedy must follow another in sequence. The powders can be individually numbered in the correct sequence and the patient instructed to take the powders in order. The powders, wrapped and usually packed in multiples of 10, are generally medicated from outside the powder paper, by dropping liquid potency on the long edge of the bundle. The alcoholic solution passes through the powder paper to medicate the lactose powder inside. The powders dry by evaporation of the alcohol. It is important to use a liquid potency made up in a high concentration of alcohol (usually 90%) to facilitate the medication process. Some authorities recommend strengths as high as 96% alcohol (Aubin et al., 1980). If a low concentration is used some of the lactose dissolves in the water content of the vehicle, giving a damp mass that clumps together.

A solid preparation composed of lactose and intended for oral (directly or dissolved in water) or sublingual use. Approximately 100 mg of powder is coated ('medicated') with a 95% alcohol preparation of one or more homeopathic potencies and enclosed in a paper sachet to form a single dose unit. Individual powders are shown in Figure 4.7.

Powder – bulk. Bulk powders have a pure lactose base and are impregnated with liquid potency. Their use has largely fallen out of currency.

Figure 4.7   Powders

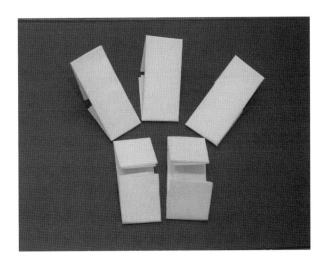

Tablets. A solid dose unit preparation, typically white and biconvex in nature, about the same in appearance as a 75 mg dispersible aspirin tablet, and composed of lactose or a compound of lactose/sucrose intended for oral or sublingual use. Usually prepared by compression of a uniform volume of the excipients and then coated ('medicated') with a 95% alcohol preparation of one or more homeopathic potencies. An alternative method of preparation exists in large scale manufacture whereby homeopathic granules are medicated and then compressed to form the tablet in a method similar to allopathic manufacture. Size and composition vary by manufacturer, but lactose tablets of approximately 100 mg weight are most common in the UK. Dispensed in clear or amber glass vials with screw cap.

Soft tablet. A solid dosage form prepared by loose compression of lactose, intended to dissolve readily when administered by the oral or sublingual route. Coated ('medicated') with a 95% alcohol preparation of one or more homeopathic potencies. Dispensed in clear or amber glass vials with screw cap.

Trituration tablet. A solid dose form containing largely insoluble remedies (e.g. Sulphir, Graphites at low potencies) and compressed directly with excipients into a tablet. Few examples of trituration tablets exist but historically they were used widely.

The medicating process for solid dose forms

On a large scale, blank lactose tablets, granules or sucrose pills can be surface inoculated by spraying on the liquid remedy in alcoholic tincture or as a syrup in a revolving pan, rather like the old method of sugar coating. The exact amount of remedy to be applied to ensure an even covering is determined using dyes.

In smaller scale production the solid dose forms are placed in glass vials and medicated by placing drops of high alcohol medicating potency on the

Figure 4.8 Medicating tablets in a 14 g vial

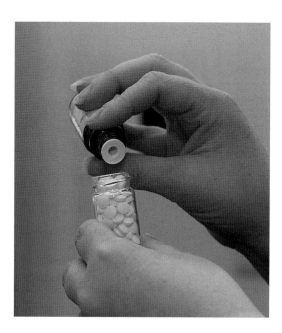

surface, depending on the amount of solid dose form being medicated. This process is shown in Figure 4.8.

Two drops of medicating potency (0.2 ml) to about 10 g of dose form is normally used, giving a final remedy content of between 1 and 2% of the raw material. In place of the traditional 'cork' method (see p. 93), a capillary dropper can be used. We will return to this technique when we discuss extemporaneous dispensing in the next chapter. As with the medication of individual powders, it is vital that a high concentration of medicating potency (sometimes called a 'strong spirit' or just 'ss') is used in this process, as otherwise the tablets can aggregate. The container is agitated in a manner similar to succussion to disperse the remedy throughout the dose form. The most frequently asked question about this process must surely be: 'How can you ensure all the tablets receive medicament?' To illustrate this point the reader is invited to take a bottle of unmedicated tablets and introduce a couple of drops of any alcohol-based perfume. If the tablets are shaken and then turned out on a clean surface, it will be found that every one of the tablets will smell of the perfume. Similarly, when the high concentration alcoholic liquid potency is applied to blank lactose tablets, the vapour is carried throughout the container and this can be checked using an alcohol meter. It is not necessary for every tablet to be coated to the same uniform extent.

In treating a patient we are seeking the smallest dose of medicine that will elicit a therapeutic response. Years of clinical observation have shown that this medicating technique does produce remedies that are active. A rather simplistic way of looking at this involves a key. Providing the design is such that the key will enter the lock and turn, the length of the shank is not important. Thus, providing we have chosen the right remedy and potency, the amount (within limits, of course) is not important. In allopathic terms this is tantamount to saying that diazepam 2 mg = diazepam 5 mg = diazepam 10 mg – a totally absurd suggestion. It is the number of times we turn the key (i.e. the frequency of administration) that is the most important factor in homeopathy, not the size of individual doses. In acute or first aid situations the remedy is given far more frequently – up to every 10–15 minutes in some cases – whereas in chronic conditions frequencies of once or twice a day (or even once a month) are more appropriate. We will return to the topic of posology in Chapter 8.

Topical preparations

Cream. A preparation for application to the skin consisting of a lipophilic and an aqueous phase in which may be dispersed one or more homeopathic mother tinctures or 95% alcohol preparations of a homeopathic potency to the required concentration. The concentration of liquid component varies by manufacturer, but 5% is most common in the UK.

Gel. A semi-solid preparation for application to the skin consisting of liquids gelled by means of a suitable gelling agent in which may be dispersed one or more homeopathic mother tinctures or 95% alcohol preparations of a homeopathic potency to the required concentration. The concentration of liquid component varies by manufacturer, but 5% is most common in the UK.

Ointment. A semi-solid single phase preparation usually based on soft paraffin and for application to the skin in which may be dispersed one or more homeopathic mother tinctures or 95% alcohol preparations of a homeopathic potency to the required concentration. The concentration of liquid component varies by manufacturer, but 5% is most common in the UK.

Liniment. An oil based preparation (typically arachis oil or light liquid paraffin) for application to the skin in which may be dispersed one or more homeopathic mother tinctures or 95% alcohol preparations of a homeopathic potency to the required concentration. The concentration of liquid component varies by manufacturer, but 5% is most common in the UK.

Lotion. An aqueous preparation for application to the skin in which may be dispersed one or more homeopathic mother tinctures or 95% alcohol preparations of a homeopathic potency to the required concentration. The concentration of liquid component varies by manufacturer, but 5% is most common in the UK.

Mother tinctures, either singly (e.g. Arnica for bruising, Thuja for warts or Tamus for chilblains) or in mixtures (e.g. Hypericum and Calendula), can be applied topically.

The clinical applications of topical products are dealt with in Chapter 9.

Other dose forms

Eye drops. A sterile solution containing a homeopathic dilution intended to be applied to the eye by means of a suitable dropper mechanism. These have caused UK manufacturers difficulties recently because of the existence of unlicensed ingredients in the formulae and have been restricted to prescription on a named-patient basis. Eye drops containing Calendula (minor infections), Cineraria (certain corneal opacities) and particularly Euphrasia (allergies) are all extremely useful when they are available. There is a tendency for older clients to use Euphrasia mother tincture in the eyes. In former times it was common practice to add a couple of drops of the liquid, also known as 'eyebright', to a wine glass of tepid water and the resulting solution used regularly as a wash or lotion to keep the eyes 'bright and healthy'. Eye lotions have fallen out of favour because of a lack of sterility, and the sterile drops are to be preferred.

It should be made clear that the mother tincture must *not* be placed in the eye undiluted. There have been several cases of lingering discomfort caused by this action. I have used Euphrasia 30c in oral form at the first aid level for conjunctivitis in an emergency situation over a holiday weekend. Although an Indian trial on this treatment came up with an insignificant result (Mokkapatti, 1992), I have certainly had some success with the remedy. It remains a possible option. One customer of mine has used steroid eye drops together with Euphrasia for years to control a recurring conjunctivitis, despite the potential incompatibility (see Ch. 8).

Injections. These are especially popular in Continental Europe and in the USA. Potencies of Ruta and Rhus tox are injected directly into painful muscles and joints respectively. Some are available on a named-patient basis in the UK. Preparations of Mistletoe grown on different hosts (oak, willow and apple) and combined with different metals (copper, mercury, etc.) are used to treat cancerous conditions. The dose regimes are often complicated, involving a number of different strengths in each course of treatment. Examples shown in Figure 4.9 are Abnobaviscum (Abnova Pforsheim) and Iscador (Weleda Ilkeston). The latter is an anthroposophical product (see Ch. 10).

Nasal sprays. These offer a convenient route of administration. There are none currently available in the UK.

Suppositories. These are not common in the UK nowadays, but are still available from some manufacturers. The base is solid semi-synthetic glyceride or cocoa butter (Belgian Pharmaceutical Society, 1995).

Figure 4.9 Mistletoe injections

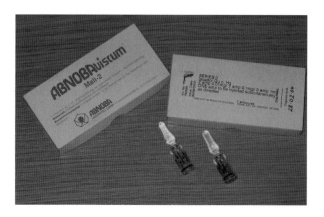

confusion is difficult to avoid. To add to the confusion, some remedies masquerade under different names. The remedies Actaea racemosa and Cimicifuga are one and the same remedy, as are Syphilinum and Lueticum and the rather unusual pair Turneria and Damiana. A selection of common remedies and their abbreviations is included in Table 4.4.

Osteoarthritic nosode is abbreviated to OAN and there are some mixtures (or 'complexes') each containing three different remedies with abbreviations like ABC, AGE and SSC. These are dealt with in Chapter 8. Complexes produced by manufacturers are currently being licensed using the name of a main ingredient followed by the abbreviation Co (for compound or complex) and the company name, for example Arnica Co (Smith).

Other sources of potential confusion have been highlighted in a report prepared by Dellmour et al. under the auspices of the European Committee for Homeopathy (Dellmour et al., 1999). Most botanical names currently used in homeopathy are still similar to the current botanical nomenclature used for the source material. However, other remedies have other synonyms that do not correspond with either the pharmacopoeias or the current botanical names. For example Belladonna (Atropa belladonna), Cactus grandiflorus (Cercus grandiflorus) and Chamomilla (Matricaria chamomilla) all have commonly used homeopathic names that are not correct. Homeopathic Pulsatilla is not *Pulsatilla vulgaris* as often stated, but *Pulsatilla pratensis*, (synonym *Pulsatilla nigricans*). The German pharmacopoeia correctly mentions *Pulsatilla pratensis* as being the species that has undergone provings. Although *Pulsatilla vulgaris* appears in both the French and German pharmacopoeias it does not appear to have a published drug picture. Further, the botanical nomenclature used in homeopathy does not indicate the part of the plant that has been used. In some countries the whole plant is used, in other countries it can be the root, the seeds, the leaves, the flower or the fruits. An annotated checklist of currently accepted names in common use has been produced by the Department of Botany at the UK Natural History Museum, London (Bharatan et al., 2002).

Most zoological names currently used in homeopathy are still similar to the current zoological nomenclature such as Apis mellifica (Bee), Latrodectus mactans (Spider) and Vespa cabro (Wasp). Some, however, are not. For example, Cantharis would be more correctly called Lytta vesicatoria.

Remedies from chemical sources have their problems too. Compounds with F, Ca, Br, 1, 0, S ions are usually called fluoratums, bromatums, iodatums, sulphuratums, etc. But calcium fluoride is called Calcarea fluorica in some countries and Calcium fluoricum in others, which is not consistent (Calcium fluoratum would be more logical).

Many of the nosode names currently used in homeopathy are insufficiently specified names, for example Psorinum, Carcinosinum, Tuberculinum, Medorrhinum. The nosodes often show different starting materials and manufacturing methods in different communities.

In fact difficulties with nomenclature are not confined just to naming remedies. A group of Latin American and European authors have pointed out that international confusion also exists as to the exact meaning of many words used routinely in homeopathy and they suggest that many inaccurate or imprecise terms should be replaced (Guajardo et al., 1999). The

Table 4.4 Examples of the nomenclature of some homeopathic remedies

Full homeopathic name	Homeopathic abbreviation	Common (trivial) name
Aconite napellus	Acon	Monkshood
Arnica montana	Arn	Leopard's bane
Agaricus muscarius	Agar or Ag mus	Toadstool
Allium cepa	Allium c. or All-c	Red onion
Apis mellifica	Apis	Honey bee
Arsenicum album	Arsen alb. or Ars	Arsenic trioxide
Aurum metallicum	Aurum met	Gold
Belladonna	Bell	Deadly nightshade
Cantharis	Canth	Spanish fly
Coccus cacti	Cocc cact or Coc-c	Cochineal
Cuprum metallicum	Cuprum met or Cu met	Copper
Euphrasia officianalis	Euphr	Eyebright
Gelsemium sempervirens	Gels	Yellow jasmine
Hypericum perforatum	Hyp, Hyper	St John's wort
Ipecacuanha	Ipecac, Ipec, Ip	Ipecacuanha root
Lachesis	Lach	Bushmaster venom
Natrum muriaticum	Natrum mur, Nat mur, Nat-m	Sodium chloride
Nux vomica	Nux vom, Nux-v	Nux vomica bean
Pulsatilla nigricans	Puls	Wind flower
Rhus toxicodendron	Rhus tox	Poison ivy
Symphytum officinale	Symph	Knitbone or comfrey
Tabacum	Tabac or Tab	Tobacco
Thuja occidentalis	Thuja	Arbor vitae
Vespa crabro	Vespa or Vesp	Wasp

International Dictionary of Homeopathy was produced with this in mind (Swayne, 2000).

Traditionally remedies are described by an abbreviation with an indication of the potency. Remedies such as Staphylococcus and Staphisagria are both shortened to 'Staph' and Euphorbium and Euphrasia both to 'Euph', so care is needed to ensure the correct remedy is ordered and supplied. With acids the word 'acid' may come before the name rather than after it (e.g. acid phos rather than phosphoric acid). There is an extensive list of abbreviated names at the beginning of some editions of Kent's *Repertory*.

Homeopathy needs a consistent international abbreviation system to ensure the accurate supply of currently available remedies and the logical incorporation of new remedies in the future. One proposal would be to take the first four letters of each part of the Latin name of the raw material; thus Aconite would become Acon. nape. and Arnica, Arni. mont. Something similar has been suggested by Patel (1994). So far, however, this suggestion has not met with widespread enthusiasm.

Attempts have been made to standardise names of common remedies across the EU member states and an approved list is in existence but irregularities still occur. For the reasons outlined above, patients are well advised to take any prescribed medication with them when they travel because the remedy obtained abroad may be different from the remedy they are used to buying in their own country. Within a particular country, it is unlikely that any conflict will arise.

LEGAL STATUS OF HOMEOPATHIC REMEDIES

On 22 September 1992 the European Parliament adopted Directive Number 92/73/EEC designed to harmonise the regulations concerning homeopathic medicinal products for human use throughout what was then called the EC, but which is now known as the European Union (EU). The Directive is divided into four chapters and 11 articles covering the scope, manufacture, control and inspection, placing on the market and final provisions. It passed into UK Law on 1 January 1994.

Article 1 defines a homeopathic medicinal product as: 'any medicinal product prepared from products, substances or compositions called homeopathic stocks in accordance with procedures described in any recognised pharmacopoeia'. In the absence of a European pharmacopoeia standard, monographs from the *BHomP, FrHomP, HAB* and *HPUS* are presently being used.

Article 2 deals with the labelling requirements of registered homeopathic medicinal products.

Articles 3 and 4 apply the provisions for controlling the import, export and manufacture of homeopathic medicinal products.

Article 5 states that all member states shall communicate to each other all the information necessary to guarantee the quality and safety of homeopathic medicinal products within the Union.

Articles 6, 7, 8 and 9 cover the registration and labelling requirements for placing a product on the market. It is probably in this area that pharmacists are most likely to become involved with the legislation.

The Directive acknowledges the special nature of homeopathic remedies and permits an abbreviated system of registration under Article 7, based on quality and safety only, providing that:

1. the remedies are intended for oral or external use
2. the remedies are sufficiently dilute to guarantee safety. A minimum dilution of 1:10 000 (4x) is specified for most remedies. Products derived from substances classified as prescription only medicines must contain no more than 1% of the smallest allopathic recommended dose. (This represents a UK interpretation of the Article; it varies across the EU)
3. no claims for therapeutic efficacy are made.

Under Section 2 of Article 7 no trade name is allowable and the label must state:

- the scientific name of the constituent stock plus the dilution
- the name and address of the supplier and if appropriate the manufacturer
- the method of administration and whether oral or topical
- the expiry date
- the pharmaceutical form and contents of the sales presentation
- any special storage requirements or warnings
- the batch number and product registration number
- the words: 'Homeopathic medicinal product without approved therapeutic indications'
- advice to consult a doctor if symptoms persist.

The remedy must therefore be sold as a generic, and the customer is obliged to choose the correct product by whatever method he or she can. Advice from health professionals, from the media or from leaflets in the retail outlet are the main sources of information.

There appear to be areas where the licensing authorities will allow some latitude in the Article 7 regulations, particularly with respect to the naming of homeopathic complexes. Following representations from manufacturers on the basis of safety, complex remedies containing several ingredients are being licensed in the UK with names of the type 'Remedy X Co' to obviate the necessity of writing long lists of ingredients on a prescription, and to prevent confusion among potential purchasers. This is similar to the approved name system for allopathic medicines (e.g. co-proxamol, co-dydramol, etc.). Brand names, and names that indicate possible uses ('fantasy names'), are still banned. In France negotiations are taking place on the naming of complexes containing ingredients including the 1x to 4x range.

Article 9 applies to products of 3x potency and below, products with claims of efficacy and injections. Such claims must be substantiated by the same range of biological and chemical testing as that required for conventional medicines in EU member states. It is unlikely that any homeopathic remedy will be able to satisfy this requirement in the foreseeable future.

There is provision for another route of registration under Article 16.2 of Directive 2001/83/EC. Individual member states can introduce a set of National Rules allowing limited claims of efficacy and the registration of products not covered by existing legislation (e.g. injections). At the time of writing (August 2005) the UK is still consulting on its national rules so registration is currently proceeding on the basis of the abbreviated Article 7 scheme alone. There has been considerable concern about the position of mother tinctures that currently do not fall under Article 7 legislation, being lower than the stipulated level of 4x. Manufacturers are keen to bring these remedies into homeopathic legislation rather than resort to the herbal regulations and there are signs that this will be accommodated before too long. The legislative position for homeopathic remedies from 1992–2001 is summarised in Figure 4.11. Subsequent legislation has changed the current Directive (See p 116), changing the numbers of effective Articles, but these same basic historic principles remain.

The presence of a registration scheme was initially optional for member states, reflecting the awareness and acceptability of homeopathy across Europe. Those member states that do not introduce a registration scheme are obliged to accept on to their market remedies registered in other member states, so there is a strong incentive to do something positive. With no announcement on any possible final transition date for discontinuing the PLRs of homeopathic remedies, companies were generally rather slow to incur the expense involved in redesigning packs and labels to satisfy the new regulations in respect of their existing products. In many cases it is

Figure 4.11   Routes for licensing homeopathic remedies 1992–2001. (Adapted with permission from a diagram supplied by Weleda, UK Ltd.)

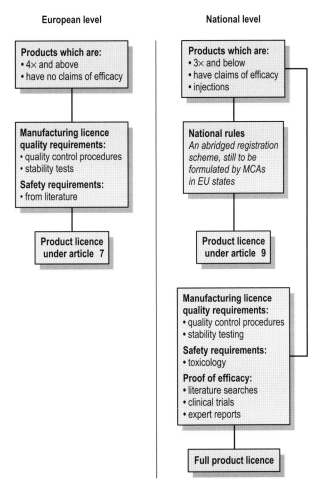

permissible to give more information on the label under the old PLRs (e.g. dose, indications for use, brand names, etc.) than on remedies licensed under Article 7. This remains a potential source of considerable confusion among consumers, especially when old and new packs are being sold side by side. A multidisciplinary expert committee, known as the Advisory Board on the Registration of Homeopathic Products, was established in 1993 to give advice to the MHRA with respect to safety and quality in relation to human, and where appropriate animal, use of any registerable homeopathic product or service.

Some countries tried to extend Article 7 into areas not originally intended to be covered by the Directive; others attempted to adapt Article 9 in such a way as to favour their own nationals. The Directive has now been implemented across all established EU member states New entrants to the enlarged EU are taking necessary action. There is still work to be done in the area of nosodes, presently under threat in a number of member states.

In July 2001, the Commission adopted a proposal for a comprehensive reform ('codification') of the EU pharmaceutical legislation, rationalising many different regulations. It involved three important documents:

- Regulation 2309/93 that provided the legislative framework for regulating medicinal products
- Directive 2001/93 on human medicines (in which the provisions associated with marketing homeopathic medicines were reorganised)
- Directive 2001/82 on veterinary medicines.

The main benefits of the new legislation to homeopathy were (T. Nicolai, personal communication, 20 January 2005):

- An obligation for member states to establish a simplified registration procedure for the registration of homeopathic medicines (the old Directive left it up to the national governments to decide).
- A procedure to have low potencies follow the simplified registration procedure providing safety can be guaranteed.
- A mutual recognition procedure making registration easier and facilitating free circulation of homeopathic products through the EU. Member states are required to agree on the registration requirements (there are multiple interpretations of the Directive leading to registration requirements that differ slightly from one member state to another).
- In view of their increased use in organic farming, homeopathic medicinal products intended for food producing animals are now eligible for the simplified registration procedure (Directive 2004/28/EC).
- The industrial production of 'homeopathic medicinal products that are placed on the market without therapeutic indications in a pharmaceutical form and dosage which do not present a risk for the patient' are allowed. Single homeopathic medicines in potencies above 2c/4x for oral or external administration will thus continue to be safeguarded.
- Directive 2004/27/EC formalises regulations for the registration of homeopathic kits containing more than one homeopathic medicine.

With input from numerous stakeholders, including input from the European Coalition on Homeopathic and Anthroposophical Medicinal

Products (ECHAMP) and the Pharmacy Subcommittee of the European Homeopathic Committee, a number of homeopathic monographs appeared in Supplement 4.1 of the *European Pharmacopoeia* (4th edition) for the first time and became active on 1 April 2002. These included herbal drugs for homeopathic preparations, iron for homeopathic preparations and mother tinctures for homeopathic preparations.

In 2005 veterinary medicines were taken out of the overarching UK Medicines Act 1968 and made the subject of separate legislation, with changes in classification and supply channels for many veterinary products. The production, licensing and supply of homeopathic remedies are included in the Veterinary Medicines Regulations 2005 and comply with the European codified pharmaceutical legislation mentioned above.

Elsewhere in the world, New Zealand currently does not require remedies to be licensed per se, although a Code of Good Manufacturing Practice must be observed in their manufacture. Israel is following the European legislative pattern. In the USA homeopathic products are regulated as drugs under federal law, regulation being the purview of the FDA and the Homeopathic Pharmacopoeia Convention of the United States (HPCUS). The legal and regulatory status of homeopathic drugs is considered to be stable.

In addition to full or abbreviated manufacturing licences under the EU Directive, there exists in the UK another system of licensing that allows the manufacture of remedies on a 'one-off' basis. Special Manufacturing Licences enable producers (usually registered pharmacies) to supply other professional outlets – pharmacies, hospitals, doctors, etc. – in addition to the public. The remedies are considered to be 'unlicensed products' under the EU Directive (i.e. they do not have a product licence obtained under the abbreviated or full scheme outlined above) and wholesale purchasers should be made aware of this fact, for there are certain obligations placed upon the buyers of such products. No claims of efficacy can be made. The facility is designed to allow a homeopathic pharmacy to prepare remedies for colleagues who are unable to do it themselves; it is not designed for the large-scale production of remedies for stock. Special Licence holders are subject to regular inspections by Medicines' Inspectors from the MHRA, must keep manufacturing records, and are obliged to carry out limited quality control procedures on raw materials and finished products.

FURTHER INFORMATION FOR PHARMACISTS

The Royal Pharmaceutical Society of Great Britain has a fact sheet for pharmacists giving guidance on the preparation and use of homeopathic remedies. It may be accessed at www.rpsgb.org.uk/members/pdf/scifactsheethomeo.pdf.

REFERENCES

Aabel, S, Fossheim, S and Rise, F (2001) Nuclear magnetic resonance (NMR) studies of homeopathic solutions. *Homeopathy*, 90: 14–20.

Acier, A, Boiron, J and Vingert, C (1965) Essais pharmacologiques de nouvelles dilutions Korsakoviennes. *Les Annales Homoeopathiques*, 7(8): 597–600. (In: Homeopathic Compendium, trans. JA Underwood, 1995, Ainsworth, Hastings.)

Ainsworth, JB (1991) Homoeopathy and the community pharmacist, part two. *Homeopathy*, 41(1): 5–7.

Anon. (1980) How about plastics? [Editorial] *J Am Inst Homoeopath*, 73(3): 7.

Anon. (1991) Question time. *Homeopathy*, 41: 32.

Aubin, M, Baronnet, S, Baronnet, A et al. (1980) Etude d'une forme galénique particulière à l'homéopathie. *Annales Homéopathiques Françaises*, 22(3): 7–22.

Banerjee, DD (1991) *Textbook of Homeopathic Pharmacy*. B Jain & Co, New Delhi, pp 6–7.

Barker, R (1997) *LM Potencies*. Homeopathic Supply Company, Bodham, Norfolk.

Barthel, P (1993) Hahnemannian legacy: quality standards for homeopathic medicines. *Homeopathic Links*, 6(3): 30–33.

Belgian Pharmaceutical Society (1995) *Belgian Homeopathic Compendium for Pharmacists*, trans. JA Underwood. Ainsworth, Hastings.

Bharatan, V, Humphries, CJ and Barnett, JR (2002) *Plant Names in Homeopathy*. National History Museum, London.

Birch, K and Rockwell, J (1994) A homeopathic proving of *Sequoia sempervirens* (redwood). *Simillimum*, 4: 80–91.

Bonnet, MS (1996) The Laxosceles spider. *Br Homeopath J*, 85: 205–213.

Bonnet, MS (1997) Toxicology of Androctonus scorpion. *Br Homeopath J*, 86: 142–151.

British Homeopathic Pharmacopoeia (BHomP) (1870, 1876, 1882) E Gould and Son, London.

British Homeopathic Pharmacopoeia (BHomP) (1993) British Association of Homeopathic Manufacturers, Ilkeston, vol. 1.

Brunner, H (1992) Modification of Korsakoff's method of producing high potencies by hand [in German]. *Documenta Homoeopathica*, 12: 271–282.

Conte, RR, Berliocchi, H, Lasne, Y and Vernot, G (1996) *Theory of High Dilutions and Experimenta*. Aspects Polytechnica, Paris, trans. Dynsol Limited, Huddersfield. (Cited in: Milgrom, L, King, K, Lee, J and Pinkus, A (2001) On the investigation of homeopathic potencies using low resolution NMR T2 relaxation times: an experimental and critical survey of the work of Roland Conte et al. *Br Homeopath J*, 90: 5–13.)

Davey, R, McGregor, JA and Grange, JM (1992a) Quality control of homeopathic medicines (1). *Br Homeopath J*, 81: 78–81.

Davey, R, McGregor, JA and Grange, JM (1992b) Quality control of homeopathic medicines (2). *Br Homeopath J*, 81: 82–85.

Dellmour, F (1994) Importance of 3c trituration in the manufacture of homeopathic medicines. *Br Homeopath J*, 83: 8–13.

Dellmour F, Jansen, Nicolai T et al. (1999) *The Proposal for a Revised International Nomenclature System of Homeopathic Remedies and their Abbreviations*. European Committee for Homeopathy, Brussels.

Dynamis School (1994a) *Proving of Chocolate*. Dynamis School of Homoeopathy, Northampton.

Dynamis School (1994b) *Proving of Hydrogen*. Dynamis School of Homoeopathy, Northampton.

Elia, V, Baiano, S, Duro, L, Napoli, E, Niccoli, M and Nonatelli, L (2004) Permanent physicochemical properties of extremely diluted aqueous solutions of homeopathic medicines. *Homeopathy*, 93: 144–150.

Fisher, P (1993) More on magnetic resonance. *Br Homeopath J*, 82: 60–61.

French Homeopathic Pharmacopoeia (FHomP) (1982) Supplement to the Pharmacopée Française. L'Adrapharm, Paris.

Gaier, HC (1991) *Encyclopaedic Dictionary of Homoeopathy*. Thorsons, London, p 461.

German Homeopathic Pharmacopoeia (HAB) (1825) Dr Caspari, Leipzig (also 1872, Schwabe).

German Homeopathic Pharmacopoeia (HAB) (1990) Deutscher Apotheker Verlag/Govi Verlag, Stuttgart/Frankfurt.

Griffiths, E (1993) Some chemical and biological approaches to quality control of homeopathic medicines. PhD thesis, University of London.

Guajardo, G, Bellavite, P, Wynn, S, Searcy, R, Fernandez, R and Kayne, S (1999) Homeopathic terminology: a consensus quest. *Br Homeopath J*, 88: 135–141.

Guajardo-Bernal, G (1994) Letters to the Editor. *Br Homeopath J*, 83: 12–14.

Guedes, JRP, Ferreira, CM, Guimarães, HMB, Saldiva, PHN and Capelozzi, VL (2004) Homeopathically prepared dilution of *Rana catesbeiana* thyroid glands modifies its rate of metamorphosis. *Homeopathy*, 93: 132–137.

Hahnemann, S (1935) *Organon of Medicine*, 6th edn. Boericke and Tafel, Philadelphia.

Harries, D (1991) Review of packaging for homeopathic remedies. Project in the Faculty of Homoeopathy, Scottish Branch. British Homeopathic Library, Glasgow.

Hering, C (1879) *Guiding Symptoms of our Materia Medica*. American Homeopathic Publishing Society, Philadelphia, vol 1.

Hofmeyr, D (2004) A nuclear magnetic resonance study of potencies of Natrum muriaticum 15CH prepared by trituration and succussion versus Natrum muriaticum 15CH prepared by succussion alone. MTech diss., Durban Institute of Technology.

Joliffe, GH (1977) Thin layer chromatographic examination of mother tinctures. *Br Homeopath J*, 66: 197–202.

Jones, RL and Jenkins, MD (1983) Effects of hand and machine succussion on the in vitro activity of potencies of Pulsatilla. *Br Homeopath J*, 72: 217–223.

Julian, OA (1979) *Materia Medica of the New Homeopathic Remedies*. Beaconsfield Publishers, Beaconsfield.

Kayne, SB (1992) Report on Russian Homeopathic Congress, Moscow, 1992. *Br Homeopath J*, 81: 203–204.

Kennedy, B (1997) Homoeopathy in the Irish potato famine [Book review]. *Br Homeopath J*, 86: 40.

Kent, J (1969) *Repertory of the Homeopathic Materia Medica*. S Dey, Calcutta.

King, L and Lawrence, B (1993) Luna: a proving. *Helios Homeopathic Pharmacy*, Tunbridge Wells.

Leary, B (1994) Cholera 1854: update. *Br Homeopath J*, 83: 117–121.

Lorenz, I, Schneider, EM, Stolz, P, Brack, A and Strube, AJ 2003 Influence of the diluent on the effect of highly diluted histamine on basophil activation. *Homeopathy*, 92: 11–18.

Milgrom, L, King, K, Lee, J and Pinkus, A (2001) On the investigation of homeopathic potencies using low resolution NMR T2 relaxation times: an experimental and critical survey of the work of Roland Conte et al. *Br Homeopath J*, 90: 5–13.

Mokkapatti, R (1992) An experimental double-blind study to evaluate the use of Euphrasia in preventing conjunctivitis. *Br Homeopath J*, 81: 22–24.

Murphy, F (1980) Preliminary report of materials used in packaging homeopathic pharmaceuticals. *J Am Inst Hom*, 73(2): 33.

Nandi, M (2002) Alcohol, concentration in the preparation of mother tinctures of vegetable origin. The example of Holarrhena antidysenterica. *Homeopathy*, 81: 85–88.

Patel, RP (1994) Systems of abbreviations of drug names. *Z Klass Homöopathie*, 38: 236–239.

Riley, D and Zagon, A (2005) Clinical homeopathic use of RNA: evidence from two provings. *Homeopathy*, 94: 33–36.

Roder, E and Frisse, R (1981) On the stability of homeopathic dilutions in glass and plastic containers. *Pharmazie*, 36: H9.

Sacks, A (1983) Nuclear magnetic resonance spectroscopy of homeopathic remedies. *J Holistic Med*, 5: 172–175.

Satti, JA (1997) Sanicula aqua [Letter]. *Br Homeopath J*, 86: 60.

Schober, U and Luckert, G (1994) Homeopathic curiosities. *J LMHI*, Autumn: 26–27.

Sherr, J (1990) *Homeopathic Proving of Scorpion*, 2nd edn. Society of Homoeopaths, Northampton.

Smith, R and Boericke, GW (1968) Changes caused by succussion on NMR patterns and bioassay of bradykinin triacetate succussions and dilutions. *J Am Inst Hom*, 61: 197–212.

Sukul, NC, De, A, Dutta, R, Sukul, A and Sinhababu, SP (2001) Nux vomica 30 prepared with and without succussion shows antialcoholic effect on toads and distinctive molecular association. *Homeopathy*, 90: 79–85.

Sukul NC, De, A, Sukul, A and Sinhababu SP (2002) Potentized Mercuric chloride and Mercuric iodide enhance α-amylase activity in vitro. *Homeopathy*, 91: 217–220.

Swayne, J (1992) [Letters to the Editor]. *Br Homeopath J*, 81: 159–160.

Swayne, J (2000) *International Dictionary of Homeopathy*. Churchill Livingstone, Edinburgh.

Torres, J-L (2002) On the physical basis of succussion. *Homeopathy*, 91: 221–224.

Treuherz, F (1995) *Homoeopathy in the Irish Potato Famine*. Samuel Press, London.

US: Homeopathic Pharmacopoeia of the US (1979) American Institute of Homeopathy, Washington DC.

Verma, PN (1995) *Vaid Indu, Indian Encyclopaedia of Homeopathic Pharmacopoeia*. B Jain, New Delhi. [Incorporates vols 1–6 of *Indian Homeopathic Pharmacopoeia*.)

Vithoulkas, G (1980) *The Science of Homeopathy*. Grove Press, New York, pp 103–104.

Walker, E (1995) Some observations on the behaviour and pharmacology of snakes and their venoms. *The Homoeopath*, 57: 385–386.

Weingärtner, O (1990) NMR-features that relate to homeopathic sulphur-potencies. *Berlin J Res Homoeopathy*, 1(1): 61–68.

Young, TM (1975) Nuclear magnetic resonance studies of succussed solutions. A preliminary report. *J Am Inst Hom*, 68: 8–16.

Zacharias, CR (1995) Contaminants in commercial homeopathic medicines. *Br Homeopath J*, 84: 71–74.

Chapter 5

Supply of a named remedy

CHAPTER CONTENTS

Over the counter supply of a
  named remedy   121
Source of request   122
Characteristics of request   122
Interventions   122
Supply on prescription   123
Format of a prescription   125
Details of the prescribed medicine   125
  1. Name of remedy   125
  2. Potency   126
  3. Dose form   126
  4. Quantity   127
  5. Dose   127
Dispensing a remedy   130

1. Original pack dispensing   130
2. Broken bulk dispensing   131
3. Extemporaneous dispensing   131
Labelling the remedy   132
Informing the patient   133
Method of administration   133
Storage   134
Supply under the UK National
  Health Service   134
Pricing for private prescriptions   135
Product availability   136
Responding to requests for
  recommending a practitioner   136

OVER THE COUNTER SUPPLY OF A NAMED REMEDY

With the exception of the traditional poisons in very low potencies (for example Aconite, Belladonna or Nux vom; see Table 5.1), homeopathic remedies in the UK are not restricted to prescription and can be bought freely over the counter in pharmacies, health shops and even cash and carry stores. This is not the case in other countries, where medical prescriptions may be required for remedies above the 30c potency.

Source of request

Requests to suppliers for named remedies come from a number of different groups of people.

1. **Professional customers.** This group contains healthcare professionals (registered medical practitioners, dentists, vets, midwives, etc.) who have studied homeopathy at postgraduate level and non-medically qualified professional practitioners (homeopaths, chiropractors, herbalists, etc.) who may well have had several years' intensive training at colleges of homeopathy. These customers usually know exactly what they want and there is no difficulty in interpreting the remedies involved, although newcomers to the practice of homeopathy may need some help.
2. **Non-professional customers.** Lay homeopaths may include people with little or no formal training but who have acquired a very large amount of experience, earn their livelihood by practising homeopathy and, again, usually know exactly what they want. Similarly, there are the enthusiastic amateurs, who treat family and friends and have a good working knowledge of homeopathy.
3. **Members of the public.** Members of the public may know what they want, think they know what they want, or want to use homeopathy but have little idea of how to go about it.

Characteristics of request

Kayne et al. (2000) identified a predominance of polychrests among homeopathic remedies bought OTC by a sample of 407 clients in 100 British pharmacies. This was not unexpected since this type of remedy is well suited to the OTC environment. The results also suggested that homeopathic medicines are being used in an alternative way in the OTC environment, that is, as substitutes for allopathic medicines.

Reid (2002) surveyed 75 users of OTC homeopathy who completed questionnaires while purchasing OTC homeopathic remedies in three health food shops in central Manchester. The most frequently treated conditions were respiratory, mental/psychological and bruises/injuries. Respondents perceived OTC homeopathy to be effective for relieving these conditions. There was a trend for a respondent to have first used OTC homeopathy 4 or more years previously. About 13% combined homeopathy with prescription drugs. The most strongly endorsed reasons for using an OTC homeopathy remedy were that it was a natural treatment and was perceived as harmless.

Interventions

One of the most difficult decisions to make for a knowledgeable supplier is how and when to intervene in a sale. The delicate balance between antagonising the customer and losing a sale and satisfying one's professional integrity is generally only achieved after several years' experience. The fact that the questions are for the customer's safety and not for the supplier's benefit is not always obvious to a busy customer. The classic example is meeting what is ostensibly a simple request for a cough remedy in a pharmacy. By the time the requirements of the appropriate written protocol for selling medicines have been met, some patients may feel that an interrogation is in progress. If customers are aware of the principles of homeopathy, then such difficulties should not arise. As in all OTC sales, the pharmacist has a responsibility to ensure as far as possible that customers buy the correct medicine and take it according to instructions.

Requests for the following remedies may give cause for concern:

1. Inconsistent potencies, for example, purchases of 6c and 30c tablets at the same time. As a general rule in the OTC environment the lower potency is often (but not exclusively) used for chronic conditions while the higher is more suited to acute conditions. Mixing these potencies might well be inappropriate.

2. High potencies, especially M and 10M. Many homeopathic pharmacies will not sell such potencies without evidence that the customer will use them 'correctly'. These potencies are mainly used in small courses of treatment (1–3 days), so a request for 200 tablets should be viewed with caution.

3. Very low potencies. Table 5.1 summarises most of the remedies that are restricted to prescription in the UK. This list is not exhaustive; suppliers will advise on the up-to-date position. Such remedies are used extremely rarely; some (e.g. Aconite 1x) are potent poisons.

4. Purchase of many different remedies in an attempt to treat several conditions at once. Astute observation may mean that one or two carefully chosen remedies will deal with several different symptoms, obviating the necessity to use polypharmacy.

5. Purchases that involve homeopathic and allopathic remedies obviously being used for the same purpose. There may be potential difficulties in taking the two side by side owing to aromatic flavouring agents in the allopathic medicines inactivating the homeopathic remedy.

6. Purchases that involve homeopathic and aromatherapy products for use concurrently. Aromatic oils are thought to inactivate homeopathic remedies.

7. Large quantities of a remedy. Most homeopathic remedies offered for OTC sale are designed for short-term administration. Long-term chronic conditions are best treated under the guidance of a practitioner. One factor that allows patients to continue to use the medicines much longer than necessary is the number of tablets in a typical container. Taken at a rate of three per day, a single container may well last for a month or more, which could be too long for an acute condition.

SUPPLY ON PRESCRIPTION

In the UK, requests for supply by prescription may originate from a number of sources:

Table 5.1 Examples of homeopathic remedies classified as prescription only in the UK

Remedy	Potency below which remedy POM
Aconite (and mixtures containing Aconite)	3c or 6x
Ammonium bromatum	3c or 6x
Antimonium tartaricum	3c or 6x
Arsenicum album	3c or 6x
Arsenicum salts	3c or 6x
Atropine	1c or 2x
Belladonna	3x (2c nearest centesimal)
Cocculus	3c or 6x
Colchicum	4c or 8x
Croton tiglium	3c or 6x
Folliculinum	3c or 6x
Gelsemium (and mixtures containing Gels)	3x (2c nearest centesimal)
Hyoscymus	3x (2c nearest centesimal)
Ignatia	3c or 6x
Kali arsenicum	2c or 4x
Kali bromatum	3c or 6x
Natrum arsenicum	3c or 6x
Natrum bromatum	3c or 6x
Nux vomica	3c or 6x
Penicillin (tautopathic remedy)	3c or 6x
Prednisolone (tautopathic remedy)	3c or 6x
Strychnine salts	3c or 6x
Thyroid	3c or 6x
Vaccine derivatives	3c or 6x
Veratrum album	3c or 6x
Veratrum viride	3c or 6x

1. A registered medical practitioner or a supplementary prescriber pharmacist working under an agreed clinical management plan may issue a National Health Service (NHS) prescription for homeopathic remedies and this will be fully reimbursed by the Common Services Agencies throughout the four UK jurisdictions. Homeopathic remedies are not included in the Dental Formulary and are not therefore reimbursable under the NHS. The position with prescribing nurses and other health professionals is unclear at the present time but practitioners with appropriate training are likely to be authorized at a future date. In cases where the prescription tax is payable by the patient and exceeds the retail cost of the remedy, pharmacists should make this known to the patient and sell the remedy over the counter. In Scotland, registered medical practitioners may issue an NHS stock order form for homeopathic remedies for use in their practice.

2. Private prescriptions represent a convenient way for homeopathic practitioners, including professional homeopaths (also known as non-medically qualified practitioners), to convey remedy requests to the pharmacist. They can be written by doctors, vets or dentists in the case of the prescription-only medicines (POM) (see Table 5.1) or by any health professional or homeopath for all other remedies. VAT concessions are allowable in the UK only on prescriptions written by qualified medical or dental practitioners.

Format of a prescription

In order for a pharmacist to dispense a NHS prescription a number of elements should be present on the form:

- Name and address of patient (and age if a minor)
- Full details of the remedy or remedies to be supplied
- Practitioner's signature
- In addition, private prescriptions should give the practitioner's name, address and qualifications.

Details of the prescribed medicine

1. Name of remedy

We have already seen that the names of remedies are usually Latin abbreviations and that care must be taken to ensure that remedies with similar names are not confused. There are several ways of identifying remedies:

- **The index in a materia medica may point out likely candidates.** The materia medica contains a list of drug pictures of all the main remedies and therefore is a good source of information. There are a few mixtures of remedies that have been found useful over the years (e.g. ABC, comprising Aconite, Belladonna and Chamomilla, for teething). These complex remedies are not included in the materia medica and it may be necessary to resort to telephoning the prescriber to identify the remedy.

A further complication is that the elements making up the mixtures may vary. AGE may contain Arsenicum iodum, or Aconite or Arsen alb plus Gelsemium and Eupatorium for influenza. Another example we have met is SSC (Silica, Sulphur and Carbo veg). Many of the isopathic remedies (e.g. some of the nosodes and allergodes mentioned in Ch. 4) do not have drug pictures and cannot be found in the materia medica.

- **The prescriber can be contacted in the case of a prescription.** You should not be coy about telephoning the prescriber to confirm a badly written prescription or one that uses a non-standard abbreviation.
- **The client may be asked to clarify the situation** if he or she has used the remedy before. Such a request might well invoke a lack of confidence if an allopathic medicine is involved; experience shows that homeopathic customers rarely worry about requests being clarified in this way.

2. Potency

The potency level should be stated, together with an indication of the dilution scale required. Most often it is given as the centesimal scale, expressed as the letters c or cH after the potency number, or the decimal scale, expressed as x after the number (or D before it in some Continental European countries). Remember that if there is no letter after the potency number, then by convention the centesimal scale is implied. Thus: 6, 6c or 6cH all represent a 1 : 100 dilution serially carried out with succussion six times and 12x or D12 both represent a 1:10 dilution serially carried out with succussion 12 times.

High potencies such as M (1 : 100 dilution carried out 1000 times), 10M (1 : 100 dilution carried out 10 000 times) and CM (1 : 100 dilution carried out 100 000 times) are expressed as Latin numerals without the letter 'c' being present. Certain potencies are used more routinely than others. On the centesimal scale 6c, 12c, 30c and 200c are seen frequently in the UK; in France remedies such as 3x, 6x, 4c, 6c, 7c, 9c, 12c, 15c and 30c are common. The decimal scale is more frequently prescribed in Germany (6x, 8x, 10x, etc.). On the decimal scale 6x, 12x and 30x are seen most regularly in the UK. The remedy mixtures referred to above are sometimes used in high potencies, so be on the look-out for prescriptions written as AGEM calling for the remedy AGE at M potency, and not a single remedy with that abbreviated name.

3. Dose form

The part played by the dose form in delivering the medicine has already been discussed. From time to time there are suggestions that the dose form is important in determining the speed of onset of remedy activity, but this aspect of homeopharmaceutics has been largely ignored by researchers. In the meantime, it is generally accepted that the choice of dose form is therapeutically insignificant, although there may be psychological or other reasons why particular dose forms are chosen. Ideally the prescription or request should state the dose form, but given the lack of therapeutic significance the pharmacist does have some discretion in this matter.

Tablets and powders are prepared with lactose ('milk sugar') and cannot be used in cases where the client reports the possibility of an allergic reaction or intolerance. There may be religious concerns from Jewish patients whose dietary customs would be compromised by taking a milk-based product after food.

Pillules and crystals are sucrose. Diabetic patients may express concern if instructed to take pills, although if they are well stabilised and the course of treatment lasts only 2 or 3 days there is unlikely to be a problem.

For longer treatments, the remedy can be supplied in liquid potency form. Liquids include both mother tinctures and liquid potencies. The latter are made up in alcohol, varying from a concentration of 20% to one of 40%. If the alcohol presents a problem, then the remedies can be made up in water for short courses of treatment.

4. Quantity

Solid dose forms dispensed or OTC prescribed in the UK are often sold in 7 g, 14 g or 25 g glass vials. This indicates the capacity of the container, not the actual weight of the contents, and corresponds to approximately 55, 125 and 250 tablets respectively. Depending on the size of the tablets (or pills), which may differ according to the manufacturer, there may be slight variations in these numbers. The remedies were traditionally sold in old apothecary measures of 2 drachms, 4 drachms and 8 drachms and the rather unusual size of modern packs reflects the metric equivalents.

Glass bottles and plastic tubes are also used by the larger suppliers.

Over-the-counter packs specify numbers of tablets rather than weights and vary from 50 to 125 tablets. Requests may use either notation in stating the quantity required. Homeopathic suppliers will be able to help out in cases of uncertainty when placing an order. Liquids are usually supplied in 5 ml, 10 ml, 30 ml or 50 ml dropper bottles. Larger quantities are available to trade customers.

5. Dose

Counter packs will often give suggested doses and, despite such information also being present on a prescription, advice may be sought by the client. This is yet another area of homeopathy where differences of opinion occur. By convention it is generally stated that an adult dose should comprise two tablets or pillules and the dose for a child under 12 years should be one tablet or pillule. The patient expects this from exposure to allopathic medicine and is comfortable with the notion of minors being given less than adults. However, there is no homeopathic reason for this, for we know from clinical observation that one unit dose will provide enough medicament to elicit a response. Thus, both an adult and a child can be given a single unit as a dose. As we have already seen it is the frequency of dose that is significant, rather than the size of dose. The frequency of dosing will be dealt with in greater detail in due course in a discussion on counter prescribing. In general terms, it depends on whether the condition being treated is acute

---

Box 5.1   Some example prescriptions for homeopathic remedies

Tablets/granules	Powders	Mixed powders	Liquids
Prescription 1	*Prescription 6*	*Prescription 7*	*Prescription 9*
Arn 6 pills	H	Arnica 30 1–10	Crataegus 6x LP
Mitte 14 g	AGE 200 powders	SL 11–16	5 drops ex aq om
Sig: 1 b.d.	Mitte 10	Belladonna 30c 17–26	30 ml
	One 4 hrly	SL 27–36	
Prescription 2		Take in order as directed	
Bell 30c			
Mitte 50		*Prescription 8*	*Prescription 10*
Sig: 2 t.i.d.		Arnica 30 1–6	Thuja MT
		7 g SL tablet	Apply 2 drops daily
Prescription 3		1 twice daily	10 ml
Sulph 6x tabs			
Mitte 7 g			
Sig: 1 b.d.			
Prescription 4			
Arn 10M – 200 tabs			
1 q.i.d.			
Bell 6x – 50 tabs			
2 b.d.			
Prescription 5			
Cham 6c grans			
1 × OP			
One dose ac for teething			

(frequent dosing) or chronic (less frequent dosing). Liquids are usually prescribed as 'x number of drops in water'.

Tablets and pillules. Some examples of prescriptions for tablets or pillules are shown in Box 5.1.

Prescription 1 is for a 14 g vial of Arnica 6c pills (i.e. a 1 : 100 serial dilution carried out six times). Note that the letter 'c' denoting a centesimal potency is not included, but is implied. The dose is one tablet twice daily.

Prescription 2 calls for the remedy Belladonna 30c. No dose form is indicated, but from the quantity ordered we know it must be tablets or pillules. You might consult the prescriber or patient as to his or her preference. The dose here is stated as two, taken three times daily; a dose of one would be equally effective.

Prescription 3 is for a 7 g vial of Sulphur 6x (i.e. a 1 : 10 dilution six times) in tablet form. The dose is one tablet twice daily.

Prescription 4 is a little more complicated. Here the prescriber has ordered 200 tablets (equivalent to a 25 g vial) of Arnica 10M potency (a 1 : 100 dilution carried out serially 10 000 times) together with 50 tablets of Belladonna 6x potency (a 1 : 10 dilution six times). In addition the dose of the first remedy is one tablet four times a day and of the second two tablets twice a day. This example serves to highlight the sort of gross inconsistencies that can be identified occasionally. High potencies such as 10M are usually given in short courses of treatment – one to three doses are not uncommon. A 2-month course would be highly unusual and warrant further investigation. The size of dose should be standardised at either one or two tablets.

Granules, crystals and powders. In comparison with tablets, doses of granules, crystals and powder sound imprecise, but are actually quite reproducible. The cap of a 7 g vial provides a useful means of transferring a suitable amount of medicament. The patient should be instructed to just cover the cap liner by gently tapping out the medicated product until the cap liner is just obscured. The amount thus obtained constitutes a dose. When the remedy is packed in containers other than 7 g vials, another measure is provided by using a salt spoon, filled and levelled off with a knife or other suitable implement. Traditionally homeopaths used the small depression on the side of the wrist formed by crooking the thumb and first finger as a measure. This has been called the 'anatomical snuff box'.

Prescription 5 shows how granules are ordered. It is for Chamomilla 6c granules, one original pack, with one dose twice daily before food for teething. The original pack may be a 7 g glass vial, available in the UK from two or three small suppliers, or the larger glass and plastic containers produced by the major manufacturers. Occasionally one sees prescriptions giving 'five granules' as a dose. This is not meant to be taken literally – the patient is not expected to count out five tiny granules! It should be taken as the equivalent of a 'small pinch'. Again, remember we are seeking the smallest amount of remedy that will 'turn the key in the lock'. Nothing is to be gained from taking larger amounts.

Prescription 6 shows the position of the helpful letter 'H' when it is used to signify a homeopathic prescription, with a dose of one powder every 4 hours. Individual powders provide a useful means of controlling single doses. The remedy here is the complex AGE, a mixture of three remedies required as a set of 10 powders in the 200c potency. Unfortunately, as I have already mentioned, the ingredients making up AGE are not consistent throughout the homeopathic community; sometimes the 'A' stands for Aconite and sometimes Arsen alb, so it is advisable to check exactly what is required. Other combinations to look out for are: SSC (Silica, Sulphur and Carbo veg) and CGP (Carbo veg, Gelsemium and Phosphorus).

Powders are particularly useful where complicated dose regimens are involved. The technique here is to use sets of numbered powders. Consider, for instance, the following instructions: '10 Arnica 30c powders. Take one twice daily. When finished, wait 3 days, then take 10 Belladonna 30c powders. Wait a further 5 days and return to prescriber'. An elderly person might find these instructions difficult to follow. To make things easier for them, we can assemble a set of 36 powders, physically numbered in sequence in the top corner. The first 10 powders would be Arnica 30c, the next six placebo (plain unmedicated lactose), the next 10 Belladonna 30c and the final 10 placebo again. The patient could then be instructed to take the powders twice daily in sequence until the course is complete and then return to the prescriber. These numbered sets of powders can be ordered from homeopathic suppliers. If dispensing extemporaneously, care must be taken to ensure the medicated powders are perfectly dry before combining them into the set. A similar use of placebo is made when only one or two medicated powders are indicated (often these are of a very high potency like 10M). To satisfy the expectations of the patient, the course of treatment may be extended by several days with the addition of plain lactose powders.

Prescription 7 shows how numbered powders might be prescribed. Note that the prescription may not even mention the word 'powders' so unless you appreciate what is required, interpretation is rather difficult to say the least! Commonly, the abbreviation SL standing for Sacc lach, or milk sugar, is used to denote placebo in any dose form, thus obviating the necessity of writing the dreaded word on the prescription. Another commonly used pseudonym for placebo is 110/P. Occasionally the prescriber may issue a prescription containing different potencies of the same remedy with the aim of treating the physical symptoms first, and then a few days later the mental symptoms, filling the intervening days with placebo.

Prescription 8 shows another variation, with the inclusion of 7 g tablets. Here the prescriber requires six powders of Arnica 30c and 7 g of unmedicated placebo tablets, the patient being instructed to take one powder twice a day until the powders are finished, following on with one tablet twice daily. Placebo tablets may be prescribed alone, in which case they appear on the form written just as SL tablets.

Liquids. In quantities up to 50 ml, liquids are usually dispensed in dropper bottles, and a dose here can vary from one or two drops up to about 10 drops. It is not usual to give homeopathic liquids (other than products like cough mixtures) in 5 ml spoonfuls.

Prescription 9 is for 30 ml Crataegus 6x liquid potency, directions five drops in water each morning. In the absence of instructions to the contrary, the medicine should be placed into half a cup of tepid water that has been recently boiled and cooled, and sipped slowly.

Prescription 10 demonstrates how a prescription for a topical mother tincture might look. This is for 10 ml of Thuja mother tincture, with the instructions 'apply two drops (to the affected part) daily'.

DISPENSING A REMEDY

After interpreting the prescription the prescription may be dispensed. There are three approaches that can be taken, depending on the degree of expertise available.

1. Original pack dispensing

In the early days of homeopathic experience this alternative is to be recommended, particularly with the wide availability of supplies. Chances of contamination are zero and in the case of a remedy supplied on prescription all that is required is a label to be attached with the necessary instructions. A brief discussion between practitioners and a local pharmacy will ensure that appropriate stocks are held. Where there is no original pack size to match the quantity ordered on NHS prescriptions exactly, UK pricing authorities will normally allow pharmacists to claim the nearest size available.

2. Broken bulk dispensing

The transfer of quantities of tablets or liquid from a large container to a smaller one is a process that requires considerable care. Tablets and pills should not be counted using a counting machine or a triangle, because these implements cannot be cleaned sufficiently to prevent contamination from previous medicines that have been counted. Solid unit dose forms are best transferred by gently shaking small quantities at a time into the lid of the stock bottle and tipping them into the final container without touching. Liquids should ideally be transferred without the intervention of a measuring cylinder, but if the latter is necessary it must be cleaned, rinsed out with 50% alcohol and purified water and dried before use.

3. Extemporaneous dispensing

For the more experienced homeopathic pharmacist or practitioner, remedies may be prepared by adding drops of liquid potency to a bottle of blank carriers. A number of precautions must be taken, however:

- the area used to prepare medicated products should be clean and well away from allopathic dispensing areas
- the liquid potencies used to medicate solid dose forms should be made up in 95% ethyl alcohol, otherwise the water in the tincture will dissolve some of the lactose or sucrose and the finished product will end up as a soggy mass. This is especially important for granules and crystals
- to ensure reproducibility of product the remedies should be prepared by the same operator(s)
- a written protocol should be available to standardise the procedures to be followed
- practise using blank tablets and alcohol until you have perfected the technique before considering the method for dispensing prescriptions.

The medication process may be carried out in one of several ways:

Solid dose forms. A container, preferably glass, should be filled with blank carrier (tablets, pills, etc.) and, for a 7 g vial, two drops of strong spirit liquid potency introduced on the top with a dropper. The bottle is then capped and agitated with a similar action to that used for succussing liquid potencies for between 20 and 30 'strikes'. With a 14 g vial three drops of liquid potency are used; with a 25 g vial four drops are sufficient.

With larger quantities of tablets and pills and for granules, crystals and powder it is usual to introduce a second oversize container in which to medicate. Thus 7 g of granules will be tipped into a 50 g clean glass bottle, shaken as above until medicated, and then transferred back to the original container. The number of drops given for medicating tablets and pills can be reduced by one drop for granules, crystals and 'bulk' powder. Whenever possible the container used for solid dose forms should be glass, ideally amber to minimise discoloration of product owing to light. For short-term courses of treatment, clear glass or plastic is acceptable. Larger quantities of remedies (i.e. above 25 g, equivalent to 250 tablets) require amber screw cap bottles.

Individual powders are made by bundling together the required number of wrapped blank lactose powders (usually in multiples of three, 10 or 12) and then placing a drop of strong spirit liquid potency on the outside edge of each powder. The medicament passes through the paper and can then be allowed to dry off. Powders are packed in a powder envelope or box.

Oral liquids. Liquid potencies and small quantities of mother tinctures should be dispensed in glass dropper bottles. For short-term treatments, teat droppers will not experience undue deterioration from contact with alcohol in the liquids and are acceptable. The major suppliers use elegant amber screw cap bottles of capacities up to 50 ml with a plug in the neck. This plug has a small channel in it, and if the bottle is held at an angle of about 45° and gently tapped, exactly one drop (0.1 ml) will emerge. Unless you are able to locate a source of these bottles for your own use (your homeopathic wholesaler may be able to help), there is a considerable advantage to be gained from dispensing original packs.

Mother tinctures are sometimes ordered in relatively large volumes. Crataegus, for example, may be prescribed in quantities of 200 ml. Here an amber screw cap medicine bottle should be used and a separate teat dropper given out to facilitate dosing.

Topicals are best bought in, but they can be made up for short-term use by incorporating a mother tincture or liquid potency into a base. Wool alcohols ointment BP and the Crookes products Unguentum M and E45 are examples of suitable vehicles.

LABELLING THE REMEDY

Homeopathic remedies are considered to be medicines in the UK, and dispensed items should be treated the same as any other prescribed items with respect to labelling. An appropriate label is illustrated in Figure 5.1.

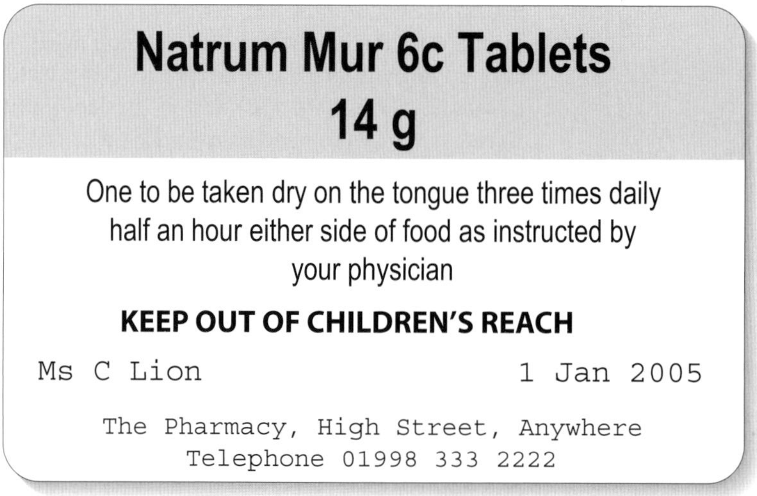

Figure 5.1 Example of label on dispensed remedy

Natrum Mur 6c Tablets
14 g

One to be taken dry on the tongue three times daily
half an hour either side of food as instructed by
your physician

KEEP OUT OF CHILDREN'S REACH

Ms C Lion   1 Jan 2005

The Pharmacy, High Street, Anywhere
Telephone 01998 333 2222

INFORMING THE PATIENT

If the patient answers 'No' to either of the questions 'Have you used homeopathy before?' or 'Do you know what homeopathy is?' it is appropriate to say a few words about the discipline. It is well known that patients are much more likely to comply with what can be quite complicated dose regimens if they have some input into the management of their disease. Understanding how they are being treated is a major influence in this area. There are several areas in which counselling should be given.

You might say: 'Homeopathy is a form of medicine that helps your body heal itself' or 'This homeopathic medicine is safe and has been chosen for you individually, so it should not be given to anyone else, even if they have similar symptoms.' Advising on exactly what to say is difficult, because demographic characteristics vary widely with geographic areas; what is appropriate in one area might be inappropriate in another. It is a good plan to have one or two stock phrases up your sleeve to be able to reassure patients whenever necessary. A leaflet similar to that shown in Box 5.2 should help.

The possibility of an aggravation should be considered when counselling patients. It was mentioned briefly in Chapter 2, and will be explained more fully in Chapter 8.

Method of administration

Because homeopathic medicines are thought to be absorbed in the mouth, they should be taken on a clean palate. Many homeopaths insist that patients do not eat and drink for an hour or more either side of taking a remedy. Indeed, some state that coffee and tea must not be taken throughout the course of treatment. There is no absolute evidence that reasonable consumption of coffee (three to four cups per day) has a detrimental effect. The compromise that is generally adopted is to say that food and drink, tobacco and products containing aromatic flavourings (for example, toothpaste) should be avoided for at least 30 minutes either side of a dose.

It is also important that patients are made aware of the fact that homeopathic medicines in solid dose forms are not handled, so as to minimise the possibility of bacterial or chemical contamination. The appropriate dose should be tipped into the cap and (holding on to the cap tightly!) transferred into the mouth without touching. Sometimes more than one remedy is prescribed – for example Arnica and Ruta for a soft tissue injury – and the question arises of how they should be taken (concurrently or sequentially). Once again, there are no hard and fast rules, but allowing about half an hour between the different remedies would seem to be sensible. Two or even more ingredients can be combined into one complex dose form, which solves the problem nicely but at the expense of offending those of a classical point of view. As the remedy is absorbed in the mouth through the mucosa, it is important that it is sucked slowly and not chewed. Liquid remedies can be taken in water, and should be held in the mouth for 15 seconds to allow absorption.

Box 5.2   Example of an appropriate patient information leaflet

Advice for patients on the storage and taking of homeopathic remedies

- Keep the remedies in the original container.
- Keep the remedies away from strong-smelling substances such as camphor, peppermint, perfumes, paint, etc. and from high temperatures and direct sunlight.
- Your mouth should be free of other tastes. It is best not to take remedies within 30 minutes of food, drink, tobacco, toothpaste or sweets.
- Homeopathic remedies should not be handled. Tablets and granules should be tipped into the cap of the container and then administered onto the tongue. A dose of granules is a quantity sufficient to just cover the base of the cap.
- The remedies are absorbed from the mouth and so should not be swallowed, but allowed to dissolve. Liquids should be held in the mouth for several seconds before swallowing.
- If any remedies are spilled do not put them back into the bottle.
- Do not stop any orthodox medication unless advised to do so by the doctor who prescribed it.
- If stored correctly and not handled, homeopathic remedies are thought to remain active almost indefinitely.

What is homeopathy?
Homeopathy is essentially a natural healing process, providing remedies to help patients regain health by stimulating the body's natural forces of recovery.

It concentrates on the patient rather than on the disease in isolation.

For many years, homeopathic medicines (or 'remedies' as they are often called) have been recognized as being a safe and effective means of treating illnesses. There are no side-effects.

The main principle of homeopathy – let like treat like – refers to the procedure of giving patients minute quantities of medicines that in much larger quantities actually cause the symptoms being treated.

Homeopathy has developed in many countries and is now accepted widely as a credible therapy. It may be used alone or to support other orthodox treatments in a complementary role.

In the UK it has been favoured by the Royal Family. It is recognised by an Act of Parliament.

All homeopathic remedies are available under the National Health Service. If you have any questions about your medicine, please ask the pharmacist.

XYZ Pharmacy, Anytown
Telephone: 09980 333222

Storage

The remedies should be stored in a dry cool atmosphere away from aromatic odours and out of direct sunlight. Refrigeration is unnecessary, but they should not be kept away in steamy kitchen cabinets. Providing that there are no obvious signs of physical deterioration, remedies should remain efficacious indefinitely, despite the requirement to place an expiry date on the label.

SUPPLY UNDER THE UK NATIONAL HEALTH SERVICE

The right of patients to undergo homeopathic treatment was accepted in 1948 when the NHS came into being, and for many years it remained the

Box 5.3	Examples of prescription charging					

Example 1

Arnica 30c	1–5
SL	6–10
Arnica 200c	11–20
SL	21–30

Example 2

Arnica 10M	1–3
SL	4–20

Example 3

Arnica 30	1–5
SL	6–10
Symphytum 30c	11–20
SL	21–30

only complementary discipline available to the public in this way. Increasingly other treatments are becoming available. Although homeopathy is available under the NHS it is necessary to have access to the service to use it, and that is not quite as simple as it sounds, for the availability of homeopathic treatment is limited to certain active geographic areas. Thus while a patient living in Bristol, Glasgow, London or Tunbridge Wells might have access to a hospital, an outpatients' clinic and a number of homeopathic physicians under the NHS, a patient living elsewhere in the country might not be so lucky. The training courses held for physicians are producing more and more practitioners, so the position is certainly improving. The UK pricing bureaux keep price lists from all the main suppliers of homeopathic remedies and endeavour to price prescriptions accurately. It helps the clerks immeasurably if the prescriptions are endorsed with what has been dispensed and the net cost price. Homeopathic supplies are not subject to a 'clawback' discount, so the prescriptions should be marked 'ZD' for zero discount.

Patients who are not claiming exemption from prescription tax by signing the back of the prescription form must be charged the appropriate fee per item. In many cases the retail price of the remedy will be less than the tax, and under these circumstances pharmacists should adopt the normal allopathic practice of selling the remedy off the shelf, rather than dispensing it. In the case of a set of numbered powders if one remedy is involved (even if it is in more than one strength) with the placebo, the prescription counts as one item, attracting one charge (see Examples 1 and 2 in Box 5.3).

However, if more than one remedy is involved (see Example 3) then each attracts a charge. In this case it will nearly always be cheaper for the set of powders to be sold to the patient rather than dispensed, bearing in mind that it will probably have been bought in from a supplier at an all-inclusive price (i.e. the elements of the set will not be charged at individual prices).

It is not possible to cover all possible situations with respect to charging prescription tax for homeopathic preparations. In cases of uncertainty a telephone call to your supplier or local pricing office will often resolve the situation.

PRICING FOR PRIVATE PRESCRIPTIONS

Private prescriptions, where the patient bears the full cost of the item dispensed, may be priced using whatever scale is favoured. The calculation should be based on what has been charged by the supplier, and not on an arbitrary basis. Records should be kept as for allopathic medicines. Increasingly, private insurance schemes are accepting receipts for the reimbursement of homeopathic medication. The situation is changing month by month, and queries on this matter should be referred back to the insurance provider.

PRODUCT AVAILABILITY

There is an efficient network of manufacturers and wholesalers in the UK, all of whom will be delighted to advise and supply homeopathic remedies. Many offer next-day delivery, so there is no reason why a client should need to wait more that 24 hours for a remedy except at weekends or on national holidays. A limited range of homeopathic remedies is available from some mainline allopathic wholesalers; special or unusual remedies can be obtained from pharmacies with Special Manufacturing Licences.

A list of suppliers is included in Appendix 1.

RESPONDING TO REQUESTS FOR RECOMMENDING A PRACTITIONER

One of the most difficult enquiries to satisfy is 'Where can I get treatment?' or knowing to whom referrals can be made. The British Homeopathic Association has geographic lists of medical, dental and veterinary practitioners in the UK, and the Faculty in London and Glasgow can also supply names of members and licentiates. Their addresses can be found in Appendix 1. Governing bodies abroad can also supply lists of suitably qualified practitioners. Patients who wish to consult privately should have no hesitation in phoning their chosen practitioner and asking about the costs involved.

Deciding on a competent non-medical qualified practitioner can be more difficult because the degree of training can vary widely with different colleges and the qualifications may appear unfamiliar. Trained homeopaths may be recognised by initials such as MCH (Member of the College of Homeopathy), LCH (Licentiate of the College of Homeopathy), LCPH (Licentiate of the College of Practical Homeopathy), etc. Homeopaths registered with the Society of Homeopaths may use the initials RSH or FSH.

Unless you have personal experience of a particular practitioner, it is best to direct potential patients to the governing body of the complementary discipline in which they are interested. Thus, patients seeking homeopathic treatment can contact the Society of Homeopaths (see Appendix 1) for the address of a local homeopath who is registered with the Society.

REFERENCES

Kayne, S, Beattie, N and Reeves, A (2000) Self-treatment using homeopathic remedies bought over the counter (OTC) in a sample of British pharmacies. *Br Homeopath J*, 89(Suppl): S50.

Reid, SA (2002) Survey of the use of over-the-counter homeopathic medicines purchased in health stores in central Manchester. *Homeopathy*, 91: 225–229.

Chapter 6

The provision of homeopathic treatment

CHAPTER CONTENTS

Problems associated with treatment
   provision   137
Facilities   137
Obtaining the right information   138
Patient deciding diagnosis and treatment   138
Lack of records   139
Patient expectations   139

Decisions to make before treating   139
Am I competent to deal with this case?   140
Should I treat or refer to an appropriate
   colleague?   141
Should I treat with allopathy or
   homeopathy?   141

PROBLEMS ASSOCIATED WITH TREATMENT PROVISION

Before discussing the opportunities that do exist (see Ch. 8), it would be appropriate to consider the constraints that effectively govern what can be achieved in day-to-day practice by an intermediate level prescriber. These difficulties are also a feature of orthodox counter prescribing in a pharmacy but because of the holistic nature of homeopathy they are even more of a problem in this area.

Facilities

Gathering information requires an environment that allows interaction with the client. This may be a problem in a community pharmacy setting. Fortunately the chance of an intervention by other clients (a common feature of open discussions across a pharmacy counter for so many years) has now been effectively stopped in most premises. As the role of the pharmacist has expanded in recent years, and with the move towards providing enhanced services such as medicines management and pharmaceutical care, the provision of facilities for a private consultation has become necessary and clients are generally happy to discuss their healthcare problems with pharmacists. However, in some pharmacies the provision of such facilities is impractical due to building restrictions and so the problem persists.

Obtaining the right information

Obtaining the right information is often based on asking the right questions. Questions such as 'Are you taking any medicaments?' can be met with a negative response because the contraceptive tablet or antibiotic eye drops, for instance, may not be considered by customers as 'medicaments'. It may be necessary to ask specific questions about other complementary medicines, for example Chinese and Indian medicine where the term 'herb' includes more than just vegetable material. Elderly patients may forget one or more of a long list of drugs they are taking. The other big problem is remedies sought for a third party. Typically a wife may be seeking help for her husband or a mother for her teenage son. Here the well-meaning messenger and the sufferer may have totally different interpretations of what is wrong. For example, a child's diarrhoea may be attributed to 'food poisoning' by a parent when anxiety may be the cause. In homeopathic treatment this would involve two quite different remedies: in the first case Arsen alb might be prescribed, in the second Argent nit (if the diarrhoea came directly after food) or Gelsemium (if a fright or bad news were involved). A famous surgeon once said 'Never believe what a patient tells you his doctor has said', and while this might sound too sceptical, there is probably some truth in the warning.

Patient deciding diagnosis and treatment

All pharmacists can relate stories of customers asking for their advice on an OTC medicine to treat a condition, only to reject it in favour of a product of their own choice following several suggestions. We have already mentioned the difficulty of knowing when to intervene in an OTC purchase. The examples of cases from the author's case book illustrate some of the problems.

Case Study 1: A DIY diagnosis

Customer: 'I'm suffering from acute gastroenteritis. Could you give me something gentle so I can have a good bevvy [a considerable quantity of alcoholic beverage] at my sister's wedding this afternoon?'

Pharmacist: 'Sir, if you had acute gastroenteritis you'd probably be in hospital. Perhaps you have a tummy upset?'
Customer: 'Don't get smart with me – just give me something NOW.'

Case Study 2: Foot and nose disease?

Boy: My mother says I've got a wee verruca on my nose and can I please have some homeopathic medicine.'

Pharmacist: 'How does you mother know it's a verruca?'
Boy: 'Because she says she once had one like it on her foot.'

Case Study 3: Mistaken identity?

Customer: 'Do you have some Belladonna for scabies? I think that's what the remedy is called. It was recommended by a friend who is into this natural stuff in a big way.'

These requests all present the problem of knowing whether the customer is actually suffering from the condition that has been self-diagnosed. In Case 3 in particular, uncertainty as to whether the remedy is appropriate may exist, especially in the early days of homeopathic prescribing. These problems may be difficult to resolve without antagonising the customer.

Lack of records

Patient Medication Records (PMR) systems in pharmacies make it possible to check up on the history of regular patients and ensure that any OTC products – whether homeopathic or allopathic, prescribed or requested – do not conflict with other concurrent medication. The situation is rather different with casual 'walk-in' clients whose details are not held by the pharmacy. The pharmacist then has to resort to asking questions and there is always the risk that important information will be withheld. One solution is to have people carry a health smartcard with their medical history encoded on a magnetic strip. Access to selected information can be obtained with a special electronic reader. Access to the NHS net for pharmacists is proceeding in Scotland and this will make it much easier to access clients' records and communicate with GPs electronically in the not too distant future

Patient expections

An important reason for people turning towards complementary medicine is a hope that it will succeed where orthodox medicine has failed. 'Miracle cures' reported in the media stoke up an expectation among customers. Care must be taken to remain within one's limits of competency.

DECISIONS TO MAKE BEFORE TREATING

There are three important questions to answer before proceeding to the treatment stage in a consultation:

- Am I competent to deal with this case?
- Should I treat or refer to an appropriate colleague?
- Should I treat with allopathy or homeopathy?

Am I competent to deal with this case?

At this point, before moving on to deal with prescribing techniques in detail it would be appropriate to pause for a moment or two to reflect on the issue of professional competence (Ernst, 1995). In orthodox prescribing, therapeutic decisions are usually based on an assessment of the risk:benefit ratio. This is also one of the factors considered by members of the public when purchasing homeopathic remedies (see Ch. 1). It means that the effectiveness of a given course of treatment must be viewed within the context of patients' overall safety. Generally, concerns centre on adverse drug reactions and other potential direct hazards.

There are those colleagues who ask: 'Does it all matter anyway? Homeopathic remedies are so dilute that they cannot possibly do any direct harm.' Certainly a patient's life is unlikely be threatened directly by the use of an inappropriate remedy or potency in an OTC situation, although the homeopathic symptom picture could be sufficiently confused as to make continuing treatment difficult.

Equally important, however, is the possibility of an indirect hazard due to a prescriber's incompetence. Patients need to be protected from the effects of inadequate training. The rigorous standards of education for orthodox health professionals largely ensures that such risks are minimised, although sadly this does not guarantee absolutely that there are no incompetent pharmacists or doctors around. With complementary medicine no such universal standards apply and minimum levels of competence cannot be guaranteed across either health professionals or non-medically qualified practitioners. The practice of operating within one's own established limits of competence is thus very important, not only to ensure that a client receives the right remedy, but also to ensure that more serious underlying conditions are identified promptly and referred on.

Ernst (1995) has pointed out that competence cannot be discussed without linking it to responsibility that a given practitioner may take on with respect to patients. For example, if a pharmacist seeks to dispense remedies in response to requests from others without initiating a new treatment proactively, the professional responsibility involved would be rather different from that assumed by a colleague counter prescribing on a daily basis. Notice the use of the word 'different' and not 'less'.

There are two basic principles to guide practitioners in the practice of homeopathy:

1. The normally accepted limits of competence of one's own professional discipline must be maintained at all times.
2. One must remain within the current clearly defined limits of one's own homeopathic knowledge and confidence. In this regard most patients will assume quite legitimately that provided practitioners are registered their *bona fides* is guaranteed (Stone and Mathews, 1996).

Unfortunately this has not been the case in the past, given that each registering body claimed to ensure high standards. With control now being taken over many health professions by the Health Professions Council, the stimulus for standardising practice is growing.

Finally, remember that it is a complementary approach that is being advocated. We are seeking to give the patient the best treatment available; this may mean referring on to a more appropriately qualified colleague in the healthcare team, or making decisions over whether allopathic or homeopathic remedies (or both) should be offered in a given set of circumstances.

Should I treat or refer to an appropriate colleague?

A useful acronym to use when assessing a case, whether you intend to treat or refer or use allopathy or homeopathy, is LOAD, standing for **L**isten, **O**bserve, **A**sk and **D**ecide:

Listen to what the client has to say. They will tell you why they are asking for help and the most obvious symptoms, usually without prompting. This gives an indication of the sort of problem they have.

Observe the customer's appearance, demeanour and any obvious symptoms. We have already briefly mentioned the importance of obtaining information in this way using the painter and student cases in Chapter 1. As we shall see in Part 3 in much greater detail, observations of whether a patient is agitated, pale or flushed are often vital in choosing the correct homeopathic remedy.

Ask appropriate questions to gather in enough relevant information. Here there is another well-worn acronym – W-WHAM (Box 6.1) – which can act as a guide, but other more specialised questions may also be necessary.

Decide what should be done. A good guideline is that if you would not attempt to treat a condition with allopathic medicines then you would not treat it with homeopathy – with a few notable exceptions. Having decided that the condition can be treated safely, then the next decision is whether allopathic or homeopathic medicine should be offered.

Should I treat with allopathy or homeopathy?

It is difficult to give a set of firm pointers to making a decision one way or the other; in time, with experience, one tends to get a 'gut feeling' about

---

Box 6.1   The W-WHAM process

The W-wham questions:
WHO is the patient?
WHAT are the symptoms?
HOW long have the symptoms been present?
ANY action taken so far?
MEDICATION any being taken?

which method is likely to be the more beneficial for the customer. However, a number of factors need to be considered.

Situations where one might consider offering allopathic treatment include the following:

- where the condition is caused by an invader to the body – e.g. antifungals or antimalarials
- where there is a need to treat a lack of vitamins or minerals
- where the patient is taking steroids that interfere with homeopathic remedies
- where the patient expresses a wish for allopathic medicines
- where a customer is unlikely to observe necessary precautions when taking homeopathics
- where you are uncertain of the correct homeopathic remedy
- where the patient is in a low-risk group
- where the customer is sceptical
- where the customer requests a widely advertised product.

Situations where one might consider offering homeopathic treatment include the following:

- where there is no suitable allopathic medicine – e.g. for 'exam nerves' or anxiety
- when the customer is pregnant and worried about adverse drug reactions
- where there are worries about interaction with prescribed medication
- where the patient specifically asks for a homeopathic remedy
- where there are worries about dope testing in sport
- where allopathic medicines appear to be losing their effectiveness over time
- where customers are constantly buying the same analgesics and cough medicines
- where infants are being treated
- where there are worries about the cost of allopathic treatments.

Assuming that it has been decided to treat the customer, and then to treat the customer using homeopathy, we can now move on to the next group of decisions, affecting the type of treatment and the frequency of administration. Remember in this chapter we have been looking at the general procedures for acute prescribing; the actual choice of a specific remedy will be covered with other clinical topics in Part 3, Clinical Applications.

REFERENCES

Ernst, E (1995) Competence in complementary medicine. *Complement Ther Med*, 3: 6–8.
Stone, J and Matthews, J (1996) *Complementary Medicine and the Law*. Oxford University Press, Oxford, p 123.

Placebo side-effects occur when expectations of healing produce sickness, however minor; a positive expectation has a negative outcome (Hahn, 1997).

Physicians have known for several centuries that patients often display marked improvement of symptoms when given a sugar pill or some other substance having no known medicinal properties, believing that it is an active drug. In 1651, the great English scholar Robert Burton wrote: 'An empiric oftentimes, and a silly chirurgeon, doth more strange cures than a rational physician – because the patient puts confidence in him.'

Anecdotal experience suggests that perhaps as many as 30% of patients improve initially because their orthodox drug looks, smells or tastes 'medicinal' in their estimation. It has been shown that placebos are often used in modern medicine (Nitzan and Lichtenberg, 2004). Nitzan and Lichtenberg's survey of 89 doctors and nurses providing hospital based and ambulatory care in Israel found that 60% used placebos in their practice, most often (43%) to fend off an 'unjustified' demand for medication, to calm a patient (38%), as an analgesic (38%), or as a diagnostic tool (28%).

The main current application of placebo is in clinical research. With the advent of large-scale clinical drug trials, placebos have taken on the role of eliminating bias, although some doubt has been cast on the technique (Keine, 1993). It has been suggested that placebo treatment might be considered as an ethical obligation subject to the following provisos (De Deyn and D'Hooge, 2004):

- no adequate therapy for the disease should exist and/or (presumed) active therapy should have serious side-effects
- placebo treatment should not last too long
- placebo treatment should not inflict unacceptable risks
- the experimental subject should be adequately informed and informed consent given.

There are of course ethical issues raised by the use of placebos. Practitioners are obliged both by Codes of Ethics and morally to use interventions that they know to be effective in treating the particular condition presented. 'Effective' is usually taken to mean in a pharmacological sense. However, this is not always the case, even in orthodox medicines.

There have been calls for trials on well-established OTC products to determine whether reasonable grounds exist to assume that these products are safe and effective (Chaplin and Blenkinsopp, 1992). On the one hand, many of the newer OTC products, particularly those that have switched from a prescription-only to a pharmacy-only classification, have extremely well-documented evidence available to those wishing to make an informed decision as to the suitability of a particular medicine. The older traditional products, on the other hand, have little or no supporting literature. The embarrassing question that immediately springs to mind is: 'Why then do pharmacists continue to adopt an empirical approach and counter prescribe these products if proof of efficacy is critical?' For example, why do we still recommend certain antitussives when the British National Formulary clearly states: 'there is no evidence that any drugs can specifically facilitate expectoration; the assumption that subemetic doses promote expectoration is a myth'. It goes on to say that a simple expectorant may serve a useful placebo function (British National Formulary, 2005). It further states that 'the rationale for some compound cough preparations is dubious'. If there are elements of modern pharmacy practice that are no better than placebo, why is it that the placebo portion of the response to homeopathy is dismissed so contemptuously by sceptics? There is a belief that if a patient gets better it can only be the medicine that caused it (Paisley, 1979), when the healing powers of nature and the mind must be, at the very least, an important contributory factor, and at best, as with the cough preparations mentioned above, perhaps the main reason for recovery.

It seems homeopathy is not alone with its conceptual problems!

A first step towards making the distinction between homeopathy and the placebo effect may be to compare characteristic aspects and factors of the placebo effect with the action of homeopathic medicines, establishing the pharmacodynamics of placebo (Richter, 1993). This would include evolution of the placebo effect in time, dose–effect relationship and cumulative effects following repeated application.

Placebos have been classified as 'passive', containing no medicament and achieving no result, and 'active', also containing no active principle, but nevertheless achieving some clinical effect (Harrison, 1990). A fluctuation in blood pressure is a common response. An analysis of the elements of a practitioner–patient relationship during the consultation has suggested that a clinical approach that makes the illness experience more understandable to the patient, instilling a sense of caring and interest in the problem, is likely to create a placebo response and improve the symptoms (Brody, 1982). There is little doubt that a measure of the response to homeopathic treatment is due to a placebo response based on this factor. Indeed, as we have already stated, the lengthy sympathetic consultation is one reason for patients moving from orthodox to homeopathic practitioners. After all, the word 'placebo' does mean 'I shall please'. However, that is not the whole story of how homeopathic remedies might work. If that were the case, remedies could not be expected to work according to the various Laws of Cure (see below), nor would it matter which remedy was administered for any given condition.

One of the most frequently quoted pieces of clinical research was carried out by Dr David Reilly and co-workers on allergy patients (Reilly et al., 1986); it showed that homeopathy cannot be due purely to a placebo effect (see Ch. 11). Other research has not been so rewarding. In a double-blind crossover proving carried out by Walach (1993), 4 weeks of Belladonna 30c were compared with 4 weeks of placebo in 47 healthy volunteers. Single-case evaluation showed differences between the two experimental phases for 21 subjects, but group evaluation showed no clear-cut differences. Walach concluded that the results were 'promising' but that further studies were required to test the claim that homeopathic potencies can produce symptoms other than placebo in healthy subjects. The subject of research will be covered in greater detail in Chapter 11.

The well-tested phrases based on the placebo argument can be expressed as follows: 'It can't possibly work as an active medicine', say the sceptics.

'It won't work,' they go on, then, with a final flourish and a wry smile, 'and, anyway – it definitely doesn't work.'

A general characteristic of placebo effects is their relatively short duration, ranging from 2 to 6 weeks. In a two-part trial of patients with chronic rheumatic arthritis in Glasgow in 1980, in which separate groups of patients were treated with homeopathic remedies, salicylates and placebo, 60% of the patients receiving placebo withdrew from the study at 3 weeks, dissatisfied with their progress. By 6 weeks, all the placebo participants had withdrawn from the study whereas after a year the homeopathic group still had 74% of its patients and the salicylate group 15% of its patients (Gibson et al., 1980). Longstanding chronic conditions apparently cured by homeopathy cannot therefore be due entirely to a placebo effect (see Ch. 11).

Some years ago I was preparing some homeopathic teething powders and, having medicated three or four, turned to answer the telephone. In the interim my dispenser, who thought she was being helpful, folded and wrapped the complete set of 12 powders and issued them to an anxious mother who was tapping her fingers on the counter, in the way that anxious mothers often do. With the modern emphasis on audit and crisis management in the dispensary, nothing moves a centimetre without checking now, but in those 'good' old days it was a little different. Some hours later, the mother, who was not known to the staff, telephoned to ask if anything could possibly be wrong with the medicaments because they seemed to be working intermittently. This was a perfect, if unplanned, double-blind trial! The baby had received medicated powders interspersed with unmedicated placebo randomly, and apparently could tell the difference.

This anecdotal evidence is corroborated by apparent cures in animals. While small companion animals are subject to extra attention and sympathy accompanied by gentle stroking, leading to claims of a placebo response, the same claims cannot be made for a horse, cow, pig or goat, all of which respond well to homeopathy.

Undoubtedly, the placebo response does have a part to play, but is certainly not the whole story. In a wide ranging review of placebo research, Walach and Jonas conclude that the evidence emerging from the psychological literature and from experiments investigating the mechanisms of placebo effects is showing that placebo effects can be viewed as self-healing capacities of the person, qualities that are normal neglected in medicine (Walach and Jonas, 2004).

THE VITAL FORCE AND THE LAW OF SIMILARS

Let us now turn to a more traditional hypothesis of how homeopathy might work. While allopathic treatment is based on theory, logical deductions or generalisations from experimental evidence, homeopaths derive their clinical knowledge purely from observing the action of remedies on live patients. Underpinning homeopathy (and other complementary disciplines) is a vitalist philosophy, according to which the living organism is subject to 'laws' that are very different from those found in physics, chemistry or the biological sciences. These laws have also been determined by observation, not by deduction from theoretical principles.

Homeopaths consider disease to be an expression of the 'vital force' (also known as the 'life force') of each individual. Since all individuals are quite different in their expression of the vital force, patients are treated according to their idiosyncratic, rather than their common, symptoms. The symptoms are important only in that they act as an indicator for the selection of an appropriate remedy. The essential concept of homeopathy is 'self-recovery'. In order to explain this term adequately we must look at what we know about the body's regulatory mechanisms that are being targeted in homeopathic treatment. This in turn leads back to a discussion on the concept of 'vital force', a vibrating dynamic element, with an inherent, underlying bioenergetic quality that has been likened to the Chinese 'chi' or the Japanese 'ki' (Ullman, 1988). Vitalism has a long history in medicine (Wood, 2000). Hippocrates suggested that it was 'nature' in the body (he called it 'physis' from whence came 'physician') that healed the patient. The doctor could assist the physis through passive means (e.g. nutrition and removal of waste products). Galen also promoted the idea of a vital force. Paracelsus called it the 'archeus'. Hahnemann introduced the word 'dynamis' to describe the vital force. By this he meant that life was dynamic and took an active part in organising biological activity. He also called the process of potentisation 'dynamisation'. Much later a theory came into existence within biomedical research that was closely allied to it; this is the 'field concept'. The 'field' is said to be 'an organising factor in which certain reactions occur, space and time being used as a language for the continuous interactions between material elements' (van Wijk and Wiegant, 1995).

According to vitalism, the body comprises a hierarchy of parts – cells, tissues, organs – systems that are all fully interdependent in both ascending and descending order, and whose relationship to one another is controlled by a steering entity – the vital force. Under normal conditions, the vital force is thought to be responsible for the orderly and harmonious running of the body and for coordinating the body's defences against disease. It dominates life processes within the biological environment and controls the quality of the body's vibration. However, if the force becomes disturbed by factors such as emotional stress, poor diet, environmental conditions or certain inappropriate allopathic drugs, then illness results. Homeopathy views the living organism as unceasingly reacting to its environment, attempting to ward off danger and repair damage. Thus, what is called 'sickness' actually represents the organism's striving after health. The signs and symptoms of the illness are not the impact of some morbific stimulus on a patient but are the reaction to it – the body's attempts to restore order. These attempts represent the healing activity of the vital force, which can be stimulated by the administration of an appropriate remedy.

It is believed that the vital force operates on three different vibratory levels or planes, listed below in order of importance:

1. mental: where changes in understanding and consciousness are recorded; examples are confusion, delusions, lack of concentration, lethargy, absent-mindedness
2. emotional: where changes in emotional states are recorded; examples are anguish, anxiety, apathy, envy, fear, irritability, joy, love, sadness

3. physical: where changes to the body's organs and systems are recorded; examples are organ malfunctions and disease, injuries, sex, sleep.

The three planes may be depicted as a set of concentric circles with the mental plane, the most fundamental, being represented by the innermost circle. A person can survive with a physical infirmity or if emotionally disturbed, but without a measure of mental health the normal functions within the community are impossible (Vithoulkas, 1980). Sheila and Robin Gibson (Gibson and Gibson, 1987) have identified a fourth level, the spiritual, as represented in Figure 7.1.

When determining which homeopathic remedy is appropriate, classical homeopaths consider the body's functions to be an amalgam of all the planes. The principle of vibrationary resonance is the basis for the insistence of homeopathy upon the totality of the symptoms. If only a partial image of the total symptom picture is acquired, the effect of the remedy will be limited to that vibrational level only. Thus, if a patient consults a homeopath complaining of asthma and only the physical symptoms are recorded (shortage of breath, associated skin disorders, etc.), while the emotional and mental symptoms are ignored, the prescription is likely to act only locally (i.e. only on the physical vibratory plane). Such a procedure will produce only a transient cure. To find a remedy in tune with the optimum resonant frequency of the entire person, all the deviations from normality should be recorded.

Ullman (1988) has applied the analogy of music to support this idea. It is commonly known that when one plays a 'C' note on a piano, other 'C' notes reverberate. Even on another piano in another room, 'C' notes have a hypersensitivity to the 'C' resonance. They resonate because they are 'similar'. In homeopathy, medicines are chosen for their 'similarity' to the patient's total symptoms. It is postulated that the resonance of the homeopathic remedy affects the resonance of the vital force.

An attempt has been made to show how it might be possible to explain the vital force in terms of modern complexity theory, raising the possibility of a new understanding of life processes (Milgrom, 2002). Milgrom uses an interesting metaphor based on the concept of spin.

We can now define Hahnemann's Law of Similars more precisely than in Chapter 2, with reference to the totality of symptoms:

Figure 7.1
Interrelationships of the vibrational planes

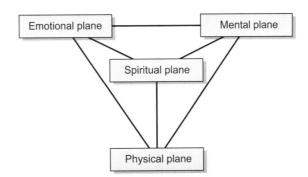

Any remedy which can produce a totality of symptoms in a healthy person, can cure the same totality of symptoms in a sick person.

It represents a method by which one can find a remedy with which an individual person's body can resonate at an optimum level. The remedy may stimulate the body's immune and defence systems to begin a self-healing process.

Most of the conditions treated in pharmacies OTC are of the first aid or acute type. They are usually of a simple self-limiting nature, where the course of action is well defined, comprising a latent period, a period of exacerbation and a period during which symptoms subside. Most will resolve on their own, given time. The rationale for prescribing polychrests in these cases on local symptoms alone, using a keynote or three-legged stool approach (see Ch. 8) is merely to hasten recovery. The vital force is temporarily depressed – with a consequent change in the resonant frequency of the body – but, rather like a trampoline, it has the ability to bounce back quickly (Lockie, 1989). This is analogous to the body's normal defence mechanisms coping with the situation. Under these circumstances Hahnemann found that one remedy could treat these conditions in a large number of different people, without the need for individualisation.

Chronic illnesses present a completely different scenario. We will look at them more closely in the next section. Here the analogy is the creeping bank overdraft that rises and falls over the course of a year, but always maintains a trend towards insolvency, necessitating a request to the bank manager for a higher limit at each annual review. What is required is an injection of sufficient capital to restore the balance to normality so that minor irregularities in spending can be accommodated once again. The administration of a homeopathic remedy seeks to provide the stimulus for the vital force to reverse its downward trend, become re-energised and bounce back to its normal resting state of well-being.

When similarity exists between remedy and patient, we can expect a biological version of resonance; the patient exhibits a hypersensitivity to the remedy. The choice of a particular potency, produced by serial dilution and succussion, is responsible for 'fine tuning' the frequency and amplitude of the resonance to such a point that the reaction is maximised. Solutions diluted beyond Avogadro's number (see Ch. 1) have no molecules left in solution that can be detected with methods available today, so how can the power of similarity be present? In fact, the current detection limit is somewhat higher than the Avogadro threshold. There must be something left in solution for the remarkable healing powers of high potencies to be achieved. This 'something' is the subject of furious debate: a resonance, a molecular pattern, an energy, mumbo-jumbo – it has been called by many names, not all of them complimentary. Certainly experiments have been conducted with nuclear magnetic resonators to reveal vibratory properties of remedies in high dilutions (Smith et al., 1968). Like many of life's ethereal mysteries we cannot be more specific about the nature of the vital force, other than to say that it is not a material phenomenon. The concept is all the more difficult to accept because a materialistic or chemical view of the world has now become the norm, and many scientists reject paradigms for which there is no rational explanation. For the time being, the reader is invited to set aside such sensibilities and adopt an open mind on the matter.

There are many receptor and keyhole theories approximating to the theory of allopathic drug mechanisms. Several workers have provided explanations of the potentisation phenomenon based on physical chemistry principles. Some seem so plausible that they are as difficult to disprove as to prove!

However, it is important to stress once again that explanations or theories of how homeopathy works are of secondary importance to most people (that is, apart from sceptical colleagues). Patients use the remedies because they work, just as they do with allopathic remedies.

THE MIASMATIC VIEW OF CHRONIC DISEASE

One of the greatest barriers limiting dialogue between orthodox and homeopathic medicine is the homeopathic classification of chronic diseases as 'miasms' (Bellavite and Pettigrew, 2004). The concept of miasms appears alien and anachronistic to contemporary Western medicine. It was based on Hahnemann's observations and influenced by the limited pathological knowledge of his time. Many homeopaths still feel miasm theory empirically observable and useful in prescribing, others prescribe with no reference to it.

Hahnemann observed that certain of his patients, whom he had treated for acute conditions, returned to him complaining of a new set of apparently unconnected symptoms. These often appeared following some stressful episode, and reappeared with increasing strength following periods of comparatively good health. He interpreted this deep-seated cyclical susceptibility towards chronic illness as indicative of a fundamental underlying problem, possibly a micro-parasitic invader, that he called a 'miasm'. Anton van Leeuwenhoek, the Dutch microscopist, had visualised protozoa and bacteria as early as 1687, and several other researchers showed the presence of microorganisms during the 19th century, but it was not until 50 years after Hahnemann that, Robert Koch and his colleagues, working with anthrax, demonstrated that specific bacteria were associated with specific infectious diseases.

In his 1828 book *The Chronic Diseases* (available online at http://homeoint.org/books/hahchrdi/index.htm) Hahnemann postulated that three primary miasms were responsible for most of the chronic weakened states that, in turn, led to acute illness in his patients (Ortega, 1983). These were the 'sycotic' miasm (also called gonorrhoea), the 'luetic' miasm (also called syphilis) and the 'psora' miasm. The last was considered to be by far the most widespread, and manifested itself as a skin eruption known simply as 'the itch' in Hahnemann's day. It is generally thought of as being synonymous with scabies although there is some evidence that Hahnemann made a distinction between the two terms, believing that scabies was a 'living eruption' that 'has its origin in small living insects or mites' while 'the itch' represented a constitutional predisposition to skin disease. In his early works Hahnemann suggested Sulphur lotion to remove the scabies mites but he later confirmed that these methods had serious side-effects which complicated chronic diseases. This led to the use of Sulphur and other remedies in homeopathic potency in the treatment of 'itch'.

Gonorrhoea and syphilis were related to the acute infections of the same name. Two further miasms, tubercular and oncotic, were added later by other homeopaths.

The classical chronic miasmata may be summarised as follows:

- luetic – the miasm of destruction – skin ulcers
- sycotic – the miasm of excess – proliferative skin changes
- psoric – the miasm of deficiency – scabies, eczema
- tubercular – the miasm of exhaustion – body sweats, weight loss
- oncotic – the miasm of cancers – changes in body characteristics (odours, discharges, warts, moles).

This doctrine of chronic disease caused much opposition among Hahnemann's colleagues. The link between chronic and acute disease in the same patient was difficult to explain in terms of the vital force. Further, accepting such a small number of chronic diseases seemed to conflict with the principle of individualisation. In due course the miasmatic concept was accepted, but it remained the source of controversy for a long time.

If any of the conditions were suppressed by inappropriate treatment, Hahnemann postulated that the miasm was driven deeper, causing additional problems with internal organs. There was then the possibility of either an underlying genetic trait being exposed, or its transmission to offspring. This idea may well be yet another difficult concept to accept, but if one thinks of the treatment of syphilis in the first half of the 19th century, it was not uncommon for patients to experience some effects of the disease for the rest of their lives even after treatment with mercury. Any children could also suffer from hereditary effects of their parents' condition.

Modern public health procedures have largely eradicated these historical miasms, but the idea continues to be discussed widely by homeopaths, many of whom define a miasm as follows:

> *a blockage or distortion of the normal flow of energy in the self-regulatory mechanism of the organism, causing a disposition towards long-standing illness and resulting from*
> - *infection*
> - *previous medical treatment 'going wrong'*
> - *poor hygiene and environmental influences*
> - *occupational hazards*
> - *hereditary transmission.*

Many acute bacterial and viral infections, including chickenpox, cholera, glandular fever, influenza, malaria, measles, scarlet fever and mumps, seem to predispose sufferers to other seemingly unconnected conditions and can be considered to be associated with the existence of rather shorter-acting miasms. Depression and anxiety accompany many physical complaints. Hereditary conditions also have a miasmatic strand to them. The experienced homeopath will be able to recognise the disease patterns of many types similar to those described above, and prescribe remedies that are effective on a deeper miasmatic level. If a person self-treats for an acute condition on two or three occasions, but the condition persists or returns, then it can be assumed that a deeper-acting 'miasmatic remedy' may be necessary. It is important that such patients are referred to a fully qualified homeopath for investigation.

Miasmatic theory has been adapted by many modern practitioners, having become a metaphor for a class of diseases of like nature, requiring similar medication, rather than specific diseases with the same origin. An attempt has been made recently to explain the existence of miasms in terms of molecular biology (Blass, 1993). There appear to be critical sites on the DNA molecule that, when activated, trigger the production of gene products. The stretches of DNA that act as switches are called 'promoters', and the function of these promoters can be increased by other areas of DNA known as 'enhancers'. It is suggested that a normal gene, or group of genes, could be 'switched off' in response to a pathogen, resulting in hypofunction (psoric mode), or 'switched on' so that the cell overfunctions (sycotic mode) or causes an aberrant gene to start working (syphilitic mode). At meiosis, when sperm and ova are produced, the miasmatic factors would be passed on in the DNA, establishing a hereditary link. The regulation of genes is a highly complex process, and only a simplified version of this hypothesis is given here. It is certainly worthy of closer scrutiny.

Cellular pathology has led to an understanding of the basic repair mechanisms of every cell and tissue. These mechanisms exist in order to avoid necrosis or cell death. The main mechanisms are molecular repair, apoptosis (programmed cell death) and cell proliferation. Failure of any or all of these mechanisms leads to what might be called states of 'dysrepair' that are probably the basis of miasms or reactional modes.

Montfort-Cabello (2004) has proposed a new interpretation of miasms:

- The psoric reactional mode can be understood as a defect in molecular repair (e.g. asthma, epilepsy and high blood pressure).
- The syphilitic reactional mode can be understood as a defect in the apoptotic process, which leads cells to an anticipated death (e.g. Alzheimer) or to necrosis, producing ulcerative and destructive lesions (e.g. ulcerative colitis).
- The sycosic reactional mode can be understood as a defect in control of cell division and extracellular matrix production, due to mutation in DNA repair mechanisms The consequences are excessive cell proliferation with tumour production and fibrous tissue formation.

Hahnemann recognised that there were separate groups of fixed, recurring symptoms that appeared in each of the different miasmatic pictures. On the basis of these symptoms he allocated specific remedies and nosodes that could be used to obtain an effective cure. They are listed in Table 7.1. Each has a full drug picture set out in the various materia medica.

THE DIRECTION OF CURE – HERING'S LAW

Generally speaking, as stated earlier in this chapter, mental symptoms are regarded as the deepest level of an individual's health, with emotional problems next in line, then followed by physical symptoms. The depth of a par-

Table 7.1 Specific treatments for chronic miasma

Miasma	Remedy	Nosode
Luetic (Syphilitic)	Mercurius	Syphilinum
Oncotic	Lapis alb, Aurum met nat	Carcinosin
Psoric	Sulphur	Psorinum
Sycotic (Gonorrhoea)	Thuja	Medorrhinum
Tubercular	Calc carb, Phosphorus	Tuberculinum

ticular symptom depends on its severity, frequency and degree of impact on that person's ability to maintain their own normal state of wellness. In 1845 the American homeopath Constantine Hering (1800–1880) published in the preface to the first American edition of Hahnemann's *Chronic Diseases* an extract of an essay (never published again elsewhere) in which he wrote: 'Every homeopathic physician must have observed that the improvement in pain takes place from above downward, and in diseases from within, outward' (Hering, 1845). In an article some 20 years later Hering made further mention of this 'rule', suggesting that it represented what might be expected to happen rather than what will definitely happen. The earliest reference to Hering's Law by name is to be found in an article written by his fellow countryman James Tyler Kent in 1911. These general guiding principles of the way in which people recover from disease are extremely useful to homeopaths in deciding whether a particular remedy is working or not. It is widely accepted that Hering's Law is second only to Hahnemann's 'similia similibus curentur' in importance.

Hering's observations were:

● **The healing body tends to direct disease from inner more serious levels to outer, more superficial levels. Conversely, the deteriorating body will internalise disease, moving it to deeper levels.** A patient with asthma may thus develop eczema as part of the curative process. A classical homeopath would not use a topical preparation to treat this condition, as such preparations are considered to act suppressively, rooting the illness into the organism and causing it to assume a chronic form. If the asthmatic's eczema is treated with a steroid it will probably clear up, but the likelihood is that, in suppressing the condition, the asthma may be exacerbated. A person with emotional problems may experience more superficial physical 'side-effects' as a cure proceeds. In allopathic treatment, symptoms are often dealt with in isolation, and not always seen to be connected with other concurrent conditions. Homeopathic principles do not normally allow the suppression of symptoms, except in the case of postoperative pain where the symptoms do not reflect a response to illness by the vital force and also in terminal disease. In the latter case, where the vital force is hopelessly overwhelmed, the 'like to treat like' approach is contraindicated because there may either be no response at all, or if an overstimulation should occur the ensuing aggravation could actually hasten death. In such situations the most troublesome individual symptoms may be treated in isolation with polychrests.

- **Healing proceeds from the top of the body to the bottom.** A person with arthritis in many joints will normally experience relief first in the upper part of the body before the lower part.
- **Healing proceeds in the reverse order to the onset of symptoms.** The most recent symptoms will resolve before the older ones, and may cause symptoms that have been suppressed to reappear. The pattern of disease resolves rather like a cassette tape playing in reverse.

Hering's Law is demonstrated by the following case.

Case Study: 10-year-old girl

A girl aged 10 was bought to an allergy clinic by her mother who had requested referral from her GP so that the child's asthma could be treated homeopathically. During the consultation it emerged that the child also suffered from a 'touch of eczema', but that this was not worrying either the patient or her mother. A skin test revealed an allergy to the house dust mite and an isopathic preparation of this in 30c was prescribed. After a month the child returned to the clinic. Mother was incensed; her daughter now had only 'a touch of asthma', but a worsening of the eczema. The child's body had externalized the disease. After a further period, without medication, both eczema (and mother) had thankfully quietened down.

Hering's Law is extremely important for homeopathic practice since it outlines the natural course that must be followed by morbific and curative processes (Coulter, 1980). Failure to respect the natural process of illness and recovery will cause harm to the patient. Specifically, practitioners have found that the improper treatment of acute illness may engraft on to the patient an incurable chronic illness.

THE CONSTITUTIONAL TYPE

In any given population the following may be observed:

1. People react to homeopathic remedies with different levels of intensity.
2. Some people respond especially well to a particular remedy.
3. Among people in this unique group, certain physical and mental characteristics appear to be common (e.g. skin texture, hair colour, height and weight). Further, these people also tend to suffer from similar complaints (e.g. premenstrual syndrome, or PMS).
4. Parallels can often be drawn between certain characteristics shared by people in this group and the physical or chemical properties of a remedy.

Constitutions have been described as 'constellations of mental, physical and general features' (Davidson et al., 2001). The constitutional characteristics of the patient prevail in the absence of illness just as the usual constitution of a country or state does in the absence of crisis (Swayne, 1998). They are also aspects of the individual that may intensify during illness to become symptoms. Particular physical characteristics, body functions and psychological traits may become exaggerated.

James Tyler Kent called the groups associated with particular remedies 'constitutional types'. Constitution is really a symptom pattern rather than a physical type, though characteristics have been described. For example, we may talk of a person being a 'Phosphorus' or 'Pulsatilla person' or a 'Natrum mur type'. This means that the person reacts especially strongly to these particular remedies in early undifferentiated stages of disease, after an acute episode, and also in chronic complaints.

The concept of constitutional response is known in allopathic medicine, where gender and ethnic differences may be linked to the efficacy of treatment, albeit for pharmacologically identifiable reasons (Lamba et al., 2003).

The determination of a patient's constitutional type may be facilitated with the aid of a Constitutional Type Questionnaire (CTQ). A 152 item CTQ was shown to display a high degree of reliability and validity when assessed in a sample of 472 patients attending clinics at the Royal London Homeopathic Hospital (Van Haselen et al., 2001). The correlation between CTQ results and the medicine prescribed by homeopathic physicians following a traditional consultation was 75.8%. The results gave some support to the homeopathic concept of constitution (Davidson et al., 2001).

Examples of homeopathic constitutional remedies are:

A *Phosphorus person* tends to be volatile, tall and slim, often with freckles and red hair. They tend to 'explode' on occasions when they are under mental strain – a bit like phosphorus bursting into flame if not kept under the right conditions. Despite this possibility, an Indian doctor has suggested that a man would be very lucky to marry a woman with a Phosphorus constitution (James, 1992). She would be good looking, fastidious, sensitive, sympathetic and loving. In addition she would be romantic, sociable and sexy!

A *Pulsatilla person* is said to be very changeable. The remedy comes from the 'wind flower', a plant so named because it sways in the wind from one side to another, changing its direction frequently. This characteristic is often reflected in uses of the remedy; for example, Pulsatilla can be used to treat a cough that tends to be dry at night but productive in the morning, or hoarseness that comes and goes – two conditions that may be described as being changeable.

A *Natrum mur person* tends to be 'pear-shaped', likes lots of salt and often suffers from constipation. They often have a withdrawn or introverted personality and a liking for their own company.

A *Sepia person* might be portrayed as being a tired mother on a washing day with a painful back, perspiring profusely and with a headache. She is tall and slim with a sallow complexion. One of her five children is screaming but she takes no notice; when her husband appears home and tries to give her a kiss she turns away.

A *Sulphur person* is characterized by: a lean body and stooping shoulders; likes fresh air and hates tight clothes; has cold feet and warm head; hot sweaty hands. 'Absent-minded professor' image.

Douglas Borland applied the idea of constitutional prescribing to children, identifying five main types, against each of which he set about six remedies with appropriate drug pictures especially applicable to children.

These are set out in Table 7.2. For a full account the reader is referred to a booklet by Borland entitled *Children's Types*, published by the British Homeopathic Association (Borland, 1940).

There is also a constitutional response associated with miasms. The miasms are not always associated with specific diseases, but rather with types of constitutional states that affect the way a person experiences disease. For example, people with syphilitic miasms tend to suffer from ulcers in the stomach, duodenum or mucous membranes, bone and tissue deformities and be prone to alcoholism.

There are other constitutional classifications used in France and Germany (Gaier, 1991). Some veterinary surgeons acknowledge the presence of constitutional groups among animals. My good friend Francis Hunter assures me that he can recognise a Pulsatilla cow, and the late George Macleod, a pioneer in veterinary homeopathy, once stated that in his experience the Irish Setter often responded well to Phosphorus – and indeed it might be expected that this was so. German Shepherd dogs often respond well to Lycopodium, while Spaniels fit the Sulphur picture.

The Irish Statesman Dr Garrett Fitzgerald was once reported in *The Scotsman* newspaper as saying to a colleague: 'Well that's all very well in practice – but does it work in theory?' It would seem to be reasonable to explain the action of constitutional remedies theoretically in terms of a harmonisation process between the normal resonance of the patient's body and the resonance of the remedy.

The use of constitutional remedies in homeopathic treatments is discussed in Chapter 8.

A COMPARISON BETWEEN ALLOPATHIC AND HOMEOPATHIC TREATMENT

At this point, before we start choosing remedies, it would be opportune to sum up the main features of the allopathic and homeopathic approach to therapeutics.

In general terms, allopathy sets out to treat the disease. It involves the use of chemical compounds administered in large enough quantities to (hope-

Table 7.2 Borland's classification of children's types (in each case the first-named remedy represents the main constitutional type) (Borland, 1940)

No	Characteristics of group	Examples of likely constitutional type remedies
1	Fat, fair, chilly, lethargic	Calc carb, Calc phos, Lycopodium, Phos, Silica
2	Backward, development delayed	Baryta carb, Carbo veg, Natrum mur, Sepia
3	With skin problems	Graphites, Psorinum, Antim crud, Petroleum
4	Warm blooded, affectionate	Pulsatilla, Kali sulph, Sulphur, Thuja
5	Nervous disposition	Arsen alb, Chamomilla, Cina, Mag carb, Ignatia

fully) achieve an overall beneficial pharmacological effect. The medicine chosen on the basis of 'one cure for all' may perform one of the following:

- directly suppress the symptoms without addressing the cause (e.g. analgesics or replacement therapy)
- ameliorate the symptoms by reducing the cause of disease (e.g. expelling tapeworms from the gut or the removal of infection by antibiotics)
- block a symptomatic pathway with an antagonistic treatment (e.g. antihistamines).

The majority of drugs used today fall into the third group. They are used in the highest dose possible to suppress the patient's symptoms and may initiate adverse reactions or even drug-induced damage. Often, an illness may require a portfolio of drugs to elicit a response. Hypertension and diabetes are typically treated with several drugs concurrently.

Homeopathy seeks to treat the patient as an individual, stimulating the body's powers of self-healing and often taking little account of the cause. Thus, in the case of hay fever, where the allopath is concerned with the underlying cause, the release of histamine, the homeopath is more interested in stopping the symptoms of red, itchy eyes and a runny nose. The choice of remedy is based on recording the symptoms and prescribing on a 'like treats like' basis. Homeopathy is accordingly not an analytical but a phenomenological method (Steinbach, 1981). This contrasts directly with allopathy, where most medicines block or destroy biochemical pathways.

A further difference between the two disciplines relates to posology. In allopathy it is frequently necessary to use different formulations, tablets, capsules, suspensions, etc., sometimes because of the physical characteristics of the active ingredients, and sometimes to accommodate dosing requirements. In homeopathy the choice of carrier is merely a matter of convenience. In allopathic medicine the magnitude of drug effect is usually related to its concentration at the site of action within limits in a smooth graded manner. Thus, a section of intestinal smooth muscle may shorten progressively as the concentration of spasmodic drug is increased. The relationship between drug concentration and effect is generally hyperbolic. This results in concentration/effect curves that are generally sigmoid in appearance, containing a central portion, between 20% and 80% of the maximum effect, where the effect is linearly related to the concentration of drug. One might postulate that if the curve were to be extrapolated back beyond the origin, it could be expected to rise (and perhaps fall again) in continuing cycles of activity (Fig. 7.2). Given the right conditions (whatever they might be), could a therapeutic result be expected at negative concentrations? It is necessary to accept for this discussion that the term 'negative concentrations' means there could be molecules present, but that they cannot be detected with current techniques. This would put them in the homeopathic range. This is an interesting academic thought to address!

Many criticisms of homeopathy are countered by its proponents who state that the difference between homeopathy and orthodox medicine can be expressed in terms of the 'art of healing' and the 'science of healing'. The former implies a measure of innovation, flexibility and tailoring the response to particular circumstances. It can be very personal and creative.

Figure 7.2 Drug–response curve extrapolated back to negative drug concentrations

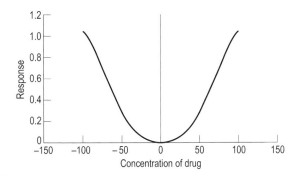

It is *my way* of doing things, a statement that is akin to saying 'in my opinion'. The opinion may be considered inappropriate by many, but it is still one person's assessment of a situation. The erroneous assumption is that what has been labelled a matter of art or philosophy is thereby exempt from rigorous evaluation. The terms are a screen behind which short cuts, muddled thinking and uncritically accepted prejudices can be hidden. They are particularly misleading when applied to aspects of medical practice that are amenable to empirical study, but about which sufficient data have not yet accumulated.

Vithoulkas (1995) has predicted that homeopathy is: 'doomed to take a downward turn toward a point of degeneration, confusion and finally, even oblivion; homeopathy's eventual downfall will be due mainly to a number of "artistic distortions" that are injected into the main body of knowledge by the "imagination" and "projections" of some "teachers" of homeopathy.' There are, however, situations where the term 'art' may be appropriately applied to all aspects of medicine, demonstrating that it can never be totally reduced to an empirical science. The scientific method of healing implies that the remedy is tried and well tested, and that the mechanisms of action are understood. Scientific methods tend to be restrictive in that they must often be used in given sets of circumstances and have specific applications. This description certainly does not fit homeopathy. There is no clear-cut boundary between the two arguments. What can be said is that an ability to adopt disciplined procedures similar to those followed by scientists in problem solving, together with a measure of informed intuition, are two of the most important qualities required by successful homeopaths. It is within this context that Vithoulkas maintains homeopathy is a science. The mechanisms of action are a well-documented stumbling block for homeopathy, particularly with the high potencies. In allopathic medicine, mechanisms of drug action are widely (though not by any means completely) understood. A drug competes for attachment to receptors for neurotransmitters or hormones based on a mutually complementary isometric structure, or it interacts with enzymes and membranes. Homeopathy is thought to be effected through interaction with a nebulous 'vital force' that cannot be demonstrated.

There are a number of similarities between allopathy and homeopathy that are not always recognised. Some were mentioned in Chapter 2 when the principles of homeopathy were discussed. Other examples are as follows:

1. It has been suggested by Savage (1980) that the concentrations of quinine in blood after conventional dosing of 650 mg 8 hourly do not reach the level required to kill the malaria parasite. Could it be that the quinine stimulates the natural defence mechanisms? This 'evidence' is often quoted by devotees of homeopathy, but unfortunately Savage does not quote any reference for his statement.

2. Notwithstanding the comments made in the BNF about the efficacy of expectorants, Ipecacuanha is included in minute doses in cough mixtures because of its supposed expectorant properties. In high doses the agent is poisonous.

3. Between 1956 and 1958 scientists formulated a vaccine with an emulsifying agent, the aim being to reduce local irritation caused by the standard preparation (Himmelweit, 1960). The force exerted to bring about emulsification of the water in oil represented succussion. The saline vaccine had been through one complete stage of homeopathic potentisation. The subsequent healing power of the vaccine was enhanced and the aggravation of skin tissue at the injection site ceased to be a problem.

It is evident therefore that certain homeopathic principles are not contrary to conventional medical pharmacological science, but are in fact, in some cases, consistent with its experience. The relationship between homeopathy and allopathy is summarised in Tables 7.3 and 7.4.

Homeopathy is a method of treatment demanding a high degree of personal attention. Its use can be acceptable for non-life-threatening diseases (and some chronic diseases); however, it is incapable of treating all diseases, despite claims to the contrary by some practitioners. There do not appear to be any risks of side-effects, except for minor aggravations (see Ch. 8).

Table 7.3 Properties of allopathic and homeopathic remedies

Allopathic features	Homeopathic features
Used on basis of therapeutic action	Used on basis of a proving/drug picture, toxicology and clinical evidence
Animals and ill patients used to test	Provings on healthy humans
Size of dose sufficient to achieve blood level	Frequency of administration more important
Strength expressed by amount of drug present	Strength set by the potentisation process
Depends on metabolic activity to work	Simple absorption; metabolic activity unproven
Source of medicines is largely synthetic	Sources mainly naturally occurring

Table 7.4 Allopathic and homeopathic remedies as they affect patients

Allopathic features	Homeopathic features
Usually same drug given to all patients for similar symptoms	Individualised treatment in chronic states
Drug given to treat symptoms in isolation	Most remedies treat patient as a whole
Condition at time of consultation treated	Holistic approach
Usually requirement for course of treatment	Taken only until improvement achieved
Symptoms disappear in no apparent order	Homeopathic laws of cure are followed
Side-effects and iatrogenicity	OTC aggravations generally only transient

REFERENCES

Bellavite, P and Pettigrew, A (2004) Miasms and modern pathology. *Homeopathy*, 93: 65–66.

Bergman, J-F, Chassany, O, Gandiol, J et al. (1994) A randomized clinical trial of the effect of informed consent on the analgesic activity of placebo and naproxen in cancer patients. *Clin Trials Metaanal*, 29: 41–47. (Cited in: Walach, H and Jonas, WB (2004) Placebo research: the evidence base for harnessing self-healing capacities. *J Altern Complement Med*, 10(Suppl. 1): S103–S112.)

Blass, G (1993) Demystifying miasms [letter]. *Br Homeopath J*, 82: 223–224.

Borland, D (1940) *Children's Types*. British Homeopathic Association, London.

Brien, S (2004) Attitudes about complementary and alternative medicine did not predict outcome in a homeopathic proving trial. *J Altern Complement Med*, 3: 503–505.

British National Formulary (2005) BNF, 49th edn. British Medical Association/Royal Pharmaceutical Society of Great Britain, London, p 162.

Brody, H (1982) The lie that heals: the ethics of giving placebos. *Ann Intern Med*, 97: 112–118. (Cited in: Harrison, I (1990) Comment – a place for placebos? *Br J Pharm Pract*, July: 228.)

Bryden, H (ed.) (1999) Human healing: perspectives, alternatives and controversies. Report on the 1999 special study module for medical students. Glasgow: ADHOM, 1999. www.adhom.org (Cited in: Reilly, D (2001) Enhancing human healing. *Br Med J*, 322: 120–121.)

Burton, R (1651) *The Anatomy of Melancholy ... by Democratis Junior*, 5th edn.

Chaplin, S and Blenkinsopp, A (1992) Clinical trials in community pharmacy. *Br Med J*, 304: 63–64.

Coulter, H (1980) Homeopathy and modern medical science. *J Am Inst Homeopath*, 73: 7–28.

Davidson, J, Fisher, P, van Haselen, R, Westbury, M and Connor, K (2001) Do constitutional types really exist? A further study using grade of membership analysis. *Br Homeopath J*, 89: 138–147.

De Deyn, PP and D'Hooge, R (2004) Placebos in clinical practice and research. *J Med Ethics*, 22: 140–146.

Ernst, E (2004) Should we use 'powerful placebos'? *Pharm J*, 273: 795.

Everson, SA, Kaplan, GA, Goldberg, DE, Salonen, R and Jukka, T (1997) Hopelessness and a 4-year progression of carotid atherosclerosis: the Kuopio ischemic heart disease risk factor study. *Arterioscler Thromb Biol*, 17: 1490–1495.

Gaier, H (1991) *Encyclopaedic Dictionary of Homeopathy*. Thorsons, London, pp 108–114.

Gibson, R and Gibson, S (1987) *Homeopathy for Everyone*. Penguin, Harmondsworth.

Gibson, RG, Gibson, SL, MacNeill, AD and Watson-Buchanan, W (1980) The place for non-pharmacological therapy in chronic rheumatoid arthritis: a critical study of homeopathy. *Br Homeopath J*, 69: 121–133.

Hahn, RA (1997) The nocebo phenomenon, scope and foundations. In: Harrigton, A (ed.) *The Placebo Effect*. Harvard University Press, Cambridge MA, ch 3, p 57.

Harrison, I (1990) Comment – a place for placebos? *Br J Pharm Pract*, July: 228.

Hering, C (1845) Preface. In: Hahnemann, S *The Chronic Diseases: Their Specific Nature and Homeopathic Treatment*. William Radde, New York, vol 1.

Himmelweit, F (1960) Serological responses and clinical reactions to the influenza virus vaccines. *Br Med J*, 2: 1690–1694.

Hyland, M (2003) Using the placebo response in clinical practice. *Clin Med*, 3: 347–350. (Cited in: Brien, S (2004) Attitudes about complementary and alternative medicine did not predict outcome in a homeopathic proving trial. *J Altern Complement Med*, 3: 503–505.)

Isenberg, SA, Lehrer, PM and Hochron, S (1992) The effects of suggestion and emotional arousal on pulmonary function in asthma: a review and a hypothesis regarding vagal mediation. *Psychosom Med*, 54: 192–216. (Cited in: Reilly, D (2001) Enhancing human healing. *Br Med J*, 322: 120–121.)

James, ICJ (1992) Importance of mental symptoms. *Quinquina*, 1(3): 28–29.

Keine, H (1993) Placebo effect in clinical trials. *Allgemeine Homöopathische Zeitung*, 238: 139–146.

Lamba, V, Lamba, J, Yasuda, K, Strom, S et al. (2003) Hepatic CYP2B6 expression: gender and ethnic differences and relationship to CYP2B6 genotype and CAR (constitutive androstane receptor) expression. *J Pharmacol Exp Ther*, 307: 906–922.

Lockie, A (1989) *The Family Guide to Homeopathy*. Hamish Hamilton, London.

Milgrom, IR (2002) Vitalism, complexity and the concept of spin. *Homeopathy*, 91: 26–31.

Montfort-Cabello, H (2004) Chronic diseases: what are they? How are they inherited? *Homeopathy*, 93: 88–93.

Nitzan, U and Lichtenberg, P (2004) Questionnaire survey on use of placebo. *Br Med J*, 329: 944–946.

Ortega, P (1983) *Notes on Miasms or Hahnemann's Chronic Diseases*. National Homeopathic Pharmacy, New Delhi.

Paisley, PB (1979) Cabbages. *Med J Aust*, ii: 646–648.

Reilly, D (2001) Enhancing human healing. *Br Med J*, 322: 120–121.

Reilly, DA, Taylor, MA, McSharry, C and Aitchison, T (1986) Is homeopathy a placebo response? Controlled trial of homeopathic potency, with pollen in hayfever as model. *Lancet*, 2(8512): 881–886.

Richter, A (1993) Effect of homeopathic treatment and placebo effect. *Allgemeine Homöopathische Zeitung*, 238: 147–150, 197–202. (See abstract by Meuss, A (1994) *Br Homeopath J*, 83: 103.)

Savage, RH (1980) The unrecognised use of homeopathy in conventional medicine. *Br Homeopath J*, 69: 87–95.

Shapiro, AK and Shapiro, L (1997) *The Powerful Placebo*. Johns Hopkins University Press, Baltimore, p 1.

Smith, RB, Boericke, MT and Boericke, W (1968) Causes changed by succussion on NMR patterns and bioassay of bradykinin triacetate succussions and dilutions. *J Am Inst Homeopath*, Oct–Dec: 197–211.

Steinbach, D (1981) The pros and cons of homeopathy. *Pharm J*, 247: 384–387.

Swayne, J (1998) Constitution. *Br Homeopath J*, 87: 141–144.

Swayne, J (2000) *International Dictionary of Homeopathy*. Churchill Livingstone, Edinburgh.

Swayne, J (2005) Homeopathy, wholeness and healing. *Homeopathy*, 84: 37–43.

Taylor, M, Reilly, D, Llewellyn-Jones, RH, McSharry, C and Attchison, TC (2000) Randomised controlled trial of homeopathy versus placebo in perennial allergic rhinitis with overview of four trial series. *Br Med J*, 321: 471–476.

Ullman, D (1988) *Homeopathy – Medicine for the 21st Century*. North Atlantic Books, Berkeley, CA.

Van Haselen, R, Cinar, S, Fisher, P and Davidson, J (2001) The Constitutional Type Questionnaire: validation in the patient population of the Royal London Homeopathic Hospital. *Br Homeopath J*, 90: 131–137.

van Wijk, R and Wiegant, F (1995) Stimulation of self-recovery by similia principle? Mode of testing in fundamental research. *Br Homeopath J*, 84: 131–139.

Vithoulkas, G (1980) *The Science of Homeopathy*. Grove Press, New York.

Vithoulkas, G (1995) Homeopathy: art or science? *Classical Homeopathy*, 1(1): 3–5.

Walach, H (1993) Does a highly diluted homeopathic drug act as a placebo in healthy volunteers? Experimental study of Belladonna 30c in a double blind cross over design – a pilot study. *J Psychosom Res*, 37: 851–860.

Walach, H and Jonas, WB (2004) Placebo research: the evidence base for harnessing self-healing capacities. *J Altern Complement Med*, 10(Suppl. 1): S103–S112.

Wood, M (2000) *Vitalism: The History of Herbalism, Homeopathy, and Flower Essences*, 2nd edn. North Atlantic Books, Berkeley CA.

Chapter 8

Choosing the remedy

CHAPTER CONTENTS

The types of remedy groups available 168
Polychrests 168
Isopathic remedies 168
  The allergodes 170
  The nosodes 171
  The sarcodes 171
  Nosodes and sarcodes used as 'vaccines' 171
  Tautodes (tautopathic remedies) 173
Standard classical remedies 175
Constitutional remedies 176
Nosodes with drug pictures – the miasmatic nosodes 177
  Bowel nosodes 178
Complex remedies 180
  Why use a complex? 182
Levels of treatment and dose regimens 182
First aid 183
Acute prescribing 183
Chronic prescribing 185
  Totality of symptoms 185
  Modalities 186

Concomitants 187
Peculiars 187
Dose regimens 188
Multiple remedy prescribing 188
Choosing the remedy 192
Using the repertory 192
  Boericke's *Materia Medica with Repertory* 192
  Kent's *Repertory* 192
  Remedy grading 194
  Other repertories 196
Repertorising by computer 196
Keeping records 198
Following up 198
Reviewing the patient's progress 198
  Possible actions 199
Safety issues 200
Inappropriate treatment 200
Side-effects 200
Aggravations 201
Interactions 204

THE TYPES OF REMEDY GROUPS AVAILABLE

Polychrests

Prescribing for acute self-limiting conditions is generally, but not exclusively, based on polychrests. Polychrests are remedies whose drug pictures show a very wide spectrum of activity and which therefore have a broad range of applications. The term polychrest (meaning 'many uses') was taken from the Greek by Hahnemann and first used by him in an 1817 article on Nux vomica. The spelling varies, some authorities using the spelling 'polycrest' and others 'polychrest'. This group of 20–30 remedies (there is some debate as to what exactly constitutes a polychrest) forms the basis of most commercially available homeopathic ranges as they lend themselves to prescribing based on abbreviated drug pictures (known as keynote or 'three-legged stool' prescribing (see below) without protracted consultations. Although they are used mainly for first aid and acute situations, polychrests are often indicated in chronic disease too, because they affect so many body tissues.

The polychrests can also serve as constitutional remedies (see below) . The remedies presented in Table 8.1 together with their keynote indications are generally accepted as being polychrests among homeopaths.

Isopathic remedies

This group of remedies was mentioned briefly in Chapter 4. Isopathy (or isotherapy) involves the use of high dilutions of the allergen(s) to which the patient is sensitive (Poitevan, 1998). The prescribing technique is empirical.

Isopathy had a long history before becoming associated with homeopathy. There are many examples quoted by Gaier (1991) and Bellavite and Signorini (1995):

- Columbian folk medicine has for centuries successfully used the macerated liver of poisonous snakes to treat bites.
- Pliny the Elder (AD 23–79) recommended that the saliva of a rabid dog, if taken in drink, will guard against rabies.
- In Chinese medicine the powder of dried smallpox vesicles was used as snuff in the prevention of the disease. The Chinese also encouraged the wearing of clothes in the full suppurative phase of the disease.
- Dioscorides of Anazarbo in the first century AD stated 'where the disease is, so is the remedy'. He recommended the application of crushed scorpion to scorpion bites.
- In a book entitled *La Chimie Royale et Pratique* (1633) a treatment for excessive menstrual bleeding was described: 'Three or four drops of the same blood, the clearest available, should be given to the patient to drink without her knowledge.'
- Edward Jenner's work with live cowpox vaccinations in 1796 represented an isopathic application.

The term 'isopathy' was probably first used by the Silesian veterinarian Wilhelm Lux, Professor of Veterinary Science at the University of Leipzig,

Table 8.1 Examples of polychrest remedies with keynotes

Remedy	Main indications
Aconite	Sudden onset, hot skin with thirst, sneeze no. 1, great anxiety (= terror?)
Allium cepa	Profuse bland lachrymation, copious sneezing, worse in warm conditions
Argent nit	Anticipatory anxiety especially when with flatulence and diarrhoea
Arnica	Trauma, mental and physical exhaustion, fear of being touched
Arsen alb	Diarrhoea and vomiting
Belladonna	Intense throbbing pain, redness, sudden onset; worse lying down
Bryonia	Sharp stitching pains, dryness with thirst, cough, worse with movement
Calc carb	Increased perspiration, apprehension, severe vertigo, nausea
Calc phos	Mentally tired, forgetful, restless, chronic catarrh
Cantharis*	Urge to urinate: burning sensation; burns and scalds
Carbo veg	Flatulence; desire for fresh air; collapse (especially with 'blueness')
Chamomilla	Teething and colic; child better when carried
Euphrasia	Acid lachrymation; conjunctivitis, bland coryza
Gelsemium	Influenza, low-grade fevers; diarrhoea from fright
Hypericum	Damage to nerve endings – 'blood and crush' injuries
Ignatia	Immediate and next day effects of grief and worry
Ipecac	Frequent nausea and vomiting; persistent wheezing cough; croup
Ledum	Puncture wounds, insect bites, especially where skin cold to touch
Natrum mur	Violent sneezing with fluid coryza; cold sores
Nux vom	Gastric complaints from overeating; chronic constipation
Pulsatilla	Catarrh – bland yellow or green discharge; headache; cough
Rhus tox	Arthritic-type pain, worse on initial movement, better for heat
Ruta grav	Sprains, soft tissue injuries, eye-strain
Sepia*	Hot flushes, indifferent and easily offended, menstrual problems
Symphytum	Bone injuries – surgical intervention or fractures

* The inclusion of Cantharis and Sepia in the polychrests is the subject of some debate and is not universally accepted

about 1832. After becoming an enthusiastic homeopath, Lux became convinced that every contagious disease had the means of curing itself and subsequently used isopathic remedies prepared according to homeopathic principles (Lux, 1833).

As stated in Chapter 4, there are several different types of isopathic remedies used to treat allergies and certain chronic and contagious diseases:

Allergodes are potentised allergens derived from many sources (e.g. grass and flower pollens, moulds, house dust mite, animal hair, food products – chocolate, milk, shellfish, wheat, etc.).

Nosodes are prepared from diseased material of plant, animal and viral origin (e.g. fluid from an arthritic joint, bowel tissue, vesicles). The term is also commonly used for homeopathic preparations made from bacterial cultures, more correctly termed 'sarcodes' (see below). Auto-isopathics are similar to nosodes, but are prepared from an individual patient's own products (e.g. blood, secretions, urine, warts, verrucae, or milk from a cow or sheep suffering from mastitis).

Sarcodes are generally obtained from 'healthy' materials (e.g. bacterial cultures or secretions such as Lac can, dog's milk, or Moschus, musk oil). The term may also be applied to venoms.

Tautopathics are derived from drugs (e.g. chloramphenicol, diazepam, nitrazepam, penicillin, etc.), chemicals (e.g. pesticides, industrial fluids, biological washing powders) or synthetic products (e.g. nylon, plastics, rubber latex). One of the first tautopathic preparations was made during the Second World War from mustard gas (see Ch. 11).

The allergodes

Because of their very nature many allergodes – isopathic remedies used to treat allergies – do not have drug pictures obtained through provings, and are still prescribed on the basis of local symptoms alone. Other isopathic remedies have developed in a more classical way. Several companies produce OTC packs of allergodes, specifically Mixed pollens and Mixed grasses. These can be used effectively, providing the patient knows that he or she is allergic to that substance. There are geographic variations that need to be considered both within countries and internationally. Different species of grasses and weeds grow in different areas, so to be certain that the particular allergen is included, it is sometimes necessary to have the remedy made specially from a sample gathered fresh in the patient's home locality. Special isopathic preparations can be made to order by licensed homeopathic manufacturers, but it is always worthwhile enquiring whether your requirement is available before you place an order. Most manufacturers carry stocks of all sorts of weird and wonderful source materials. It is my experience that some isopathic remedies are cross-functional. The remedy made from Plantago major (plantain, ribwort) appears to be effective in treating an allergy to rubber latex gloves commonly found among nursing staff, and vice versa. This phenomenon has also been reported in allopathic medicine (Lavaud et al., 1992).

tective effects of LD or ULD exposures to 13 pre-identified biological and chemical agents. Two further articles of fair to good quality reported both protective and treatment efficacy from exposure of animals or humans to LD and ULD exposures to toxins of risk in biochemical warfare. Despite this paucity of evidence the researchers concluded that rapid induction of protective tolerance is a feasible but under-investigated approach to bioterrorist or biowarfare defence. In their opinion, further research into the role of induced protection with LD and ULD toxic agents is needed.

Standard classical remedies

By far the biggest group of remedies are what might be called 'standard' or 'classical' remedies. There are thousands of these remedies – perhaps as many as 7000, of which about 1250 are in regular use. These are remedies where a lengthy consultation is required, at least at the initial stage. It is necessary to try and match as many mental and physical features as possible; there may be several remedies that appear to do the job, and differentiating between them can be difficult, particularly if the symptom picture is confused by a number of overlying conditions.

In order to speed up the repertorisation process, homeopaths often identify one or more symptoms that provide a strong indication for a particular medicine – known as 'guiding symptoms' – and when combined with their knowledge of common remedy keynotes gives a feeling for the direction of their further investigation. Vermeulen has introduced a similar idea of using 'the nucleus of a remedy' representing a summary of the main keynotes and food affinities (Vermeulen, 2004).

Another less tangible pointer to the choice of a remedy is to consider its essence, defined as being 'the unique character of a remedy's materia medica'. This individuality is usually expressed in psychological or abstract terms that often reflect metaphorically the physical characteristics (Swayne, 2002). Practitioners often acquire a 'feeling' for the essence of a remedy, illustrated by the case study below (see also p. 184).

Case Study: 26-year-old woman (courtesy Frank Randall, MRPharmS, Barrow-in-Furness)

History
A 26-year-old woman had a baby 2 years ago. She had repeated laxatives from her GP with no change of functionality although passing stool with difficulty.

Prescription
1. Arnica 30c – a trauma problem? Some relief from this.
2. Constitutional remedy. She is an only child and was very pretty when younger, growing into an attractive woman. She is very intelligent but used to getting her own way and becomes very upset if this is not the case. She seems quite delicate in some way and this seemed to indicate Silica – given as 30c potency twice daily.

Follow-up
This worked perfectly and normal bowel movement was restored in 2 weeks.

Comment
Not all the pointers were obvious initially but on thought and observation, with time, one can get the 'feel' of a remedy by using it and studying its effects in practice.

Finally a choice may be confirmed if a symptom unique or peculiar to the drug picture of a certain remedy is present (see below).

Constitutional remedies

A remedy may be defined as constitutional when, by virtue of its symptomatology, it covers the basic acute or chronic symptomatology of a person throughout life (Vithoulkas, 1998). In spite of the fact that such a person may suffer from several conditions at different stages of their life the constitutional remedy generally remains the same. However, the position may be complicated by the fact that a distinction can be made between a person's true constitutional remedy and constitutional features that may be exhibited in the short term during given sets of circumstances. These features can change in the course of a disease, for example during the treatment of female patients with hormonal imbalances. The question whether a constitutional remedy exists for every individual was raised quite early in the homeopathic literature by Hahnemann himself when he stated that in order to cure completely one needs to find the 'deeper' indicated remedy according to his theory of the chronic miasms (Vithoulkas, 1998).

Bailey has published in-depth analytical descriptions of the personalities of the major constitutional remedies including an attempt to portray the 'essence' of each remedy (Bailey, 1995). For each remedy Bailey has selected a single 'keynote' based on a psychological characteristic. For example, Nux vomica is 'the conqueror' and Sepia is the 'independent woman'. This could also be considered as being the essence of the remedy (see above).

As stated in Chapter 7, because of their wide-ranging uses, many of the polychrests are also constitutional remedies. If the indicated polychrest also happens to be the patient's constitutional remedy, a remarkable cure can be effected.

Phosphorus patients commonly take on the characteristics of a Sepia constitution when they are ill and depressed. In other patients, the constitutional features may become more pronounced when they are unwell. Pulsatilla subjects may become more weepy for example.

Constitutional prescribing will stimulate the total reserve of vital energy of the person. It increases resistance, improves well-being, increases the possibility of avoiding relapses and helps recovery from diseased states.

A selection of common constitutional remedies is set out in Table 8.3.

Constitutional prescribing is used:

1. as an adjunct to standard prescribing to facilitate recovery, for example combined with a pathological remedy in 'drainage therapy' (see p. 190) or in treating allergies (see Ch. 9)
2. as a general 'tonic' to tune up the body's defences
3. where the patient is suffering from a non-specific type of illness that cannot easily be pinned down. It may be effective in the stage before a localised disease has developed.

Table 8.3 Examples of constitutional remedies

Remedy	Constitutional features
Arsen alb	Intelligent, fastidious, fussy, restless, exhaustion after slightest activity
Bryonia	Dark complexion, tendency to irritability, often thirsty, vertigo, rheumatics
Calc carb	'Chalky white' complexion, apprehensive, forgetful, mentally slow
Carbo veg	Sluggish, fat, lazy; tend to suffer from chronic conditions, faint easily
Graphites	Stout, fair complexion, tendency to skin affections
Ignatia	Nervous temperament, easily offended, erratic behaviour
Lachesis	Great loquacity; restless, uneasy; cannot bear tight clothes
Lycopodium	Pale complexion, afraid to be alone; often has urinary or digestive ills
Natrum mur	Irritable, hasty; likes salt on food; often diabetic; gouty pains
Nux vom	Thin, nervous, irritable, sullen; overbearing; stomach problems
Phosphorus	Tall, slim, reddish hair, freckles; vivid imagination; volatile
Pulsatilla	Fair, warm hearted; changeable nature; weeps easily; female remedy
Sepia	Tall, slim, dark; waxy skin, shuns affection; feels cold in warm room
Silica	Nervous, excitable, cold and chilly people; subject to purulent lesions
Sulphur	'Poseurish' outlook, dishevelled, grubby; dislike of water; eye problems

Nosodes with drug pictures – the miasmatic nosodes

In the early days of homeopathy, all the isopathic remedies were used on the basis of *Aequalia aequalibus curentur* ('let same be treated by same') rather than the classical *Similia similibus curentur* ('let like be treated by like'). In the 1830s, however, causative similarity was rejected in favour of the symptomatic similarity now recognised, and the drug pictures of a few so-called 'miasmic nosodes' were obtained by provings.

Most of these remedies have the suffix 'inum'. Medorrhinum (derived from gonorrhoeal material), Psorinum (from the scabies vesicle), Syphilinum (from syphilitic material) and Tuberculinum (from a tubercular abscess), together with the bowel nosodes (see below), are examples of nosodes that have been used successfully in cases where there is a long-standing infection. When a carefully selected remedy fails to act, an appropriate nosode can be given, based on the patient's (or sometimes their parents') medical history. They have a drug picture and most can be found in the materia medica like other standard remedies.

Dr Constantine Hering was among the first to investigate Psorinum, potentised matter derived from a scabies vesicle (Banerjee, 1991). He reported his investigations thus:

> In the Autumn of 1880 I collected the pus from the itch pustule of a young and otherwise healthy negro, who had been infected . . . The pustules were full, large and yellow, particularly between the fingers, on the hands and forearms. I opened all the mature unscratched pustules for several days in succession and collected the pus in a vial with alcohol. After shaking it well, allowing it to stand, I commenced my provings with the tincture on the healthy. Its effects were striking and decided. I administered it to the sick with good results . . .

Note that the drug picture of Psorinum was found by clinical observation during treatment and not by a classic proving with healthy volunteers. It occupies more than two pages in Boericke's *Materia Medica*, 12 in Allen's *Encyclopedia* and no fewer than 28 pages in Hering's *Materia Medica*. In common with other nosodes it has a constitutional picture (see Ch. 7 and below). Indications include 'offensive discharges, profuse sweating, debility and bad taste in the mouth'. A really dirty, smelly drug picture, it is sometimes called 'the great unwashed' remedy.

Bowel nosodes

The 'bowel nosodes' form an important subgroup of the nosodes. Edward Bach was a man best known for his discovery of the range of 38 Bach flower remedies (see Ch. 10), but in fact a number of his discoveries in bacteriology parallelled those of Hahnemann. In the years immediately after he qualified as a doctor in 1912, Bach examined the flora of the colon, and found that the number of certain flora normally present in the large intestine seemed to increase greatly in the sick. This led him to utilise these bacteria as nosodes. These organisms were various types of non-lactose-fermenting bacilli, belonging to the coli-typhoid group, very closely allied to such organisms as the typhoids, dysenteries and paratyphoids, yet not giving rise to acute disease. Eventually, having become interested in homeopathy and teamed up with Dr John Paterson at Glasgow Homeopathic Hospital, he used the bowel nosodes in dilution on the basis of both mental and physical symptomatology. In 1936 Dr John Paterson presented a paper to the British Homeopathic Society in which he reported on the clinical and bacteriological observations on some 12 000 cases (Paterson, 1936).

A brief summary of the findings is as follows:

In addition to the normal *Escherichia coli* (*E. coli*) found in the bowel, a quantity of non-lactose-fermenting bacilli were isolated in 25% of the stool specimens examined. According to the accepted theories of Pasteur and Koch the appearance of these 'abnormal' organisms should be associated with disease, yet clinical observations revealed quite the opposite. Patients not only did not feel unwell, but many had experienced a distinct feeling of well-being. Since the non-lactose-fermenting bacteria were shown to have appeared 10–14 days following administration of a homeopathic remedy it was concluded that the change in bowel flora was due to the remedy. The organisms were therefore the result not of disease but of the vital action set up in the patient by the potentised remedy.

The appearance of the non-lactose-fermenting bacilli often followed, and seemed to bear a relationship to, a previously administered homeopathic remedy that had been potentised and chosen according to the Law of Similars.

Dr Paterson concluded that (Paterson, 1950):

- the specific type of organism found in the bowel is related to the patient's disease
- the specific organism is related to the remedy given to treat the disease (not all remedies affect the bowel flora). The change in bowel flora has been noted to follow the whole range of more commonly used potencies from mother tincture right up to CM
- the homeopathic remedy given is related to the disease.

From his observations Dr Paterson was able to compile a list of bowel organisms with their related homeopathic remedies, and to describe a drug picture for each. This picture was not obtained from a true 'proving' in the classical sense but from observation of a sick person's symptom picture. The use of antibiotics and other powerful allopathic drugs over the last 40 years or so has resulted in a change in the average patient's bowel flora, so the application of these nosodes today may not be as effective as Bach and Paterson reported. Originally each nosode was an autogenous preparation, that is, the individual patient's own organism was potentised and administered. This was comparatively simple when the organism had been isolated. Unfortunately this is not always possible, although the patient may present symptoms. Thus, a nosode was used from a case showing similar symptoms. Over the years, many nosodes were accumulated and combined in a composite remedy of each organism, which contained many hundreds of different strains of the organism. These nosodes were potentised and form

Table 8.4 Examples of bowel nosodes

Bowel nosode	Indication	Equivalent remedy
Bacillus no. 7	Exhaustion	Kali carb; other Kali salts
Dysentery Co	Anticipatory tension	Arg nit, Arsen alb
Gaertner	Malnutrition	Phos, Silica, Merc viv
Morgan pure	Congestion	Chelidonium, Lycopodium, Sulphur
Morgan Gaertner	Calculi	Lycopodium
Mutabile	Urinary conditions	Pulsatilla, Ferrum phos
Proteus	Mental irritability	Natrum mur, Ignatia
Sycotic Co	Irritation	Rhus tox, Thuja

the basis of the nosodes available from manufacturers today (Paterson, 1960).

Examples of the bowel nosodes, adapted from Laing (1995), are summarised in Table 8.4.

The bowel nosodes are used (Laing, 1995):

- when an associated homeopathic medicine fails
- as a 'fallback' in complicated or confused cases
- in combination with the indicated homeopathic remedy
- as a medicine with its own drug picture.

Routine prescribing of nosodes along isopathic lines is not considered good homeopathic practice by classical homeopaths, but they can be useful in the treatment of chronic diseases ranging from influenza to tuberculosis, particularly in breaking up cycles of recurrence.

Complex remedies

Although classical homeopaths keep true to Hahnemann's principles in prescribing only single remedies, it has been found by clinical experience that some homeopathic remedies can be mixed together and administered successfully as a complex. This method of treatment has become very popular. In Belgium, France, Germany and the Netherlands there is a collective market of over 450 such branded products.

Complexes may also be mixtures of generic remedies in the same dose form, for example ABC (Aconite, Belladonna and Chamomilla) for teething, AGE (Arsen iod or Arsen alb, Gelsemium and Eupatorium) for influenza, SSC (Silica, Sulphur and Carbo veg) for stomach problems, usually in one potency, or patented mixtures sold under a trade name.

The last may contain many ingredients – in the case of some French and German products as many as 20 different remedies are present in potencies ranging from 3x to 30c. The complex remedies usually have specific indications, making them rather easier to prescribe. Weleda have a product in the UK comprising Feverfew, Nat Mur and Silica that is promoted for the treatment of headaches and migraine. Another, for nausea, contains Arsen alb, Cocculus and Ipecac.

There are combination remedies in the New Era Tissue Salt range (known by the letters A to S) with specific indications for use. Combination R, for teething, comprises Calc fluor, Calc phos, Ferr phos, Mag phos and Silica.

In New Zealand, Naturo Pharm of Rotorua have sports care and baby care ranges of complex remedies and Miers Laboratories of Wellington an OTC preparation called 'No-Jet-Lag'. The South Australian producer Brauer also has a large range of complexes. Soluble constituents are usually potentised individually and then mixed to give the required liquid potency prior to medication. Insoluble ingredients are individually triturated with lactose.

Some of the French manufacturers combine zoological material within their complexes (e.g. Fel tauri, ox gall). The extremely popular Oscillococcinun (also called Oscillo) is a cold and flu remedy (Papp et al., 1998) that contains elements derived from Muscovy duck liver. None of these products is licensed or can be supplied legally in the UK by OTC sale. They could, however, be available on a named patient basis with a medical prescription as an unlicensed product, the responsibility for the safety of the product passing to the prescriber.

Group remedy prescribing is claimed to represent a pragmatic (although some may say heretical) approach to homeopathy. Aware of the limitations of classical homeopathy and his own inability to repertorise accurately, Eric Powell hit upon the idea of administering a combination of plant or plant and mineral remedies that together met the totality of symptoms. He describes a total of over 60 different formulae, most with around eight different remedies (Powell, 1982). Formula P5, recommended for 'sinusitis, tonsilitis and throat disorders generally', comprises Ferrum phos 6x, Calc iod 6x, Silica 6x, Baryta carb 6x, Bryonia 3x, Guaiacum 3x, Belladonna 3x, and Lachesis 12x. P55 (Natrum phos 2x, Antim crud 3x, Cuprum met 6x, Ol Cade 3x and Santonium 3x) is said to be particularly effective in eradicating parasites in hedgehogs (Sykes and Durrant, 1995)! It is indicated for pin worms and thread worms in all species. When prescribed, the remedy mixtures are written as 'Powell PX', where X represents a number from 1 to 64. Some remedies have letters as well; for example, there is a 2B, a 3B and 28B and C. Potencies at the 3x level contain concentrations of remedy comparable to the orthodox dose of 0.1 mg/100 ml, and have few indications in classical homeopathy.

Another range of complexes with specific indications is produced by the Dr Reckeweg Company in Bensheim, Germany. They have various agents around the world; in the UK the remedies are distributed by Complex Homeopathy Limited of Bolton (address in Appendix 1). The Reckeweg range comprises oral liquids, injections, topicals and eye drops, all with multiple ingredients. The formulae are referred to by the letter 'R' followed by a number – most also have product names. The following are examples:

- R1 ('Anginacid') comprises 10 different remedies in a range of potencies and is indicated for 'local inflammations of a catarrhal nature'
- R9 ('Jutussin'), available as syrup and drops, also comprises 10 different remedies; it is claimed to be an effective expectorant
- R77 (anti-smoking drops) comprises six remedies for the withdrawal of smoking
- R95 ('Alfalfa tonic') comprises six different mother tinctures and four remedies in low potencies. It is recommended for anaemia, convalescence and after a debilitating fever or surgery.

The manufacturers recommend that the oral drops are taken in a teaspoonful of water and always on an empty stomach. A frequency of around three times a day is usually indicated, but this dose can be increased, especially at the start of treatment. Reckeweg also have a range of veterinary complexes sold under the ReVet label. In some countries it may be necessary to comply with certain legal directives before Reckeweg's products can be supplied. The requirements are changing from month to month and the current situation should be checked carefully with the supplier at the time of purchase.

The Pascoe range of complex products is made by a German company called Pharma-zeutische Präparate GmbH of Giessen. They are usually described by a product name with the word 'Pascoe' following in parentheses, for example Lymphdiaral (Pascoe). The UK distributors are Noma

(Complex Homeopathy) Limited of Southampton (address in Appendix 1). Noma also supply a similar German range of complexes called Kernpharma® (Kern, Buhl). The same comments on legal status given for Reckeweg's products apply to Pascoe and Kern. Another range of complexes from Europe is marketed under the brand name 'Dr Vogel'.

Why use a complex?

There are three main reasons why a complex is used. One may be that the prescriber is uncertain as to which remedy is the most appropriate. Giving a complex is seen as increasing the chance of a correct prescription. Thus if a prescriber cannot ascertain whether a sports injury is due to damaged soft tissue involving muscles (Ruta) or ligaments (Rhus tox) he or she may give both remedies, either as a complex or separately. The second reason is to treat more than one symptom of the same condition, or more than one complaint at the same time. The complex AGE given for flu comprises the following three remedies with their keynotes in parentheses: Arsen iod (thin watery discharge, swollen nose), Gelsemium (dull headache and fever) and Eupatorium perf (the 'sore muscles and bones' often associated with flu) and is given to mount a three-pronged attack against the disease. The final reason for using complexes is merely for convenience, to save time and trouble.

Opponents of this type of therapy maintain that even if this strategy works, the prescriber will not know which of the remedies cured the patient. Some clinical trials have yielded positive effects (Ferley et al., 1989) but no provings have been carried out with complexes, and there is little information available to indicate how remedies might interact. The imprecise nature of this type of prescribing does not instil confidence in the practitioner's ability. The remedies chosen may each be partial similars, but none of them the best match or similimum. In this case there may be an improvement of some symptoms but also the possibility that new symptoms will appear. My colleague Dr Stuart Semple of Edinburgh tells me that in his experience unnecessary components can give violent aggravations (often when least needed) and that he uses mixtures in less than 1% of his prescriptions. When devising formulae it is important to note that certain remedies are more suited to inclusion in a complex than others. There is also the possibility of incompatibilities arising.

LEVELS OF TREATMENT AND DOSE REGIMENS

The choice of dose frequency depends on whether the treatment is first aid, acute or chronic. Opinions on appropriate posology vary widely. For instance Argent nit (for anticipatory anxiety) and Arnica (for mental and physical tiredness and bruising) are used in over 30 different potencies ranging from 3x to 1M. Belladonna is quoted as being used in an even greater spread of potencies, from the mother tincture to MM (Rawat, 1991). In an audit carried out at Glasgow Homeopathic Hospital (Kayne and Beattie, 1998) no less than 13 different sets of instructions were given to patients for taking one particular remedy. The dose regimens suggested are not 'set in stone'. They represent suitable guidelines and can be altered to fit individual circumstances. Throughout this book any remedies indicated may be administered according to the regimens outlined below, except where otherwise indicated.

First aid

In the context of OTC supply, the term 'first aid' is being used literally (i.e. meaning 'first treatment') rather than its more usual meaning, associated with injury following an accident of some description. Thus it might as well be applied to treating the first stages of a cold as to treating bruises resulting from a blow or fall. When choosing a polychrest for first aid prescribing it is possible to reduce the drug picture right down to the smallest match possible on which to support the choice of remedy.

If one were to see an unfortunate person knocked down in the street one would be unlikely to kneel down beside the victim and whisper gently in his or her ear: 'What sort of food do you like? Are you happy when it rains? Do you like to be alone?' By the time you had conducted a 2-hour interview the poor patient could have passed away! It would be pretty obvious from your observations that Arnica was needed for trauma and bruising or perhaps Aconite for shock, without even talking to the patient. This is an example of what is known as 'keynote prescribing', that is, using one or two very characteristic features or symptoms, including the aetiology, and is appropriate in first aid type situations. The choice of polychrest can often be made by using the first two elements of the acronym LOAD (Listen, Observe) (see also Ch. 6).

Homeopathic remedies are administered frequently under these circumstances – the 30c potency or even higher (200c) is appropriate perhaps as often as every 10–15 minutes for six doses. The response can be extremely rapid (within minutes). If necessary, where troublesome symptoms are still present, dosing can then be continued on the acute scale (see below). In some extreme cases one or two doses of the M or even the 10M potency may be used. The late Margery Blackie often prescribed Arnica 10M in first aid situations like this. If uncertain it is wise to stick to 30c. It is also possible to use the 6c potency, but higher potencies are generally found to be more efficient.

Some conditions merit different remedies according to the stage of illness. Aconite is often used at the very start of a cold at first aid level dosing, whereas once the cold has taken hold Gelsemium might be more appropriate.

Acute prescribing

With acute prescribing, it may be necessary to seek a little more information from the patient than with the first aid approach, but a choice can still be made from an abbreviated drug picture that includes just the key characteristics ('keynotes') of the remedy. For example, although the materia medica contains several pages of text under Belladonna, we can effectively choose the remedy in most patients on the basis of its keynotes:

- sudden onset of condition
- bursting headache
- flushed appearance.

This is called the **three-legged stool approach**, where the seat representing the prescription is supported by three legs representing the main symptoms. If the legs are very wide (equivalent to the symptoms being clearly defined) then the stool will still balance nicely, while if the legs are very thin (i.e. the symptoms are less well defined) then four may be required to make it balance. The polychrests are well suited to first aid and acute prescribing, where the remedy can be quickly identified without a protracted interview.

It is possible to prescribe in acute situations (and occasionally in chronic cases too) where there is more than one remedy indicated, on the basis of symptoms that make up a remedy's '**essence**'. It is difficult to explain exactly what is meant by this term. It is something more than just a simple keynote or three-legged stool approach to repertorisation, because mental symptoms are often involved too. The essence of a remedy is an essential fundamental constitutional characteristic, or group of characteristics, that is expressed in nearly all people with an affinity for the medicine. It represents an interpretation of the main qualitative aspects of the case. A number of symptoms collectively indicating a theme of 'anticipation' might suggest Argent nit, while a theme or thread representing 'suddenness of onset' might suggest Belladonna. Jealousy (especially by one sibling for another) might be associated with a need for Phosphorus. Experienced homeopaths develop a kind of intuition about what is the 'right' remedy to prescribe in given sets of circumstances, often based on the essence of a remedy. There are some remedies, like Skookum or Sanicula, which contain a mixture of different chemical salts in their source material, and are generally considered not to have an essence. Even identifying their keynotes is difficult.

The treatment of acute conditions involves dosing three or four times daily (every 4 hours). A typical acute response curve is shown in Figure 8.1. The acute level can last for 7–10 days, but often a major improvement occurs within 24 hours. If there is a substantial improvement, then dosing can be discontinued earlier. The 30c potency is usually used in the UK for acute conditions, but it is possible to use 6c as well. A sudden cold might be treated in this way, if intervention at the first aid level was not possible during the initial stages. It is usual to give a course of treatment OTC to ensure compliance, but a homeopath who maintains close contact with a patient may well dose only when improvement is not being maintained (e.g. cease dosing at 20 hours, Fig. 8.1).

Prophylaxis sometimes involves a combination of acute and first aid prescribing. For instance Arnica can be administered at acute levels 1 or 2 days prior to dental surgery and then increased to the first aid level on the day of the visit. Argent nit for worry about an examination could be administered according to a similar regimen. This is a rather different concept to prophylaxis used for immunisation.

Until now we have been mainly concerned with local symptoms in acute or first aid situations. The disadvantage of this approach is that it allows

Figure 8.1 Typical acute response pattern for homeopathic remedy: Belladonna in tonsilitis

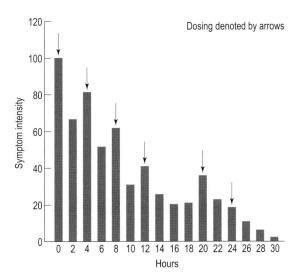

only treatment of symptoms directly associated with the local pathology, that is, not the person as a whole. Such symptoms are characterised by the patient using expressions such as 'my feet are cold', 'my eye is sore', etc. By ameliorating pain or inflammation it will produce temporary relief, but is unlikely to give a lasting cure in many cases.

Chronic prescribing

Totality of symptoms

Here we are talking of 'chronic' prescribing defined in a manner appropriate to pharmacy practice, not chronic heart problems, emphysema or asthma and the many other conditions that pharmacists would not try to treat OTC using orthodox medications. It is more the longstanding viral cough following a bout of flu or soft tissue injuries sustained some weeks ago while playing sport. Rheumatic or arthritic pain also falls into this category. In order to pick the right remedy in a chronic case, it is necessary to adopt more than the simple keynote or 'three-legged stool' approach. There are additional symptoms to consider before a choice can be made.

The classical homeopath would not dream of prescribing for chronic conditions without considering the totality of symptoms and the aetiology. If you aspire to this level of expertise then you will need more than the abbreviated introduction provided in this book. Some homeopaths prescribe in layers, starting with the local disease, before moving on to the underlying background conditions. Others place great importance on the overall state of the patient.

In the limited area of chronicity that has been defined, it is still possible to treat effectively. We can identify a marked difference between two individuals apparently suffering from the same condition, both in their mental states, often referred to just as their 'mentals' and also in their general states or 'generals'. The latter includes preferences in temperature and food, pattern of appetite, etc. Here the patient uses expressions such as 'I am frightened', 'I don't like pork', etc. These symptoms are far removed from the actual site of pathology, but nevertheless are important because they help to individualise the correct remedy.

Modalities

The extra questions to be asked are rather different from those normally posed in allopathic situations. These questions are designed to obtain information on 'modalities' – what makes a condition better or worse. This helps in differentiating between remedies that appear to have similar applications. In the materia medica entries signify those circumstances under which symptoms are worse (the symbol < signifies aggravation) or better (> signifies amelioration). It is often necessary to be more specific about the intensity of the modalities in individual cases. A series of ticks or crosses may be used to record the severity in written notes.

Examples of modalities are:

- the application of heat to the affected part makes the condition better/or worse
- movement makes the condition worse; sitting down makes it feel better
- the condition is better/worse in wet weather
- the condition is better in open air, or worse in a stuffy atmosphere.

The remedies Bryonia and Rhus tox may be used to treat deep-seated joint pain and swelling. Patients who find relief from wrapping an ice pack round their joints and for whom any movement is extremely painful will receive relief from Bryonia. Patients who find that the application of warmth to the affected joint, and for whom initial movement is painful but continued gentle movement is acceptable, will often benefit from Rhus Tox. There are a number of other rheumatic remedies ameliorated by motion including Ferrum met, Pulsatilla and Rhododendron.

Aconite, Agaricus, Calc carb, Hypericum, Phosphorus and Sepia are common remedies that are predominantly aggravated by the cold. Those affected adversely by heat include Apis, Argent nit, Natrum mur and Pulsatilla. Merc sol and Ipecac are affected by both heat and cold, depending on the situation.

There are other ways of differentiating between remedies, for instance by considering laterality – whether pain or inflammation is worse (or better) on the right or left side of the body. In an allopathic environment such questions as 'Is the condition worse on the right or left side of the body?' are likely to cause some raised eyebrows. Some homeopathic remedies may be more effective on the right or left, or if the pain radiates from top to bottom of a limb rather than the reverse direction. For example, Drosera is a remedy that treats stinging pains and coldness on the left side of the face; Belladonna tends to favour patients with a right-sided tonsillitis.

Time modalities are also significant. Some patients experience a worsening of symptoms at particular times of the day. Patients who benefit by the use of Arsen alb report symptoms being particularly troublesome between 1.00 a.m. and 2.00 a.m.; Kali iod is indicated for headaches that are at their worst during the very early morning. The modalities associated with Sulphur can be plotted by the hour. All the following rubrics are worse during the time intervals shown:

- 00.00–01.00 gastric pain, loose cough
- 01.00–02.00 insomnia (typically between 02.00 and 05.00)
- 02.00–03.00 abdominal pain and diarrhoea, urge to urinate (colourless urine)
- 03.00–04.00 pain in the extremities, dyspnoea (better for sitting up)
- 04.00–05.00 insomnia
- 05.00–06.00 diarrhoea, cramps in the legs
- 06.00–07.00 sneezing, itching in the anus, salivation, skin irritation
- 07.00–08.00 bitter taste on waking, burning sensation in eyes, urge to urinate.

The time modality also includes reference to cosmic rhythms such as the seasons, at sunrise or during full moon.

Concomitants

Yet another way one can differentiate between remedies with similar indications is to consider the concomitants. These are general effects that can be identified but which are not directly associated with the pathology caused by a particular disease. There are four types:

1. physical concomitants to mental emotions, for example a burning sensation across the shoulders experienced by some people when they become excited
2. physical concomitants to pain, for example photophobia
3. mental concomitants due to a physical complaint, for example an aggressive reaction to severe pain
4. mental concomitants to a mental complaint, for example loquacity ('he won't stop talking'), depression or accompanying grief.

Modalities and concomitants are generally listed in the materia medica and repertories and can give a guide to the sort of questions that need to be asked. Patients are often impressed when some apparently unconnected symptom is tracked down as a result of appropriate questioning to differentiate the correct remedy.

Peculiars

'Peculiars' are symptoms that are highly characteristic for a particular remedy – rather like the cough associated with taking ACE inhibitors in orthodox medicine. They are often useful in finally confirming the choice of remedy. Examples include:

- Belladonna: patients like to drink lemonade when suffering from a fever
- Calc sulph: patients have a productive cough that is worse after a bath
- Hypericum: patients who benefit from this remedy are partial to drinking wine

- Ignatia: patients with haemorrhoids find the condition ameliorated by walking
- Pulsatilla: patients often sleep with hands behind their head.

Homeopathic prescribing depends on accurate case taking and correlation of information. This can be difficult if there is a paucity of symptoms or lack of time. Two elements seem to be of use in these circumstances (Cohen, 2002). The first is the need to select the more striking singular uncommon and peculiar symptoms. The second is the reliability of the information in the homeopathic literature. At times there is only one outstanding feature in the case and nothing else to confirm the prescription.

Dose regimens

According to the British school of thought, in 'chronic' OTC treatment the patient would normally be advised initially to take a 6c remedy twice daily for a period of up to 4 weeks, except where an aggravation is experienced, when dosing is temporarily suspended as explained on page 201. Many homeopaths dose only until a marked improvement is obvious, reinstating treatment again if a plateau is reached. If the case has been carefully repertorised this works well. As with acute OTC treatments, in the pharmacy environment a course of treatment is often counter-prescribed rather than responding to 'cyclical' symptoms in this way. There are some differences in approach to homeopathy between the Kentian and British schools. Supporters of the so-called Kentian method (after the great American homeopath James Tyler Kent) use predominantly high potencies (30c to 10M), especially where mental and emotional symptoms are profound and the chosen remedy fits well. Remedies are administered sparingly. This conflicts with the classical Hahnemannian supporters who prefer to use the lower potencies (6c to 30c), repeating doses more frequently and working mainly on localised disease prescriptions. In some cases recovery is complete and the response curve reaches the baseline within days or weeks. In the majority of cases, however, a steady improvement in the condition is recorded, as depicted in the typical chronic response pattern illustrated in Figure 8.2.

In only about 15% of chronic cases can one achieve success using a single remedy and one course of treatment. Most conditions are complicated and may require several courses of treatment involving the same or different remedies.

Multiple remedy prescribing

It may appear that multiple dosing regimens contradict Hahnemann's assertion that only one remedy should be used at a time. In fact, during Hahnemann's later years in Paris he began using more than one remedy under the following circumstances:

- to treat a non-miasmic acute condition arising alongside a miasmic condition (e.g. an acute remedy was interpolated without discontinuing the chronic treatment)

Figure 8.2 Typical chronic response pattern for homeopathic remedy: house dust mite in perennial rhinitis

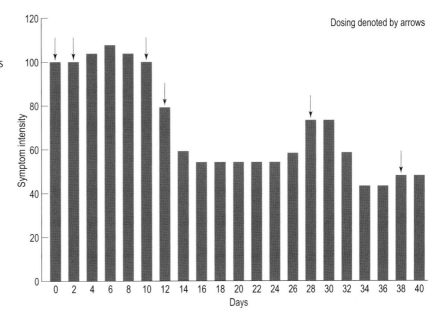

- to treat acute febrile conditions by using alternating remedies (e.g. Nux vom and Arsen alb for a cough)
- to treat conditions using an organ and a supporting remedy (e.g. digitalis for a heart condition while using other remedies at the same time)
- to treat conditions using different routes of administration (e.g. in 1836 Hahnemann prescribed Hepar sulph orally and Merc sol by inhalation for a patient).

It has been suggested that perhaps one should infer from this 'that when Hahnemann forbade the use of more than one remedy at once, he meant precisely that, not more than one remedy to be administered at exactly the same time, that is not mixed' (Hardley, 1988). Hahnemann clearly saw a place for using more than one remedy as part of a total prescription.

There is a subtle difference between using complexes, polypharmacy products with all the ingredients in one dose form, and multiple prescribing, where the remedies are administered separately. Multiple prescribing is generally more precise than using complexes, being individualised for each patient, although the same criticisms about lack of knowledge on interactions expressed earlier in this chapter might well apply.

Multiple prescribing can address different aspects of the same complaint in a course of treatment. For example, the physical and mental symptoms may be treated differently. There may be two or more remedies used, or different potencies or dose forms of the same remedy. Administration can be sequential (when half an hour should be allowed between taking different remedies), concurrent (e.g. topical and oral) or alternate. The dosing structures are often quite complicated and numbered powders offer one solution to ensure that patients comply with instructions (see Ch. 5).

One important application of dual prescribing is in **drainage therapy** (or 'detoxification'), a technique developed in France. Here the object is to attack the disease peripherally, with the appropriate indicated remedy, while at the same time encouraging the body's vital forces on a core level, by using a constitutional remedy concurrently. The more focused peripheral drug complements the wider acting constitutional remedy. The procedure is referred to as *canalisation* in French. Constitutional remedies are sometimes combined with remedies indicated in the treatment of allergies.

When using multiple prescribing it is important that practitioners realise that certain remedies complement each other and others are incompatible. Some examples of common interactions will be found in Table 8.5. They have been adapted from Underwood's translation of the *Belgian Homeopathic Compendium for Pharmacists* (Underwood, 1995), in which a more comprehensive list will be found.

In 1956, Dr R.A.F. Jack in the English West Midlands began prescribing packs of different remedies that patients could keep for use in emergencies. Initially the pack contained four remedies: Aconite, Arnica, Belladonna and Colocynth. In the early 1960s the pack was increased to nine remedies with the addition of Arsenicum, Ipecac, Nux vom, Phosphorus and Ant Tart, and finally to a set of 22 remedies prescribed routinely with a simple instruction leaflet to cover most of the problems that families were likely to experience in day-to-day living. The practice proved extremely popular with patients as well as cutting down the number of requests for visits (Ryan and Gibbs, 1998). The 'Dr Jack's Kit' idea has been adopted elsewhere in the UK and has been adapted by several rural practitioners.

The question of complex and multiple prescribing was discussed by a number of distinguished speakers during a lively debate chaired by Dr Peter Fisher at the Royal London Homeopathic Hospital in July 1992. At the end of the debate the 'unitarians' triumphed over the 'pluralists', with the audience of 60 voting two to one in favour of single remedy prescribing (report in *British Homeopathic Journal*; Debate, 1993).

The case study below involves the use of three concurrent prescriptions.

Case Study: 63-year-old man (courtesy Frank Randall, MRPharmS, Barrow-in-Furness)

History
A 63-year-old man presented in July 2004 with a tight chest having had pneumonia and two courses of antibiotics. Sweating and breathlessness on exertion. Florid in the face and moderately overweight.

Prescription
1. Ipecac 30c twice daily – for his wheeziness
2. Bacillinum 200c weekly – to help clear the chest of phlegm and give some protection from COPD
3. Echinacea tincture – 15 drops three times daily for 5 days then b.d. for 3 weeks, repeating the course as directed (3 weeks on 1 week off)

Follow-up
1. Early September – repeat of Ipecac. Patient much better and more positive. Lots of phlegm production and his wheeziness was easing.
2. November – chest better and patient dancing three times a week, some occasional sweats but much improved. Still taking all remedies.

Table 8.5 Examples of common complementary and incompatible remedies

Remedy	Complementary with	Incompatible with
Aconite	Arn, Bry, Coffea, Sulph	Glonoinum
Allium cepa	Phos, Puls, Sulph, Thuja	Allium sat
Ambra gris	Ign, Nat mur	Staphysagria
Ammon carb	Bell, Bry, Caust, Lycopod, Phos, Sepia	Lachesis
Antim crud	Baryta carb, Ipecac, Sulph	
Antim tart	Ipecac, Nat sulph, Sulph	Moschus
Apis mel	Barta carb, Bell, Canth, Lycopod, Nat mur, Sulph	Phosphorus, Rhus tox
Argent nit		Coffea
Arsen alb	All sat, Carbo veg, Nat sulph, Phos, Psor, Pyrog, Sulph, Thuja	Pulsatilla
Baryta carb	Ant tart, Dulc, Silica, Sulph	Calc carb, Calc phos
Belladonna	Calc carb, Hepar sulp, Lach, Nux vom, Sulph	Ac acetic, Dulc
Bryonia	Bell, Phos, Puls, Rhus tox, Sulph	Calc carb
Calc carb	Bell, Lycopod, Puls, Rhus tox	Baryta carb, Bry, Kali bich, Ac nit, Sulph
Cantharis	Bell, Phos	Coffea
Carbo veg	Caust, China, Dros, Kali carb, Lach, Phos, Sepia, Sulph	Carbo anim, Kreosotum
Chamomilla	Bell, Bry, Lycopod, Mag carb, Silica, Sulph	Kreosotum, Zinc met
Coffea	Acon	Camph, Canth, Caust, Cocc, Ign
Colocynth	Mag phos	Caust
Gelsemium	Sepia	
Graphites	Ars alb, Caust, Hepar sulph, Lycopod	
Hepar sulph	Calend, Merc sol, Psor, Silica	
Ignatia	Nat mur	Coffea, Nux vom, Tabac
Ipecac	Ant tart, Arn, Ars alb, Cuprum met	China
Kali bich	Ars alb, Phos, Psor	Calc carb
Ledum	Puls	China
Lycopod	Chel, China, Graph, Iod, Lach, Puls	Coffea, Nux mosch, Sulph
Merc sol	Bell, Podoph	Ac acetic, Lach, Silica
Nat mur	Apis, Arb nit, Ign, Lycopod, Sepia	
Nux vom	Aesc, Kali carb, Sepia, Sulph	Ac acetic, Ign, Puls, Zinc met
Phosphorus	All cepa, Ars alb, Carbo veg, Lycopod, Sepia	
Pulsatilla	All cepa, Ars alb, Lycopod, Nat mur, Sepia, Silica	Lach, Nux mosch, Nux vom
Rhus tox	Ars alb, Calc fluor	Apis, Bryonia
Ruta	Calc phos	
Sepia	Nat mur, Nux vom, Sulph	Bryonia, Lachesis, Pulsatilla
Silica (Silicea)	Puls, Thuja	Merc sol, Nux mosch
Sulphur	Acon, Nux vom	Lycopod
Thuja	Ars alb, Lach, Silica	

CHOOSING THE REMEDY

Using the repertory

Repertories have been a natural outgrowth of the materia medica and were developed to organise the vast amount of information. They are decidedly the key to the materia medica.

Most practitioners keep the drug pictures of 20 or 30 remedies in their memory and can often prescribe a polychrest quickly for simple problems using an abbreviated drug picture. In order to seek a match between a patient's symptoms and the correct drug picture for other conditions, especially longstanding chronic diseases, it is necessary to use a repertory. Here the remedy drug pictures are all classified with reference to symptoms, rather than just listed in alphabetical order as in a materia medica. Although all the many repertories essentially perform the same task they do have different biases. Probably the best known are Boericke's *Materia Medica with Repertory* and Kent's *Repertory of the Homeopathic Materia Medica*.

Boericke's *Materia Medica with Repertory*

Boericke's *Repertory* is divided into sections or chapters, the various conditions being listed in alphabetical order under a general heading. Boericke lists remedies for headache under cause (Box 8.1 is an illustration of this subsection), type of pain (catarrhal, chronic, congestive, etc.), followed by location (frontal, occipital, etc.), character of pain (bursting, splitting, intermittant, etc.), concomitants and finally modalities (aggravation and amelioration). So if a patient is complaining principally of a headache associated with being out in the sun, one can look up the appropriate heading(s) in the repertory, moving through the various sections, eliminating remedies that do not fit with the patient's symptoms. Unfortunately, this structure is not maintained throughout the text and the information is presented in different ways in different sections. A final check on the suitability of the chosen remedy can be made by consulting the appropriate drug picture in the materia medica section of the text.

Boericke is written in Victorian English, and uses terms like 'brain fag' that are unfamiliar in modern parlance. The repertory lists only about two-thirds of the symptoms listed in the materia medica section; thus occasionally it is necessary to think laterally to locate items in the index. The text is also short on remedies compared to more modern texts and quotes some unusual potencies (e.g. 1x, etc.).

In Box 8.2 there are three remedies indicated by Boericke to treat a headache that occurs after drinking spirits. They can be differentiated quite effectively on the basis of a few symptoms.

Kent's *Repertory*

Kent's *Repertory* is more uniform in its approach. It contains a number of separate sections entitled 'mind', 'abdomen', 'cough', etc. and within every section the symptoms are arranged in the order head to foot, central to distal

Box 8.1   Boericke's *Repertory*: adapted entry for headache

HEADACHE – Causes
Altitude, high – *Coca*
Bathing – Ant. c.
Beer – Rhus t.
Candy, sweets – Ant. c.
Catarrh – *Cepa*; Hydr.; Merc.; Ouls.; Sticta.
Catarrh suppressed – Bell.; *Kali bich.*; Lach.
Coffee – Arum; Ign.; *Nux v.*; Paul.
Constipation – *Aloe*; Alum.; *Bry.*; Collins.; Hydr.; Nit. ac.; *Nux v.*; Op.; Ratanh.
Dancing – Arg. n.
Diarrhoea alternating – *Aloe*; Pod.
Emotional disturbances – Acetan.; Arg. n., Cham.; Cim.; Coff.; *Epiph.*; *Gels.*; *Ign.*; Mez.; Phos. ac.; *Picr. ac.*; Plat.; Rhus t.; Sil.
Eye strain – Acetan.; *Cim.*; *Epiph.*; *Gels.*; *Nat. m.*; Onosm.; Phos. ac.; *Ruta*; Tub.
Fasting – Ars.; Cact.; Lach.; *Lyc.*; Sil.
Gastralgia, alternating or attending – Bism.
Gastrointestinal derangements – *Ant. c.*; Bry.; Carbo v.; *Cinch.*; Ipecac.; *Iris*; Nux m.; *Nux v.*; Puls.; Rham. c.; Robin.
Hair-cut – Bell.; Bry.
Hat, pressure from – Calc. p.; Carbo v.; *Hep.*; Nat. m.; Nit. ac.
Haemorrhage, excesses, vital losses – Carbo v.; *Cinch.*; Ferr.; Pyroph.; Phos. ac.; Sil.
Haemorrhoids – Collins.; Nux v.
Ice-water – Dig.
Influenza – Camph.; Lob. purp.
Ironing – *Bry.*; Sep.
Lemonade, tea, wine – Selen.
Lumbago, alternating with it – Aloe.
Malaria – Ars.; Caps.; *China. s.;* Cinch.; Cupr. ac.; *Eup. perf.*; Gels.; *Nat. m.*
Mental exertion or nervous exhaustion – Acetan.; Agar.; *Anac.; Arg. n.;* Aur. br.; Chionanth.; Cim.; Coff.; *Epiph.*; *Gels.;* Ign.; *Kali p.;* Mag. p.; *Nat. c.;* Niccol.; Nux v.; Phasseool.; Phos. ac.; *Picr. ac.;* Sabad.; Scutel.; Sil.; Zinc m.
Narcotics, abuse – Acet. ac.
Overlifting – Calc. c.
Perspiration, suppressed – Asclep. s.; Bry.
Riding against wind – Calc. iod.; *Kali c.*
Riding in cards – *Cocc.;* Graph.; Med.; *Nit. ac.*
Sexual excitement, weakness – Cinch.; Nux v.; Onosm.; *Phos. ac.;* Sil.
Sleep, damp room – Bry.
Sleep, loss – Cim.; Cocc.; *Nux v.*
Spiritous liquors – Agar.; *Ant. c.;* Lob. infl.; *Nux v.;* Paul.; Rhod.; Ruta; *Zinc m.*
Sunlight or heat – *Bell.*; Cact.; Ferr. p.; *Gels.*; Glon.; Kal.; Lach.; Nat. c.; Nux v.; Sang.; Stram.
Tea – Nux v.; Paul.; *Selen.*; Thuja
Tobacco – Ant. c.; Calad.; Carg. ac.; *Gels.*; *Ign.*; Lob. infl.; Nux v.
Vaccination – Thuja
Weather changes – *Calc. p.*; Phyt.

Box 8.2   Comparison of four remedies for headache after drinking spirits (Boericke)

Headache after imbibing 'spiritous liquors'

Ant c. (Antimonium crudum)
Aching headache, characterised by heaviness in forehead
Worse in the evening, better for open air

Nux v. (Nux vomica)
Front headache in occiput or over the eyes, often with vertigo
Worse in the morning, better after sleep

Zinc m. (Zincum metallicum)
Occipital pain; 'roaring' sensation in the head
Better while eating, despite heartburn

---

and posterior to anterior. The sequence of rubrics is always the same. First the symptoms are listed in full; this is followed by differentiation into:

- time of onset or aggravation
- concomitants and modalities in alphabetical order
- location
- type of sensation in alphabetical order
- the direction in which the pain or sensation radiates.

Box 8.3 shows an abbreviated entry for a headache.

Kent divided symptoms into two groups: 'generals' (comprising physical and mental symptoms relating to the body as a whole) and 'particulars' (relating to all other physical symptoms). General mental symptoms are called 'mentals'. The mentals are further subdivided into 'will' (loves, hates, fears, etc.), 'understanding' (delusions, sense of proportion, etc.) and symptoms relating to the memory. Rather confusingly, general physicals are referred to simply as 'generals'. The different groups of remedies are presented in a hierarchy of importance, mentals being considered the most important. Kent's system of refining and qualifying symptoms is very elaborate and requires much study and practice to become proficient. The key to a successful repertorisation is the use of an orderly method for noting the patient's characteristics and symptoms.

With Kent, particularly the edition with a handy thumb index, finding the right entry is easier than Boericke , but the amount of material presented is rather daunting to the beginner. The two texts also differ in their approach as Boxes 8.1 and 8.3 show. Even the abbreviations of the remedies differ!

Remedy grading

The remedies listed in both Boericke's and Kent's repertories are graded to indicate their importance. The remedies that have been most frequently verified and are often the most appropriate are distinguished from other less likely candidates by being shown in bold type in Kent and italics in Boericke.

Box 8.3   Kent's *Repertory* – adapted entry for physical symptoms of a headache

PAIN, headache

morning: Acon., **Agar.**, all-s., *alum.*, alumn., ambr., amm., *anac.*, ang., ant-t., arg-m., arg-n., *arn.*, ars., ars-i., asaf., asar., *aur.*, bar-c., bar-m., *bell.*, benz-ac., berb., bor., *bov.*, *bry.*, *cact.*, cadm., *calc.*, *calc-p.*, calc-s., camph., cann-s., canth., *carb-an.*, carb-s., *carb-v.*, cast-eq., caust., cham., *chel.*, chin., chin-a., chin-s., cic., cina., clem., cob., coca., coc-c., coff., *coloc.*, con., croc., *crot-t.*, cund., cupr., cycl., dios., dulc., euphr., *eupper.*, ferr., ferr-ac., ferr-i., ferr-p., *fl-ac.*, for., glon., *graph.*, grat., guaj., hell., *hep.*, hipp., *ign.*, ind., iod., ip., iris., jatr., *jug-c.*, jug-r., *kali-bic.*, *kali-c.*, kali-i., *kali-n.*, kali-p., *kali-s.*, kalm., kreos., lac-c., lac-d., *lach.*, lachn., lact., led., lil-t., lith., mag-c., mag-m., manc., *mang.*, merc., merc-i-f., merc-s., *mez.*, *murx.*, mur-ac., nat-a., nat-c., *nat-m.*, nat-p., nicc., *nit-ac.*, nux-m., nux-v., ol-an., peon., pall., petr., ph-ac., phos., phyt., *podo.*, *psor.*, *puls.*, ran-b., rheum., *rhod.*, rhus-t., rumx., ruta., sabad., samb., sang., sars., scut., *seneg.*, *sep.*, *sil.*, *spig.*, *squil.*, *stann.*, *staph.*, stram., stront., stry., *sulph.*, sul-ac., tab., *thuja.*, vat., zinc

breakfast is delayed, if: Calc

ceases toward evening: *Bry.*, calc., *kali-bi.*, kalm., *nat-m.*, plat., sang., spig., sulph.

comes and goes with the sun: Cact., kali-bi., *kalmia.*, lac-d., *nat-m.*, sang., *spig.*, sulph., tab.

increases and decreases with the sun: Acon., **Glon.**, *kalm.*, nat-m., *phos.*, sang., *spig.*, *stann.*, stram.

increases until noon, or a little later, then gradually decreases: Phos., sulph.

increases during the day: Cact.

rising, on: *Agar.*, am-c., am-m., apis, arg-n.; asc-t., aur-m., bar-c., bar-m., **Bry.**, camp., chel., chin-s., cob., colch., crot-t., **Cycl.**, dig., dulc., fabo., glon., ham., hep., hydr., ind., iod., ip., jug-c., *kali-p.*, kalm., lac-d., *lach.*, lyc., mag-c., mag-m., merc., mur-ac., nice., nux-v., petr., phos., *psor.*, ptel., puls., rhus-t., rumx., ruta., *sep.*, squil., staph., stront., **Sulph.**, tarent.

same hour, at: Kali-bi.

until noon: Ars., conv., ip., *nat-m.*, nice., phos., sep., *tab.*

waking, on: Agar., ail., *alum.*, alumn., arg-n., *arn.*, ars., benz-ac., bov., **Bry.**, bufo., calc., calc-p., calc-s., canni-i., carb-an., carb-s., caust., cham., *chel.*, chin., chin-a., cic., cob., coc-c., coff., colch., con., *croc.*, crot-h., crot-t., cupr-ar., dig., elaps, crig., euphr., *eup-per.*, fago., form., **Graph.**, hell., *hep.*, hipp., ign., ind., jug-c., *kali-bi.*, *kali-c.*, kali-n., kali-p., kali-s., *kalm.*, kreos., *lac-c.*, **Lach.**, lil-t., lob., *lyc.*, mag-c., merc-i-f., morph., murx., mur-ac., myric., *naja.*, **Nat-m.**, nice., **Nit-ac.**, **Nuv-x.**, ol-an., op., peti., *ph-ac.*, *phos.*, phys., pip-m., plan., plat., *psor.*, puls., rhus., rumx., sep., squil., stann., staph., *sulph.*, sul-ac., **Tarent.**, thuj.

First opening the eyes, on: *Bry.*, ign., kalm., *nux-v.*

Preceeded by bad dreams: Murx

Until 10 a.m.; Arn.

5 a.m., pain at: calc., kali-bi., **Kali-i.**, stann.

6 a.m. until evening, pain during: Crot-t.

until 10 a.m.: Arn., Lachn., Mag-c.

until 3 p.m.: Aur.

until 5 p.m.: Mang.

until 10 p.m.: *Phys*

Kent uses italics for second grade remedies, where symptoms have been shown by several provers and verified clinically, and plain type for a third, less valuable grade. It may be necessary to revert back to the materia medica, where the highlighted remedies can be further investigated and differentiated, until a suitable remedy emerges by considering secondary or less important symptoms and modalities.

Box 8.4   A repertorising chart

	Symptoms	A	B	C	D	E	F
1	Cough: dry	X	X	X	X	X	X
2	Pain in chest	X		X			X
3	Better in open air		X		X		X
4	Worse at night						X
5	Headache	X		X		X	
6							
7							
8							
9							
10							

A useful way to sort out the appropriate remedy from a group of several possibilities is to construct a matrix similar to the example illustrated in Box 8.4. The letters A–F refer to the various remedies under consideration. The features of the patient's condition are listed in column two, and a cross (or tick) is then placed in each remedy column as appropriate if it corresponds to the rubrics of that remedy. The remedy with most positive entries will be the medicine indicated.

Other repertories

The most widely used repertories after Boericke are Schroyen's *Synthesis*, Murphys's *Homeopathic Medical Repertory* (set out in modern, alphabetical listing rather than the traditional method of giving symptoms from top to bottom of body) and Morrisson's *Desktop Companion*. The last two books have companion materia medicas. Other well-known repertories include those attributed to Allen, Boger-Boenninghausen, Clarke and Phatak (see Appendix 2). The last of these has displaced Boericke and Kent as the suggested text on some training courses, being clearly written and easy to use.

Homeopaths have tended to embellish the drug pictures with their own observations, so Hahnemann's original provings have been greatly expanded over years since his death, sometimes with the addition of quite bizarre rubrics. There is also a suspicion that the same provings have been interpreted in different ways by different workers. In acute treatment this does not cause great difficulty, because abbreviated drug pictures are used. Details of useful remedies are included in Chapter 13.

Repertorising by computer

Despite the central role of the repertory in homeopathy, there are few resources available to instruct the student of homeopathy in the use, understanding, and methods of the repertory. Repertorising using a computer can assist in identifying potential remedies particularly in the early days of practice. However, no software package can take over the task of assessing the quality of symptoms and relating them to the essential nature of the selected drug. Nor can it deal with the logic of applying the laws of homeopathy to an individual. It is necessary to replace the present system of using qualitative terms like 'much improved', 'slight improvement', 'feel better' with quantitative numerical estimations.

The essence of repertorising is searching for a matching string of characters, so the procedure is well suited to computerisation. Computers can manipulate information and provide reports much more easily using data in this form. The computerised repertories are relatively expensive, but they do allow access to several sources of information, allowing the possibility of finding some of the so-called 'smaller' or unusual remedies that might not be considered otherwise. They have the capability of screening out the polychrests, thus allowing more weight to be given to these lesser known remedies.

Software packages have been developed to allow homeopaths to search several repertories with one keystroke, thus greatly expanding the scope for choosing remedies. A list of possible remedies is produced within a short space of time. Patients are not intimidated by the use of a computer. Indeed, in many cases they are fascinated.

There are several programs available in both PC Windows and Mac formats. The most comprehensive programs range from less than a thousand to several thousand pounds and require a minimum hard disk space of around 50 Mb. By judicious purchase of software modules, however, this memory requirement can be reduced; a laptop version is possible.

There are three main suppliers:

1. RADAR (UK Kents Road Books, Haywards Heath)
http://www.radar-uk.co.uk/
Radar UK and Ireland – various other editions and suppliers around the world

RADAR, originally an IBM program developed in Belgium, is available in Windows and MacIntosh versions. Version 9 takes advantage of a new revamped database in Synthesis 9 and has many innovative features (http://www.radar-uk.co.uk/radar9tooker.htm). It includes the *Encyclopaedia Homoeopathica*, the full version of which has 754 volumes of carefully selected homeopathic literature.

2. Kent Homeopathic Associates Inc., San Rafael, California
http://www.kenthomeopathic.com/p1b.html

MacRepertory Pro and MacRepertory Classic. The Professional version offers more advanced customization and analysis features than the Classic version. Both MacRepertory Pro and MacRepertory Classic are available with either the Core Library (six repertories, 30 materia medicas and a huge reference library) or the Full Library comprising all the core items augmented with extra material, including cases and provings.

ReferenceWorks. ReferenceWorks uses the materia medica directly to find a patient's remedy and goes straight to the cure. By simply typing in the symptom, ReferenceWorks collects every reference and creates a graph of the result. The remedies are scored based on the importance each author gave them, how many authors suggested the remedy for the symptom and the rareness of the remedy. Professional and Classic versions are available (http://www.kenthomeopathic.com/p1c.html#ReferenceWorks%20Pro).

3. Miccant Limited Nottingham
http://www.miccant.com/

Miccant hace two products for PC and Mac formats. Cara was the first homeopathic software created by David Witko for the Royal London Homeopathic Hospital who wanted to repertorise using Kent's *Repertory* (http://www.miccant.com/cara/cara_pro.shtml).

The company is now offering a product named ISIS, available as a slimmed down starter version and in a second version. Both come with an impressive array of materia medicas, repertories and reference material (http://www.miccant.com/isis/).

With ISIS it is possible to have all the literature and single remedy information available on one screen: The whole library (more than 300 volumes) – usually part of a different program – is an integral part of ISIS and always directly accessible.

A comprehensive review of the features offered by PC versions of RADAR, MacRepertory and ISIS, written by Wichmann and reprinted from the journal *Homeopathic Links*, may be found at http://www.minimum.com/reviews/macrepertory-kent-homeopathic.htm.

A wide range of less comprehensive remedy finder software is listed at http://www.homeopathyhome.com/services/computer_software.shtml.

KEEPING RECORDS

It has not been the practice in the past for pharmacists in the UK to keep records of OTC sales although it is becoming more common, particularly in practices where pharmaceutical care is offered. If records can be kept of all prescribing activities, they will be found useful as a source of reference in the future, both to follow up the case and to provide material for further study. A simple recording sheet for first aid or acute counter-prescribing is illustrated in Figure 8.3; it can be easily modified as necessary.

It will also help when the inevitable request for 'some more of those wee white tablets' is received from a satisfied customer who has lost the container and quickly becomes dissatisfied when they cannot be identified.

FOLLOWING UP
Reviewing the patient's progress

Guidelines for reviewing cases are as follows:

- first aid treatment – after six to eight doses
- acute treatment – after 5–7 days
- chronic treatment – after 3–4 weeks.

It may be that these instructions are combined in some cases, for example 'Take these tablets half hourly for six doses, then three times daily for 7 days' or 'Take two tablets three times daily for 7 days, then twice daily for 4 weeks'.

Patient name or reference number	Date	Main symptoms	Remedy given	Pot	Dose	Comments or outcome
mh/011	6/1	Flushed appearance; throbbing headache; sudden onset	Belladonna	30c	2 tabs every 15 min	Pain alleviated within 2 hours
faf/06	7/1	Muscular tiredness	Arnica	30c	2 tabs q.i.d. for 2 days	Relief

Figure 8.3   Recording sheet for first aid and acute cases

Possible actions

After the prescribed time, there are several possible courses of action based on three responses:

1. **There has been no improvement.** This may be because the patient has not complied with the dose instructions for some reason, or has returned too early. If he or she has suffered with a condition for years, then expecting a miracle from homeopathy is rather ambitious. In this case the patient should be instructed to finish out the course of treatment suggested.

2. **There has been some improvement.** The difficulty here is to know whether the remedy is working and, if so, whether the course of treatment should be continued. It is necessary to determine whether the patient is continuing to improve or has reached a plateau. Strong pathology is likely to exhaust the dose quicker than weak pathology. In the event of improvement, most homeopaths would discontinue treatment, allowing the residual effects of the remedy to continue, without further action. When there is no more improvement then dosing is recommenced. However, it is possible that an aggravation may occur (see below) if dosing is too frequent, although it is unusual once a course of remedy has been given.

3. **The patient's condition has become worse**:
   - due to the patient experiencing an aggravation (see below)
   - because the remedy has not worked
   - the choice of remedy may not have been close enough.

If the remedy does not work you could consider changing the potency, the dose frequency, or even starting afresh with a new case analysis. The potency may be changed up (e.g. from 6c to 30c with less frequent dosing) or, less often, down (more frequent dosing), or the existing potency may be given more frequently. You should not be afraid to change the remedy, but you should be absolutely sure that it is necessary before doing so. Some homeopaths sometimes use an antidote before changing remedies (see p. 206).

In the third situation, the patient has ended up proving the remedy (i.e. they have grafted on to their original symptom picture new symptoms that are characteristic of the remedy). There is a need for regular assessment so that this situation can be identified if it should arise.

SAFETY ISSUES

Potential sources of concern on safety issues include the following:

Inappropriate treatment

Most ranges of homeopathic remedies available commercially for sale over the counter are designed to be used for the treatment of simple self-limiting conditions. Some may also be used for ongoing conditions such as back pain or soft tissue injuries. Clients who request unusual remedies or who return repeatedly to purchase the same remedy on several occasions should be gently reminded that advice from a physician or registered homeopath might be appropriate to confirm that their condition lends itself to self-treatment.

It is vital that all practitioners only offer advice and treatment according to their levels of competency. Patients whose problems fall outwith these boundaries should be referred to suitably qualified colleagues. Generally pharmacists should use homeopathy to deal with conditions they would normally treat OTC and not seek to widen their portfolio extensively.

Side-effects

Homeopathic medicines are regarded as safe but practitioners report several types of healing or remedy reactions including aggravations, new symptoms and recurrence of old symptoms, some of which could be regarded as side-effects or unwanted effects. Some remedy reactions may be regarded as adverse events. A number of case reports have come from conventional physicians, particularly dermatologists, where causation is presumed rather than proven. Some reports suggest that side-effects are due to the remedy being given in material doses but do not make this distinction clear in discussion. Other reports include side-effects from preparations which have only been diluted a few times to create a decimal potency. Homeopathic Arsenic used therapeutically in homeopathic medicines may cause clinical toxicity if the medications are improperly used (Chakraborti et al., 2003).

Fox has reported adverse effects including skin rashes from Sulphur right through from 6c to 10M (A.D. Fox, personal communication, October 1994).

Caulophyllum has been suspected of causing difficulties during labour (Castro, 1992; Castro and Idarius, 2004; Swayne, 2005). Adverse reactions have been investigated using electronic databases, hand searching, searching reference lists, reviewing the bibliography of trials, and other relevant articles, contacting homeopathic pharmaceutical companies and drug regulatory agencies in the UK and the USA, and by communicating with experts in homeopathy (Dantas and Rampes, 2000). The authors reported that the mean incidence of adverse effects of homeopathic medicines was greater than placebo in controlled clinical trials (9.4 to 6.1) but effects were minor, transient and comparable. There was a large incidence of pathogenetic effects in healthy volunteers taking homeopathic medicines but the methodological quality of these studies was generally low. They found that anecdotal reports of adverse effects in homeopathic publications were not well documented and mainly reported aggravation of current symptoms. Case reports in conventional medical journals pointed more to adverse effects of mislabelled 'homeopathic products' than to true homeopathic medicines. It was concluded that homeopathic medicines in high dilutions, prescribed by trained professionals, were probably safe and unlikely to provoke severe adverse reactions. Once again it is difficult to draw definite conclusions due to the low methodological quality of reports claiming possible adverse effects of homeopathic medicines. Some isolated cases in the literature have also been highlighted by Barnes (1998). An audit was carried out in the Bristol Homeopathic Hospital Outpatient Department (Thompson et al., 2004). All patients were given a questionnaire to complete when at their first follow-up consultation approximately 6–10 weeks after their first appointment. One hundred and sixteen patients were sampled over a 2-month period. Reactions were recorded: 28 out of the 116 (24%) patients experienced an aggravation. Thirteen patients (11%) reported an adverse event even though five of those were patients who also reported an aggravation followed by an overall improvement of their symptoms. Thirty-one patients described new symptoms (27%) and 21 (18%), a return of old symptoms. Those experiencing the latter appeared to have better outcomes. The authors concluded that remedy 'reactions' were common in clinical practice; some patients experienced them as adverse events. Systematically recording side-effects would facilitate our understanding of these reactions and would enable standards to be set for audit of information and patient care.

A pilot project to issue reporting cards was launched by the Pharmacy subcommittee of the European Committee on Homeopathy (ECH) in 2004. The card is illustrated in Figure 8.4. Copies are available from the ECH Secretariat (Chaussée de Bruxelles 132, Box 1, 1190 Brussels, Belgium).

A sensitivity to lactose (used principally as the base in tablets and in small amounts in other solid dose forms) can be overcome by using a sucrose based carrier or a liquid potency.

Aggravations

Occasionally, in about 10% of chronic cases, the patient's condition may become aggravated within 2–5 days of giving a remedy, although it can take up to 10 days for such a reaction to appear. Typically a skin condition may

Adverse Drug Reaction (Yellow Card) Reporting Scheme for Homeopathic Medicines Trial

1. Patient details	2. Clinician details	3. Reporter details
Initials	First name	First name
Age	Surname	Surname
Sex	Address	Address
Weight (in kilograms)	Town	Town
Height (in metres)	Country	Country
Ethnic Group	Postcode	Postcode
Patient ID number	Telephone	Telephone
	Profession	Profession

4. Homeopathic Medicinal Product(s) Concerned

Traditional, scientific name or brand name Batch number	Dilution	Route of Admin	Posology Dose & frequency daily/week/month	Date started dd/mm/yy	Date stopped dd/mm/yy	Prescribed or self-medicated

5. Other Drugs and other Homeopathic Medicinal Products in last three months

Traditional, scientific name or brand name Batch number	Dilution or Dosage	Route of Admin	Posology Dose & frequency daily/week/month	Date started dd/mm/yy	Date stopped dd/mm/yy	Prescribed or self-medicated

6. Suspect Reactions related to the homeopathic characteristics

	Date started (dd/mm/yy)	Duration
Aggravation		
Reappearance of old symptoms		
Appearance of new symptoms		

7. Suspect Reactions (others)

	Date started (dd/mm/yy)	Duration
Toxocological		
Immunological		

Figure 8.4   ECH reporting card (With permission from the Subcommittee Pharmacy of the European Committee for Homeopathy.)

get worse. Such a reaction tends to occur on the first exposure only, and may be discounted in acute disease. In fact, it is often said of complementary medicine that one 'must expect to get worse before getting better'. This is not strictly true, but when a prescriber hits upon exactly the right remedy in exactly the right potency a transient exacerbation can result and this is taken as a positive sign. This may occur because the resonance of the remedy is higher than the resonance emanating from the diseased body.

8. Additional information - Please attach additional sheets if necessary

Have any reactions to the product concerned occurred previously?
Yes   *No*   *Unknown*   *If yes, explain*

Have any reactions been previously reported?
Yes   *No*   *Unknown*   *If yes, explain*

Reintroduction of the product concerned?
Yes   *No*   *Unknown*   *If yes, explain*

Same reaction after reintroduction?
Yes   *No*   *Unknown*   *If yes, explain*

Reactions to other drugs?
Yes   *No*   *Unknown*   *If yes, explain*

9. Reaction Treatment

a) Stop the medication?   b) Posology change?
Yes   *No*   *Yes*   *No*

c) Antidoting?   d) Other medication to relieve the symptoms?
Yes   *No*   *Yes*   *No*

10. Interaction suspected

Yes   *No*   If yes, which is it?

11. Any further details

Do you consider the reaction to be serious?   **As defined by European**
Yes   *No*   **Directive 01/083CEE**

Do you consider the reaction medically significant?
Yes   *No*

Did the patient require hospitalisation?   **Periodical Safety Update**
Yes   *No*   **Report (PSUR) necessary?**
                                                             Yes   No
Did a congenital abnormality occur?
Yes   *No*

Was the reaction life-threatening?
Yes   *No*

12. Comments
Concerns with packaging, labelling, medical history, tests, allergies, homeopathic approach, peculiars

Signature: _____   Date: _____

Thank you for your contribution. Please return completed forms to:
ECH Secretariat, Chaussée de Bruxelles 132, Box 1, 1190 Brussels, Belgium

© ECH 2004

Figure 8.4 *Continued*

Three distinct types of aggravation have been identified (Mishra, 1993):

1. Homeopathic aggravation: there is an increase in symptoms, but the patient feels better
2. Medicinal aggravation: the patient develops a new symptom characteristic of the remedy
3. Disease aggravation: no improvement, and the disease progresses.

If the dose is small, the aggravation is mild and shorter; conversely, if the dose is given more often, the aggravation is likely to be severe and prolonged.

There are differing views on how to deal with this. The favoured solution with remedies given on the basis of pathological symptoms is to instruct the patient to cease taking the remedy (in case a proving should result) until the symptoms fall back to their original intensity (2–3 days), and then to recommence the remedy but at a lower frequency (e.g. b.i.d instead of t.i.d). Other homeopaths say that the remedy should be stopped in the event of an aggravation, as before, but if the condition begins to improve after the exacerbation subsides it should not be given again, unless a plateau is reached. Administration of the remedy between meals could help the hypersensitive patient to lessen the intensity of aggravation. If aggravation recurs then it is pertinent to change the potency. For physical aggravation, increase the potency; for mental aggravation, decrease the potency. Aggravation due to constitutional prescribing may take rather longer to subside.

The whole idea of aggravation has been called into question. A systematic review compared the frequency of homeopathic aggravations in the placebo and verum groups of double-blind, randomised clinical trials (Grabia and Ernst, 2003). Eight independent literature searches were carried out to identify all such trials mentioning either adverse effects or aggravations. All studies thus found were validated and data were extracted by both authors. Twenty-four trials could be included. The average number of aggravations was low. In total, 50 aggravations were attributed to patients treated with placebo and 63 to patients treated with homeopathically diluted remedies. The authors concluded that this systematic review did not provide clear evidence that the phenomenon of homeopathic aggravations exists.

Colleagues are divided over whether patients should be warned of the possibility of an aggravation when counter-prescribing homeopathic remedies (see Ch. 5). Recent legal developments on full disclosure of side-effects in orthodox treatments would suggest that it is probably wise to mention it, despite the likelihood that symptoms may become apparent if patients are expecting them. Another option is to invite customers to telephone if they are worried about any aspect of their treatment. An appropriate explanation and reassurance can then be given if an aggravation is reported.

It is difficult to predict aggravations. In Reilly's trials of homeopathic immunotherapy (see Ch. 11) for conditions relating to inhalant allergy such as hay fever, asthma and allergic perennial rhinitis there were significantly more aggravations in the treated group than in the placebo group (Taylor et al., 2000). In Lewith's trial of homeopathic immunotherapy in asthma, there were significant differences seen in the side-effect profile for the two groups with the verum group showing an oscillatory pattern of alternating aggravation and amelioration (Lewith et al., 2002).

Interactions

As far as interactions are concerned the following should be noted:
- **There is no evidence that homeopathic remedies interfere with allopathic medicines**. Unfortunately we know little about this aspect of

complementary medicine, other than that it can be of great benefit to use allopathic and homeopathic medicines side by side.

For many patients the confirmation that they have a chronic condition such as epilepsy, diabetes or Parkinson's disease is a terrible blow that can severely undermine self-confidence, self-esteem and self-worth (Cochrane, 1995). When confidence is lost and self-image poor, patients can be helped by the use of homeopathic remedies (often constitutionals) to complement allopathic medicines. Another area where homeopathic remedies can help is in the treatment of troublesome side-effects (e.g. the cough associated with ACE inhibitors, where both medicines can be taken without fear of interaction).

Homeopathic medicines may be offered to elderly patients visiting a son or daughter locally and suffering from a bout of diarrhoea because of changes in the water or some other simple cause. Not having the benefit of the visitor's medical records means that potential allopathic interactions cannot be checked. It is good to know that the homeopathic remedy will be perfectly safe. Patients taking conventional drugs at the time they request a switch to homeopathic treatment can present unique challenges to the practitioner. There is a tendency for some non-medically qualified practitioners to interfere with medically prescribed medication; however, on no account should medication be changed without consultation with the original prescriber. For some conditions, homeopathic medicines can be given alongside allopathic medicine initially, the latter being progressively reduced (with permission) until it can be safely discontinued and replaced entirely. In other cases the two types of medication can be administered together perfectly safely.

• **Some allopathic medicines inactivate homeopathic remedies**. For instance, potent topical steroids are thought to negate the use of homeopathy in the treatment of eczema and psoriasis. There is also circumstantial evidence from the treatment of HIV-positive patients that oral steroids may interfere with homeopathic remedies. However, in the asthma trial carried out by Reilly et al. (1994) all the patients received steroid therapy, some high dosage, in addition to homeopathic remedies and significant positive results were still achieved. Experienced homeopaths do treat patients while they are taking oral steroids; the patient's symptoms tend to be masked, however, making an accurate choice of remedy much more difficult. It is said that, ideally, a period of 6 weeks should be allowed between stopping steroid preparations (including aerosols) and starting homeopathic remedies. There is no danger in taking the medicines together, but the remedies cannot be expected to be as effective as they might otherwise be. This may well be the advice needed for a woman taking synthetic oral contraceptives but wanting to take homeopathic remedies for non-related conditions. The interaction between Sepia, Pulsatilla and oral contraceptives has been discussed by Dam (1992).

Allopathic medicines containing caffeine should be avoided (see below). Other allopathic remedies formulated in strong aromatic-flavoured vehicles (e.g. antibiotic syrups) are also thought to cause a problem; patients should be instructed to rinse their mouth out well with water before taking the remedy. Products such as Vicks® and Olbas Oil® should be avoided if homeopathic medicine is being used.

- **Some homeopathic remedies inactivate other homeopathic remedies**. Those homeopathic remedies that originate from aromatic source material (e.g. Camphor, Menthol and Peppermint) are claimed to inactivate other remedies and should not be used concurrently. For a similar reason, people should be advised not to use homeopathic remedies and aromatherapy products concurrently, unless they are doing so under specialised supervision. Weleda have a rather curious 'medicinal mouthwash' that contains a mixture of aromatic oils and homeopathic remedies. It is difficult to see how such a formulation can be justified. There are certain combinations of remedies that are also incompatible, for example Baryta carb with Calc carb, Dulcamara with Belladonna and/or Lachesis, and Merc sol with Silica. Other common incompatibilities are detailed on page 191.
- **Certain foods are traditionally regarded as being able to inactivate (or 'antidote') homeopathic remedies**. Ideally, these should be avoided altogether when taking homeopathic medication. As a compromise, a 30-minute gap either side of eating is probably sufficient to prevent interference with the remedy's action. Examples are coffee, cocoa, tea, lemonade, highly flavoured or spicy foods, citric juices, peppermint-flavoured sweets and drinks. There is no good quality research to substantiate these allegations. In a Dutch survey 26 classical homeopaths were interviewed about interactions (Dam, 1993); 75% stated that, according to their experience, no interactions occurred if coffee or allopathic drugs were being taken during treatment – and indeed trials and research have seemed to confirm this. However, it is generally accepted that coffee interferes with homeopathic remedies.

An **antidote** competes for an existing remedy's area of influence by interfering with its effects on the vital force. In an article published in 1798 entitled 'Antidotes to some powerful vegetable substances', Hahnemann classified antidotes into four groups based on their mode of action:

- evacuation – vomiting and purging
- enveloping – surrounding a foreign body with an appropriate chemical mass
- chemical alteration – neutralising a poison
- chemical interference with potential influence on the body.

It is in the final group in which homeopaths are most interested. Sometimes, if a remedy has not worked completely (e.g. it has treated physical but not mental symptoms), a homeopath may instruct the patient to drink two cups of strong coffee, or administer a homeopathic antidote to 'clear the decks', as it were, and start afresh. Camphor is known as a universal antidote, and should not be used in conjunction with any other remedy. Specific antidotes are often listed in the materia medica; some examples are set out in Table 8.6. Obviously such remedies must not be combined in complexes or used in multiple prescribing.

This is a very specialised application and should not be attempted without sufficient knowledge. It is certainly not dangerous in life-threatening terms, but used injudiciously will interfere with the vibrational pattern of the vital force. This will have the effect of 'muddying the water' and preventing successful homeopathic treatment for some time. If

PART 4

Homeopathic prescribing in practice

PART CONTENTS

9. First aid and acute applications   213

10. Therapies allied to homeopathy   255

Chapter **9**

First aid and acute applications

CHAPTER CONTENTS

Principles of homeopathic first aid and
  acute treatments 214
Useful first aid treatments 214
Treatments for acute self-limiting type
  conditions 216
Topical preparations 225
Ointments and creams 225
Lotions; liniments and oils 226
Mother tinctures 226
Other topical preparations 227
Treatment of allergies 227
The options 227
Useful remedies for treating allergies 228
  Treating the condition with isopathy –
    homeopathic immunotherapy 228
  Treating allergies constitutionally 228
Treatment of bacterial and viral infections 230
Homeopathy for women 231
The advantages of using homeopathy 231
Cystitis 232
Premenstrual syndrome (PMS) 233
Menopause 234
Remedies useful during pregnancy 234
  Antenatal remedies 234
  Remedies during delivery and postnatal 234
Remedies for treating infants 236

Early stages 236
Later stages 237
Remedies for treating teenagers' problems 237
Homeopathy and sports care 239
The advantages for athletes 239
Common sports injuries and treatment 239
  Abrasions and wounds 239
  Blisters 239
  Eye injuries 240
  Fractures 240
  Muscle, tendon and ligament injuries 240
  Pain, bruising and swelling 242
Common sports-related illnesses and their
  treatment 243
Other conditions 244
Performance-enhancing preparations 244
Dental applications 244
The travelling homeopath 246
Use of nosodes and sarcodes as 'vaccines' 246
Reactions to sun 248
Reactions to insect bites 248
Effects of X-ray exposure on remedies 248
Further information 248
Agricultural and veterinary homeopathy 248
Agricultural applications 249
Veterinary applications 249

PRINCIPLES OF HOMEOPATHIC FIRST AID AND ACUTE TREATMENTS

At first sight the special nature of homeopathic prescribing would seem to preclude its use in acute and first aid situations. In fact it is possible to use homeopathy very successfully in the four conditions most frequently self-treated in the UK (coughs and colds, pain and skin problems) using poly-chrests and the 'keynote' or 'three-legged stool' approach to repertorisation outlined in Chapter 8. There are also a number of OTC complexes still available with specific indications, having been granted Product Licenses of Right (PLRs) under the old UK legislation. In more chronic situations, classical techniques can still be applied. The source of chronic diseases varies so much from person to person that more individualised care is vital in these cases. It may well be necessary to refer to a qualified homeopath. Even in acute situations, homeopathy alone cannot always provide the complete answer, but it can certainly be used to complement other methods whenever appropriate. Just because this book is about homeopathy does not mean that the many orthodox options available to health professionals should be ignored. For instance, those with lacerations can be offered a suitable remedy for trauma or shock (Aconite or Arnica), and referred to hospital for stitching or antitetanus injections if appropriate. In other, more serious cases, orthodox life-saving treatment can be given where necessary and homeopathy used at a later stage to calm the mind, relieve pain and encourage the body to heal itself. Topical preparations, such as creams and ointments or lotions, are useful for minor skin abrasions or bruising.

The easiest way to administer a remedy in a first aid situation is by way of granules or liquid straight onto the tongue. Dr Andrew Lockie has suggested that some remedies can be given as often as every 60 seconds for 10 minutes (Lockie, 1989), but usually a maximum of six doses of the 30c potency (or 6c if unavailable) is given at intervals of between 10 minutes and half an hour, depending on the severity of the situation. The more severe, the more frequent is the dosing. In cases where the patient is unconscious the remedy can still be given, by dropping it subintrabuccally.

USEFUL FIRST AID TREATMENTS

Table 9.1 provides examples of the treatment available for most of the simple first aid type situations for which advice is sought in the pharmacy. Some remedies may be combined in the same course of treatment for greater effect. Arnica may be given for almost any condition resulting from an accident, certainly during the first few hours. It may be combined with another remedy where appropriate. A strain could be treated with both Arnica and Ruta. The remedies could be combined in the same dose form or administered alternately. Other examples are Rhus tox and Ruta or Hypericum and Calendula.

BHA Book Services Glasgow publishes an excellent booklet entitled *First Aid Homeopathy* by Dr D. M. Gibson. Its popularity amongst the public and health professionals is illustrated by the fact that it has run to no less than 17 editions. It is certainly worth buying a copy to keep by your side, especially during the early days of your practice, for it covers many of the

Table 9.1 A selection of useful first aid remedies

First aid indication	Remedy
Bites and stings	Apis (red, oedema), Ledum (affected area cool to touch), Staphysagria (inflammation and itch), Urtica (violent itching, nettle rash after sting)
Bruises	Arnica (sore bruises with tiredness), Bellis (deep muscular bruises)
Burns	Belladonna (sunburn), Cantharis (blistering burns), Urtica (minor burns and urticaria)
Fainting or collapse	Carbo veg (weakness, bluish skin, limbs cold)
Fractures	Symphytum (administer after bones realigned and set)
Shock and stress, trauma	Aconite (anxiety, fear shock), Arnica (trauma – patient does not want to be touched or comforted)
Skin abrasions	Calendula (usually topical, but not where deep wound)
Soft tissue injuries – strains and sprains	Rhus tox (ligaments, joints), Ruta (muscular, tendons)
Wounds, puncture	Apis (wounds feel hot and painful), Hypericum (very painful), Ledum (wound cold, but better for application of cold)
Wounds, tips of digits	Hypericum (painful crush injuries)

common conditions you are likely to meet. Other useful publications for patients (and novice practitioners) are *Homeopathic First Aid* by Dr Anne Clover, *Homeopathy for the First Aider* by Dr Dorothy Shepherd and the booklet entitled *Homeopathy for the Family* produced by the Homeopathic Development Foundation (1991). Most homeopathic suppliers keep supplies of these (or similar) books.

A number of case studies showing practical applications of the first aid remedies are given below.

Case Studies: Applications of first aid remedies

Bee stings
Child, 6 years, stung on the face by a bee in the garden. Swollen, hot, red and painful

Remedy: Apis 30c tablets
Dosage: One tablet every 15 mins for six doses
Result: Discomfort reduced within minutes, and subsided after 70 min

Bruising – collision on sports field
Rugby player collided with member of opposing team and escorted off the pitch. No concussion, but player felt 'groggy'.

Remedy: Arnica 30c tablets
Dose: Two tablets every 5 mins for six doses
Result: Substantial improvement within 10 min

continued

continued

Burns, scalds

Woman, 46, presented in pharmacy having burnt herself on kettle. Large blister, skin red and painful.

Remedy: Cantharis 30 and usual burn management procedures
Dose: Two tablets every 15 min for six doses, then four times daily for 2 days
Result: Burn much improved after 12 hours; eventually healed without scarring

Blood and crush Case 1

Some years ago I was travelling into a Scottish airport one morning and saw a young child playing on the baggage carousel. Despite parental warnings the child noticed a bright object wedged down the side of the belt and chose to retrieve it just as the belt was switched on. His finger was badly crushed. This was an ideal situation for the frequent administration of Hypericum.

Remedy: Hypericum 30c
Dose: One dose every 5–10 min for 6–10 does, then three times daily
Result: Child stopped screaming within 2 or 3 minutes

Blood and crush Case 2

One of the more unusual items in the drug picture of this remedy is a craving for wine. I can remember attending a meeting where the speaker was President of the local Wine Appreciation Society. As he opened the wooden lid of a wine crate it shot back trapping his index finger. This was the basis of a most fulfilling repertorisation; a patient with a crushed finger who liked to drink wine!

Remedy: Hypericum 30c
Dose: Two tablets every 10–15 min for six doses, then three times daily
Result: Improvement was substantial

Wounds, puncture

Teenager with wound on the foot caused by stepping on a rusty nail on the beach.

Remedy: Ledrum 30c tablets
Dose: Two tablets every 15 min and referral to hospital for antitetanus
Result: Wound healed within 4 days without leaving a scar

Soft tissue injuries

Man aged 28. Muscular problem after playing tennis yesterday.

Remedy: Ruta 30c tablets
Dose: Two tablets four times a day
Result: Considerably easier after 6 hours

TREATMENTS FOR ACUTE SELF-LIMITING TYPE CONDITIONS

In this section, suggested treatments for a number of common self-limiting type conditions are summarised in the following tables (remedies in bold type are those generally found to be most frequently indicated):

- catarrh, colds and influenza (Table 9.2)
- constipation (Table 9.3)
- coughs (Table 9.4)
- diarrhoea (Table 9.5)
- earache (Table 9.6)
- eye problems (Table 9.7)
- headaches (Table 9.8)
- indigestion and colic (Table 9.9)
- mental states (Table 9.10)
- skin conditions (Table 9.11).

The box following the tables (p. 224) contains some brief case studies to illustrate the use of acute remedies.

Table 9.2 Remedies for treating catarrh, colds and flu

Nose	Eyes/mouth	Modalities	Other	Remedy
Frequent sneezing; nasal congestion	Patient tends to be thirsty	Worse: in a stuffy atmosphere	First stages of flu: especially after exposure to cold	**Aconite**
Runny nose; sore nostrils	'Heavy' eyes, streaming	Better: wrapped up warm	Effective from first stages right through to resolution	**AGE (Arsen iod or Ars alb + Gels + Eupatorium)**
Streaming coryza, sneezing	Streaming eyes; hot and thirsty	Better: fresh air	Sore throat common	Allium cepa
Watery discharge, sneezing painful	Thirst for sips of liquid; sore lips	Worse: cold air and after eating	Patient complains of 'being cold'	Arsen alb
Watery, excoriating discharge; swollen nose	Swollen tonsils, bad breath	Worse: cold	Slight hacking cough is common	Arsen iod
Swollen, red hot: little discharge	Painful sore throat; hoarse	Worse: lying down	Sudden onset; violent headache, flushed	Belladonna
Sneezing; 'chesty'	Red and watery eyes; great thirst	Better: lying down and keeping still	Slow onset	Bryonia
Bouts of severe sneezing	Eyes red; sore throat	Worse: cold room	Pains in back and limbs	Dulcamara
Coryza with sneezing	Corners of mouth cracked; yellow coated tongue; thirst especially in early morning	Worse: night	'Bones ache'; hoarseness with cough and soreness in chest; fever; headache	Eupatorium
Flu symptoms; sore red nostrils	Eyelids sore and drooping; tongue may be coated	Better: warmth	'Bones ache', headache, urge to urinate	**Gelsemium**
Sore inside nose; copious thick coloured mucus	Eyes swollen; mouth dry, catarrh	Worse: morning Better: from heat	Often aching joints	**Kali bich**
Stuffed-up feeling especially at night; 'snuffles'	Sore gums, ulcers; dull soreness in the throat	Better: in open air	Patient irritable; difficulty in keeping warm	Nux vom
Often right nostril stuffed up. Yellow discharge especially in morning; catarrh	Dry mouth with cracked lips	Better: in open air	Pains in head (and teeth?); neuralgia – especially right side	Pulsatilla

Table 9.3   Remedies for treating constipation

Symptoms	Modalities	Other	Remedy
Stools hard and dry	Worse: in the morning on awakening; inactivity	Sore rectum, great straining. Often indicated in children and elderly	Alumina
Stools hard, dry, thick and brown	Worse: in the morning	Nausea, thirst	Bryonia
Stools dry, crumbly	Better: without food	Rectum bleeding	Natrum mur
Frequent ineffectual urging	Worse: in the morning	Patient cold and irritable	**Nux vom**
Irregular dry pellet-like stools, round and black	Worse: in the warm	No desire to defaecate. Pain in rectum	Opium*
Stools hard, lumpy and black	Worse: in the morning	Anal spasm; colic	Plumbum met
Much straining to produce large stools	Worse: at night	Infant constipation in cold weather	Verat alb

* Opium is unavailable in UK as an OTC remedy, even in homeopathic dilution, on orders of the Medicines' Inspectorate.

Table 9.4   Remedies for treating coughs

Speed of onset	Type of cough	Modalities	Other	Remedy
Sudden	Dry, painful, croupy	Worse: at night and in warm room / Better: in open air	Hoarseness; loud, laboured breathing	Aconite
Steady	Hacking cough	Worse: inhaling cold air (cough) / Worse: warm room (headache)	Tickling sensation in larynx; catarrhal headache	Allium cepa
Slow	Constant 'rattling' cough	Worse: for warmth	Throat pain; hoarseness	Antim tart
Slow	Hacking cough with expectoration	Worse: going into warm room: also after eating or drinking	Difficult quick respiration; soreness in larynx and trachea; thirst	**Bryonia**
Steady	Spasmodic, dry irritating (cf. whooping)	Worse: at night and from warmth, lying down in bed	Deep; hoarse voice; coldness on left hand of face	Drosera
Sudden	Persistent wheezing cough with shortness of breath; croup	Worse: at night and when lying down / Better: in open air	Nasal coryza; nausea and vomiting	Ipecac
Slow	Dry tickly cough (e.g. viral cough after flu); long lasting	Worse: evenings and night, cold air; exertion / Better: lying on right side	Hoarseness; tightness in chest; thirst	**Phosphorus**
Slow	Dry cough at night; loose productive cough in the morning	Better: sitting up in bed	Hoarseness comes and goes	Pulsatilla
Sudden	Dry 'barking' croupy cough	Worse: with excitement and cold air / Better: lying down	Difficult breathing; dryness of all air passages; bursting headache	Spongia

Table 9.5 Remedies for treating diarrhoea

Cause/onset	Symptoms	Modalities	Other	Remedy
Anxiety related	Colic, watery stool, flatulence	Better: warmth	Trembling, insomnia	Argent nit (also consider Gelsemium)
Food related	Rectal pain, stools small, dark	Worse: from cold	Cold sweats	**Arsen alb**
No clear cause	Copious painless diarrhoea, especially at night	Better: warmth	Much flatulence, colic; fever	China
Usually food related – overeating. Rapid onset	Green, slimy watery stools; offensive odour	Worse: lying down	Nausea, vomiting commonly present	Ipecac
Children; ingestion foreign body?	'Explosive' profuse diarrhoea with flatulence	Better: gentle rubbing over liver region	Often in summer	Podophyllum
Caused by eating rich foods	Loose watery stools that change in appearance	Worse: night	Painful distended abdomen	Pulsatilla
No clear cause	Early morning diarrhoea	Worse: morning	Rectal itching	Sulphur

Table 9.6 Remedies for treating earache

Cause/onset	Symptoms	Modalities	Other	Remedy
Sudden onset brought on by cold wind	External ear hot, swollen Intense pain	Worse: with noise and warmth	Fever, thirst No suppuration	Aconitie
Sudden onset brought on by cold to head (no hat, haircut, etc.)	Intense throbbing or 'tearing' pain	Worse: with touching, in the afternoon, jarring motion and on right side Better: application of heat	Redness, fever, headache No suppuration	**Belladonna**
Associated with predisposition to colds and flu	Acute otitis Throbbing pain with noises in the ear	Worse: at night and early morning; right side Better: application of cold, gentle motion	Suppuration	Ferrum phos
Associated with catarrh	Swollen, with 'tearing' pains	Worse: morning and in hot weather Better: in warm	Thick yellow stingy expectoration 'Stuffed up' feeling	Kali bich

Table 9.7   Remedies for treating eye problems

Condition	Symptoms	Modalities	Other	Remedy
Conjunctivitis	Red, burning; phobia Profuse bland lachrymation	Worse: in warm and in evening Better: in the open air	Cararrhal headache; sneezing	Allium cepa
	Inflamed eye lids; photophobia, aching tired feeling in eyes Purulent discharge	Worse: with warmth and at night Better: in cold and with pressure	Anxiety, worry, headache	Argent nit
	Lids swollen, red, inflamed hot lachrymation Sudden piercing pains	Worse: with heat and touch Better: in open air	Oedema at extremities?	Apis
	Burning and swelling of lids; stinging pain, acid lachrymation; 'gritty' feeling in eyes	Worse: evening and in warm Better: in dark	Fluent bland coryza Yawns in open air	Euphrasia*
Contusion	Black eye	Worse: warmth Better: cold applications	Bruising and discolouration	Ledum (consider Arnica too)
	Injury to eyeball caused by blow from blunt object	Worse: for touch	Pain in the socket	Symphytum (consider Arnica too)
Eyestrain	Red, hot and painful after reading, sewing, etc.	Worse: from cold and lying down	Constipation	Ruta
Styes	Margin of eyes itch Recurrent styes	Worse: with touch Better: with rest	Emotional upsets	Staphysagria
	Burning and itching around the eyes, especially at margins	Worse: with warmth in bed	Nasal herpes; lips dry	Sulphur
	Itching and burning sensation; thick bland yellow/green discharge/ styes	Worse: with warmth Better: in open air	Patients with changeable disposition, weep easily and seek sympathy	Pulsatilla

*See Stass et al. (2000)

Table 9.8 Remedies for treating headaches

Cause	Type of pain	Modalities	Other	Remedy
Exertion and excitement	Burning pains that occur spasmodically	Worse: from cold Better: from heat	Patient very chilly; restless; scalp sensitive	Arsen alb
Exposure of head to the cold Sudden onset	Bursting, throbbing pain in forehead, occiput and temples	Worse: noise, touch Better: lying in dark room	Redness: flushed appearance with dilated pupils	**Belladonna**
Washing in cold water after exertion	'Splitting' or 'crushing' headache in occiput	Worse: warmth and motion Better: lying still	Patient irritable and thirsty	Bryonia
Anxiety, fear, cold	Dull, heavy, ache; especially back of head	Worse: for motion, effort Better: propped up in bed	Patient desires to be left alone No thirst	Gelsemium
Eye-strain, emotional stress Anaemia in girls	'Blinding' headache	Worse: warm room Better: open air	Thirst; nausea and vomiting possible	**Natrum mur**
Overeating and/or drinking	'Splitting' headache at back of head or over eye ('hangover')	Worse: movement or mental effort Better: warmth, lying down	Patient irritable	Nux vom
Overeating	Congestive, throbbing, 'wandering' from head to teeth; head hot	Worse: heat and after food Better: open air	Weepy, changeable person	Pulsatilla
Lack of food	'Sick' throbbing headache, occurring periodically	Worse: when standing Better: when lying on right side	Heat and burning sensation in the eyes	Sulphur

See also Muscari-Tomaioli et al. (2001), Walach et al. (2001)

Table 9.9   Remedies for treating indigestion and colic

Main symptoms	Modalities	Other	Remedy
Nausea, retching and vomiting; coated white tongue	Worse: in evening and from warmth Better: sitting up and expectorating	Abdominal distension with flatulence; thirst for cold water	Antim tart
Nausea and faintness when starting to move Vomiting after food	Worse: for taking warm drinks	Dry mouth with thirst; bitter taste in the mouth	Bryonia
Belching and offensive flatulence; nausea in the morning Bloated feeling	Worse: evening and cold air Better: after belching and cold	Cold sweat	Carbo veg
Great abdominal distension; wind passed in small quantities Infant colic	Worse: evening Better: for application of local heat	Children hot, cannot be satisfied; stools grass green or 'chopped eggs'	Chamomilla
Severe cramp-like pains in the abdomen	Better: bending double or drawing knees up	Diarrhoea often severe; also vomiting; coated tongue	Colocynth
Colic, cramps, flatulence	Worse: night Better: for warm applications	Often useful premenstrually; clean tongue	Mag phos
Pain 1–2 hours after food Nausea after overeating Patient wants to vomit but cannot; retching	Better: after stool passed, for hot food and drink Worse: for alcohol, coffee	Patient irritable, chilly and oversensitive	Nux vom

Table 9.10   Remedies for common mental states

Symptoms	Modalities	Other	Remedy
Great fear, even terror Foreboding of disaster	Worse: in warm room Better: in open air	Bursting sensation in the head; sensitive to noise	Aconite
Foreboding; anticipatory worry and anxiety and failing	Better: in the fresh air	Headache from mental exertion	Argent nit
Stage fright Worry about failing exams	Worse: in wet weather, for bad news	Desire to be left alone; good pre-exam – when 'mind goes blank'	Gelsemium
Effects of grief – immediate and next day	Worse: with external warmth and open air Better: while eating	Changes of mood – much crying and sighing	Ignatia
Ill-effects of grief	Better: in the open air	Irritable and depressed; blinding headache	Natrum mur
Highly emotional – 'highly strung'	Worse: from heat Better: open air	Timid, weeps easily; fears being alone at night	Pulsatilla

Table 9.11 Remedies for skin conditions

Condition	Symptoms	Modalities	Other	Remedy
Abrasions	Superficial cuts and scrapes Painful puncture or crush wounds			Calendula Hypericum
Acne, eczema	Itching, burning skin that is dry, rough; psoriasis	Worse: with scratching and cold Better: from heat	Disturbed sleeping pattern Chilblains (see Tamus)	Arsen alb
	Rough, hard skin with persistent dryness; oozing lesions Cracked skin in nipples, hands and behind ears	Worse: with warmth and at night Better: from wrapping up	Pain on blowing nose Pain in small of the back Itching pimples	Graphites
	Suppurating, abscesses Generally unhealthy skin	Worse: dry cold winds, touch Better: from warmth	Cold sores; sweats freely Weeping and sensitive boils	Hepar sulph
	Greasy oily skin, especially on hairy parts. Many little eruptions; bends of limbs and behind ears affected Raw, red, excema	Worse: with heat Better: cold bathing, open air	Irritable, headache	Natrum mur
	Dry, scaly, unhealthy skin; suppurating; pruritus; itching and burning	Worse: with scratching and washing and with warmth in bed	Styes	Sulphur
Allergies	Allergic reaction to sun; urticaria 'itchy blotches' (also minor burns)	Worse: from touch and scratching	Fever; rheumatism	Urtica (see Cantharis below, Euphrasia (Table 9.7) and also consider the isopathic preparations
Burns	Burns and scalds that blister	Better: with rubbing	Dermatitis and other similar skin conditions	Cantharis (see Urtica above)
	Sunburn; throbbing red rash	Worse: with touch	Throbbing headache, flushed	Belladonna
Chilblains	Burning and itching: hands and feet	Worse: with extremes of hot and cold		**Tamus** (see Arsen alb)

Case Studies: Using acute remedies

Anticipatory anxiety

Subject: Male, 17 years. Seen 2 days before driving test

Appeared very nervous – mother said she was sure her son would not turn up – 'again'

Remedy: Argent nit 30c tablets

Dose: Two tablets three times daily for the 2 days before the test, then hourly on the day of the test

Result: Boy failed on this attempt but passed next time round with same dose regimen and was absolutely delighted

Catarrh

Subject: Male patient, elderly, complaining of catarrh; greenish colour

Remedy: Pulsatilla 30c tablets

Dose: Two tablets three times daily

Results: Slight improvement; discomfort reduced after 1 week

Colic with teething

Subject: Male infant, 8 months. Very frightened with bright red cheeks, hot and flushed. 'Terrible colic': mother giving gripewater frequently. Gums very red and sore; one tooth present and obviously teething

Remedy: 10 powders of Chamomilla 30c

Dose: Discontinue gripewater; one powder to be given dry on tongue every 2 hours for six doses, 15 mins before food

Result: Redness subsided within 5 hours. Subsequent treatment: one powder 15 mins before food

Colic infant

Subject: Infant of 14 months, suffering from 'windy' colic

Remedy: Colocynth 30c granules

Dose: one dose to be given half hour before food

Result: Some improvement; eventually used to complement orthodox treatment

Grief

Subject: Elderly lady came into pharmacy, sobbing bitterly after seeing her cairn terrier run over and killed by a bus

Remedy: Ignatia 30c granule

Dose: one dose every 30 min for four doses, then twice daily for as long as required

Result: Patient felt a lot better almost immediately; discontinued powders in 2 days

Ingestion

Subject: Male aged 45 requested 'hangover' remedy

Remedy: Nux vom 30c tablets

Dose: Two tablets every 10 mins for six doses (if necessary)

Result: After four doses patient telephoned to say 'he felt like magic'

Influenza

Subject: Male, 65, complaining of flu; came on last couple of days or so; bones aching, sore all over, headache

Remedy: Gelsemium 30c tablets

Dose: Two tablets four times a day, plenty of fluids and rest

Result: Patient up and about after 30 hours

Nausea (pregnancy having been discounted)

Subject: Female, 32, complaining of persistent nausea

Remedy: Ipecac 230 liquid potency

Dose: Five drops in water, sip slowly three times daily

Result: Slight improvement after 3 days; patient referred back to GP

Sore throat/headache

Subject: Female, aged 24, complaining of sore throat of 2 days' duration, not responding to orthodox OTC medicine. Bursting headache came on suddenly

Remedy: Belladonna 30c tablets

Dose: Two tablets every 2 hours for six doses, then three times daily

Result: Progressive improvement over 2 days

TOPICAL PREPARATIONS

Although frequently described as being 'homeopathic', in most cases the topical preparations are essentially herbal in nature, being prepared by admixing a mother tincture with a suitable vehicle and used without individualisation although they may still be used on the basis of like to treat like (e.g. Urtica for urticaria). In the case of remedies that cannot be made into true mother tinctures due to their lack of solubility, low potencies (typically 6x) are used as the active ingredient. The preparations are generally applied sparingly twice daily until the symptoms subside, and can be used in conjunction with homeopathic or orthodox oral therapy. There is little therapeutic difference between the products of different manufacturers, although some patients at one of the hospital clinics in Glasgow reacted to a change of ointment base. All the ointments and creams are extremely effective. Because they are not licensed under the medicines regulations as homeopathic medicines, claims of efficacy can be made on the labels, making them easy to sell!

Ointments and creams

Ointments and creams are not sterile and should not normally be applied where the skin is broken. Under these circumstances oral medication should be used.

Preparations containing single ingredients:

- Arnica: applied after bruising. Can also be used for aching muscles after prolonged activity or an accident.
- Calendula: excellent in the treatment of minor skin abrasions, chapped skin and nappy rash.
- Hamamelis: often combined with other remedies in the treatment of haemorrhoids, Hamamelis is also used alone in the topical treatment of varicose conditions on the legs.
- Hypericum: often combined with Calendula, with which it shares many applications. It is indicated for painful crush injuries, especially when fingers and toes are involved, but not when the skin is extensively broken.
- Rhus tox: useful where there is deep arthritic-type joint pain, either alone or as an adjunct to oral treatment.
- Ruta: applied in cases of soft tissue injuries, torn tendons, split ligaments and possibly synovitis. Sometimes used in conjunction with Rhus tox.
- Tamus: specific for the treatment of chilblains; used in conjunction with oral therapy. In resistant cases and where the skin is intact, the mother tincture may be applied directly.
- Thuja: an effective treatment for warts and verrucae. A good starting point, but if treatment ineffective, can be combined with oral therapy or mother tincture, as with Tamus.
- Urtica: one manufacturer markets this as a suitable application to cool the skin after sunbathing. It can be used in cases of urticarial-type eruptions as well as to treat prickly heat rashes.

Mixed ointments/creams. The following are available from manufacturers:

- Burn ointment: contains several ingredients, but mainly Cantharis. Confers rapid relief after scalds and burns. Also useful for sunburn.
- Haemorrhoid ointment: a mixture of Aesculus, Hamamelis and Paeonia mother tinctures. One manufacturer supplies tubes with handy applicators.
- Hypericum and Calendula: widely known as Hypercal (originally from A Nelson & Co) in the UK. This product combines the indications of its two constituents and is frequently indicated.
- Arnica is often mixed with other remedies to form a compound ointment. A popular example is Arnica, Calendula and Urtica (ACU).

Other preparations. This category includes products that are not strictly homeopathic but are often used in homeopathic environments:

- marigold therapy products used in podiatry (Khan, 1997)
- tea tree cream
- vitamin E cream
- Bach rescue cream (covered in Ch. 10).

There are also small ranges of branded topical preparations on the market.

Lotions; liniments and oils

Arnica, Calendula and Hypericum are three remedies used most frequently in these forms. Rhus tox is occasionally prescribed as a liniment or oil. Verbascum oil (also known as 'Mullein') is usually used as ear drops to soften wax and treat otalgia, but I have heard of it being rubbed on the chest for catarrh. Sepia is unusual in that the 8x potency has been used as a hair lotion, the vehicle being a fearful mixture of ether and alcohol.

Mother tinctures

Mother tinctures are generally applied topically only when the skin is unbroken. They may be diluted with tepid water.

- Hypericum and Calendula mixture is used for herpes-type lesions, although patients complain bitterly that it nips the skin if applied undiluted.
- Arnica (bruises), Calendula and Hypericum (superficial abrasions) are all used in the bath water; the soothing effect is probably only a placebo effect. Patients can also make up gargles and mouthwashes by placing five drops of mother tincture in a cup of warm water, and they may also be applied to the skin, providing there is no deep wound.
- Bellis perennis is useful for blows and deep-seated muscular injuries.
- Echinacea can be applied for superficial burns.
- Ledum is suitable for insect bites – particularly puncture wounds.
- Paeonia is effective in treating externally protruding haemorrhoids.
- Phytolacca might be used in veterinary mastitis (see Ch. 11).

- Tamus and Thuja may be applied to chilblains and warts respectively. In each case one or two drops once or twice daily is the recommended dose.
- Urtica in dilution may be applied to burns.

Other topical preparations

Among other topical preparations are the insect repellant Pyrethrum, which can also be used in oral form as a prophylactic, and Calendula talc. The latter is non-sterile.

TREATMENT OF ALLERGIES

Research has shown that allergies and asthma are perceived as responding well to CAM in general (Schafer, 2004). Approximately 30% of patients with allergies report experiences with CAM in Europe. In selected inpatient populations, the prevalence reaches 50%. Users of CAM tend to be younger women with a higher educational background. Although a larger number of different CAM modalities are provided, only a few techniques account for the majority of use (e.g. acupuncture, herbalism and homeopathy).

The options

Allergic reactions can vary from a mild skin rash to streaming eyes to chronic asthma (see case study).

Case Study: Allergic reaction

Allergy
Teenager: streaming eyes, red and sore
Lachrymation acrid
Remedy: Euphrasia 30c tablets (cf. Allium cepa where lachrymation bland)

Dose: Two tablets four times daily for 3 days, then twice daily
Result: Only slight improvement. Referred to Allergy Clinic at hospital for further investigation

---

We are looking here at the type of conditions producing acute symptoms rather than the longstanding chronic conditions (asthma, eczema) that would normally be referred. Generally speaking, homeopathy offers considerable relief without the side-effects of allopathic drugs.

Allergies may be treated in several ways:

1. By instructing the patient to avoid the allergy. This may or may not be possible. If the offending allergen is dog or cat hair, then getting rid of the pet may solve the problem. If the allergen is unknown (a skin test might help), or is widely distributed in the home environment (like house dust or house dust mite), such action might not be practicable.

2. By treating the patient classically, that is, matching the patient's symptoms with the drug picture of the remedy and administering the remedy in the normal way. The most widely used remedy in this category is Euphrasia. If a 'healthy volunteer' were to be given this

drug in large quantities, then he or she would suffer the normal symp-toms of hayfever: rhinitis, streaming eyes, headache, etc.

3. By treating the patient with isopathy (a procedure also commonly called desensitisation or homeopathic specific immunotherapy).

Useful remedies for treating allergies

Poitevan (1998) has reviewed the evidence base for using homeopathy in the treatment of asthma and allergies. The most commonly prescribed are, in order of frequency: Apis mel, Allium cepa, Sabadilla and Euphrasia. Histamine can also be used. Other remedies mentioned by Poitevan for treating more complex cases include Psorinum, Sulphur, Natrum mur, Thuja, Lycopodium and Arsenicum album.

A list of suggested allergy remedies is set out in Table 9.12. The table shows how complicated homeopathic prescribing can be even when it is based on only a few physical symptoms. The main remedies to remember are in bold type, with distinguishing features in italic.

There are one or two remedies that seem to be specific for certain aller-gies. Urtica, for example, is often effective in treating a patient with an allergy to shellfish. Euphrasia seems to work well against milk allergies.

Treating the condition with isopathy – homeopathic immunotherapy

Here the actual allergen causing the condition is identified, and the patient given a homeopathic potency of this material (i.e. 'same to treat same'). The range of isopathic preparations available is huge as we saw in Chapter 8. Manufacturers will also prepare new remedies from sample material to order. The patient may be given a skin test to identify the allergen by their GP or at a hospital clinic (Fig. 9.1), but if they know the allergen (grass pollen is a common culprit) then the remedy can be supplied directly.

The dosing structure varies widely with the practitioner; however; there is no universally accepted regimen. Some practitioners find that three powders of the 10M potency given at the start of the hayfever season and repeated half way through is successful. Other practitioners suggest that a 30c or 200c should be used when necessary. Patients may also be treated throughout the season with a 6c potency on the chronic level, increasing the frequency of dosing if the incidence of allergens should rise.

A 4-year trial at Glasgow Homeopathic Hospital tested three different regimens and found two tablets of 30c potentised allergen for a month to yield the best outcome (Beattie and Kayne, 2000).

Reilly and his colleagues have demonstrated the use of the immuno-therapy technique effectively in their series of four placebo study trials (Taylor et al., 2000; see also Ch. 11). Treatment of birch pollen allergy with dilutions of Betula, however, has produced inconclusive results (Aabel, 2000, 2001; Aabel et al., 2000).

Treating allergies constitutionally

A well-indicated constitutional remedy can help an idiosyncratic hyper-sensitivity. Unfortunately the allergic symptoms may be so forceful that they

Table 9.12 Selection of allergy remedies

Remedy	Eye symptoms	Nasal symptoms	Ears/throat/chest	Other symptoms
Allium cepa	*Bland secretion, photophobic*	*Fluent watery acrid coryza*	*Tickle in throat, cough in cold air*	Better in the open air
Arsen alb	Burning eyes, tears, photophobia	Thin watery burning discharge	Burning throat Asthma	Restless, exhausted
Arsen iod	Burning sensation, watery discharge	Sneezing, watery discharge, soreness	Burning throat, dry irritating cough	Dry scaly skin
Arundo		Itching in the nostrils, sneezing	Itching in roof of mouth and ears	Early hayfever
Euphrasia	*Acrid burning discharge*	*Fluent watery coryza*	*Productive cough*	Better in the open air
Gelsemium	'Heavy' swollen eyes	Sneezing, watery discharge	Sore throat	Listless, giddy, trembling
Iodum	Inflamed swollen eyelids	Sneezing; hot watery discharge	Congested ears	Symptoms better walking about
Natrum mur	Watery, 'uncomfortable'	Violent sneezing, watery discharge	Coughing, makes eyes water	Depressed and 'touchy'
Nux vomica	Smarting feeling, photophobia	Stuffy nose, difficult breathing	Itching in inner ear	Irritable, headache of migraine type
Sabadilla	Eyelids red, burning, discharge	Sneezing spasms, runny nose	Sore throat, better for warm drink	Feeling of chilliness
Urtica		Profuse discharge		Skin: itching blotches, urticaria
Wyethia		Itch and dryness at back of nose	Dry throat and dry hacking cough	Early hayfever

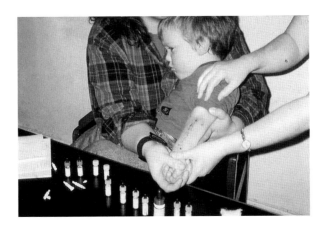

Figure 9.1 Skin testing at Glasgow Homeopathic Hospital

overwhelm the constitutional picture. In cases where it can be clearly deter-mined, Shore (1994) has suggested that it can complement a remedy chosen on the basis of allergic symptoms alone.

Allergies are conditions that often exhibit very clear emotional symptoms as well as physical symptoms. In these cases patients state that they are only seeking advice because their spouse or partner had begun complaining that they were 'difficult to live with'. Irritability or even aggression can result from an allergy. In some instances the physical aspects of an allergy are only marginally helped by homeopathy alone, but the 'feel-good' or 'well-being' factor can be substantially improved using a constitutional remedy.

TREATMENT OF BACTERIAL AND VIRAL INFECTIONS

Because of the small amounts of medicine in the remedies, homeopathy is often said to be ineffective when treating conditions involving invaders to the body.

There are notable exceptions to this statement. For example:

- Aconite, Berberis and Cantharis can be used very effectively to treat cystitis.
- Eupatorium and Gelsemium can be used to treat influenza.
- Belladonna can be used to treat throat infections.
- Hepar sulph and Silica can be used to treat boils resulting from a bacterial infection.
- Echinacea is a remedy having amongst its indications in Boericke's *Repertory* 'acute auto infection'. It is useful when the tonsils are sore and ulcerated and in the treatment of recurring boils.

John English has offered a whole raft of remedies as possibilities for the treatment of upper respiratory tract infections in general practice (English, 1995). In fact classical homeopaths claim that any infectious disease can be treated. They suggest that the presence of an invader is more the result of a prior disease than the sole cause of the illness. In order for the bacteria to gain a foothold there must be some susceptibility on the part of the patient. The choice of an appropriate remedy may remove this suscep-tibility and thereby create an environment in which the invader can no longer thrive. A similar argument supports the use of homeopathy in treat-ing viral infections, against which conventional medicine still has little to offer.

There is a story related by Sister Moira Gray of Glasgow about the late Dr Jean Hindmarch who died at the age of 93 in January 1995 (Gray, 1995). During an epidemic of diphtheria in the early 1930s, Dr Jean treated many families with homeopathy. One morning she made her return visit to two families in a Lanarkshire mining village. As she approached the tenement building where they lived, she noticed a group of weeping women huddled together. One of the women rushed towards her crying 'Oh, Dr Jean, my wee wean (child) is deid (dead)'. Dr Jean climbed the stairs, not knowing whether it was one of her patients who had died. It was a great relief to dis-cover that the four children she had treated homeopathically had survived, but equally a sadness to learn that three out of five in the block who had been treated allopathically had died during the night. It proved to her the power of the 'those wee white pills' as the children liked to call them.

According to Savage (1984), there are four ways in which homeopathy can be used in the management of bacterial infections:

1. **Prophylaxis.** In the early days of homeopathy Aconite and Ferrum phos were given to prevent the onset of influenza. Belladonna was commonly used to prevent and treat scarlet fever, while Camphor was used in the same way for cholera. All these remedies were apparently very successful in producing stronger and healthier people who did not become reinfected – so much so that in the USA many life insurance companies offered lower rates to people who went to homeopathic physicians (Ullman, 1988). Remedies such as Bacillinum and Influenzinum are now given prophylactically at the beginning of winter to guard against influenza.

2. **Treatment.** Because homeopathy treats patients on the basis of the symptoms, it is not usually necessary to identify the exact cause of a condition before treating it. This eliminates the requirement for taking swabs and cultivating the offending organism. An interesting homeopathic product called Oscillococcinum®, manufactured by Boiron Laboratories in France, is claimed to be highly successful in the treatment of influenza when taken within 48 hours of onset of symptoms. It is not licensed for supply in the UK.

3. **Recovery** from longstanding viral infections. The symptoms of certain longstanding conditions such as herpes simplex and warts can be alleviated very effectively using isopathy. Samples of affected tissue are made into medicines for administration in the 6c or 30c potencies. This aspect of homeopathy is dealt with in Chapters 4 and 8. In addition, warts respond to topical and oral treatment with Thuja. Combined treatments of Thuja, Antim crud and Acid nit have also been used (Labrecque et al., 1992).

4. **Correction of chronic after-effects of disease.** Patients often complain of being 'washed out' or 'below par' after a viral infection. It takes some people several weeks before they are back to their normal level of wellness. There are several ways of treating this discomfort, using constitutional (see Ch. 8) or isopathic prescribing.

HOMEOPATHY FOR WOMEN

The advantages of using homeopathy

There are some excellent books dealing with this topic in great detail and for more details than those presented here the reader is referred to Miranda Castro's *Homeopathy for Mother and Baby* and *A Woman's Guide to Homeopathy* by Andrew Lockie and Nicola Geddes.

Many of today's women have discovered that conventional medical treatments for numerous complaints attract unacceptable risk:benefit ratios. As women generally visit their GPs more frequently than men, their exposure to risk is correspondingly higher. Homeopathy is not always effective in treating women's problems. Conditions involving vitamin or iron deficiency or hormonal imbalance require orthodox input to restore physiological levels. This does not mean that homeopathy cannot be used alongside these medicaments to improve the body's overall well-being, and such combination treatment is quite usual. There are many instances where a full consultation is necessary to prescribe accurately on the totality of symptoms for longstanding or recurrent conditions, especially where the emotional plane is disturbed, and under these circumstances referral to a qualified homeopath is strongly advised. However, there are a number of areas where self-treatment is appropriate, and patients can be assisted by supplying homeopathic remedies with appropriate counselling.

Cystitis

This condition affects women mainly because the urethra is short and easily invaded by bacteria. The term is used to describe four different conditions with similar symptoms:

- an urge to urinate frequently
- a scanty flow that smells strongly
- a burning sensation as the urine is passed
- a dull ache in the lower abdominal region.

The causes are: infection of the bladder due to transfer of *E. coli* from the bowel; chronic irritation from causes other than bacterial infection (orthodox medication, hormonal imbalances, stress); and lastly urethritis, an inflammation of the urethra usually caused by bruising during sexual intercourse. Cystitis is said to pose little risk to general health but should be treated because of the discomfort it causes. Women who do not experience substantial improvement within 2–3 days should contact their GP.

The long-term homeopathic treatment is constitutional or with nosodes, often in association with antibiotics. In the case of isolated episodes there are several homeopathic remedies available to treat the symptoms, five of which are included in Table 9.13.

Table 9.13 Common remedies for cystitis (Lockie, 1989)

Indications	Possible remedy
Sharp stinging pains, symptom worse for heat, evidence of blood	Apis
Burning pains, frequent urge to urinate, inability to empty bladder	Cantharis
Frequent urge made worse by coughing and sneezing; 'dribbling'	Causticum
Comes on after getting wet and cold, especially in autumn, blood	Dulcamara
Frequent and painful urging with little result	Nux vom

Premenstrual syndrome (PMS)

This term covers the wide range of symptoms on both physical and emotional planes that affect many women on the days leading up to their menstrual period. The cause is thought to be due to hormonal imbalance, psychological factors (stress) or possibly allergies. There may be a tenderness and enlargement of the breasts with fluid retention, and twinges of pain referred to as 'cramps'. The intensity of the emotional symptoms can vary from a mild irritability to marked mood changes and unusually aggressive behaviour. Because of the effect on other family members it is often this aspect of the condition that prompts the patient to seek help. In severe cases the GP will prescribe hormone treatment, diuretics or anxiolytics.

There are four main remedies that can be recommended for short-term treatment on the basis of limited physical and emotional symptoms (Table 9.14).

Because of the importance of emotional involvement some attention must be given to this aspect of case analysis. The three-legged stool approach (see Ch. 8) is inappropriate in this case. If discomfort persists after two cycles, then patients should be referred to a medically qualified homeopath for investigation. There are constitutional differences that can be a guide in distinguishing the remedies, but unfortunately patients do not always match these constitutional features exactly, and may change their picture during the course of a disease. Treatment can be given at the chronic level of dosing for 3 weeks each month, starting 1 week after each cycle.

- Lachesis patients are restless and uneasy, cannot bear tight clothes, and are loquacious. They tend to be mistrustful of others, often to the point of jealousy. These patients are definitely not morning people – they are at their worst mentally and physically on waking. This is one of the three most frequently administered remedies for older women experiencing symptoms of the menopause.
- Natrum mur patients are depressed, easily upset, and are averse to sympathy. They like salt on their food and have dry mucous membranes in the mouth and vagina. They also have an oily skin, and are prone to constipation.
- Pulsatilla patients tend to be fair, shorter and plumper, with a friendly disposition, but indecisive and weepy.

Table 9.14 Remedies suggested for PMT

Indications	Possible remedy
Breasts painful, symptoms worse in morning, sad, talks a lot	Lachesis
Fluid retention, swollen breasts, depressed, wants to be left alone	Natrum mur
Breasts painful, stomach upset, irregular scanty periods, weeps easily	Pulsatilla
Abdominal pain, cystitis, flatulence, irritable, craves sweet things	Sepia

- Sepia patients are usually tall slim brunettes, with a skin that appears sallow and 'waxy'. They have a rather offhand manner, and are said to shun affection.

Menopause

Sometimes requests are received from women suffering from hot flushes and other symptoms of the menopause. Many are uncertain as to whether they should be using hormone replacement therapy given the uncertainties surrounding this treatment. In the short term, prior to a full investigation by their GP, Lachesis, Pulsatilla or Sepia may be of assistance (see Table 9.14 for indications).

Clover and Ratsey (2002) reported an uncontrolled pilot outcome study, conducted at the Tunbridge Wells Homeopathic Hospital using the remedies Amyl nit, Calc carb, Lachesis, Natrum mur, Pulsatilla and Sepia. Their results indicated useful symptomatic benefit for patients with and without breast cancer who were experiencing hot flushes.

Remedies useful during pregnancy

Antenatal remedies

It is appropriate to recommend that the patient takes her constitutional remedy before conception if possible. Homeopaths find that women who receive constitutional homeopathic treatment prior to becoming pregnant rarely seem to get morning sickness during pregnancy (Ullman, 1988). Homeopathic remedies are especially useful to treat a range of trivial self-limiting type conditions in the first trimester of pregnancy and again immediately prior to delivery, when safety to mother and her new baby is of the utmost concern to the parents (Table 9.15).

Some conditions such as morning sickness in the first trimester cannot be helped by orthodox means. In these circumstances homeopathy may be able offer support. The usual remedy of choice is Cocculus, or the rather unusual remedy Symphoricarpus (from the snowberry); several others are available (Table 9.16).

Remedies during delivery and postnatal

There are two remedies that can be given immediately prior to delivery. Caulophyllum is thought to improve the tonicity of the uterus and facilitate an easier delivery. It can be administered quite safely in the 30c potency, (although some practitioners use the 6x) once or twice daily commencing between weeks 34 and 36, and increasing to twice daily immediately prior to expected delivery. It may be continued if delivery is delayed. During labour the remedy may be given every 2–4 hours. Miranda Castro suggests that women in their first pregnancy should think carefully before taking Caulophyllum, in case a proving should occur, leading to 'a short violent labour'. In a survey carried out in Bristol, six respondents (out of 125) mentioned particular problems after taking the remedy (Webb and Gray, 1994).

Table 9.15 Remedies suggested for antenatal treatments

Indications	Possible remedy
Anxiety and emotional distress	Aconite, Argent nit
Backache	Arnica (accident), Rhus tox
Constipation	Nux vomica, Alumina
Exhaustion	Arnica
Cystitis	Cantharis (see Table 9.13)
Diarrhoea	Aloe, Podophyllum
Haemorrhoids	Esculus, Hamamelis (bleeding)
Heartburn	Carbo veg, Conium (sore breasts)
Incontinence of pregnancy	Causticum
Indigestion, flatulence	China
Indigestion, vomiting especially after fatty foods	Pulsatilla
Indigestion	Nux vom
Insomnia	Coffea
Morning sickness	See Table 9.16

Table 9.16 Remedies suggested for morning sickness

Indications	Possible remedy
Nausea with faintness and vomiting, aversion to food	Cocculus
Nausea, heartburn with sore breasts	Conium
Persistent vomiting of food and mucus, much saliva	Ipecac
Nausea in morning before eating, flatulence, constipation	Sepia
Persistent vomiting, aversion to all food, constipation	Symphoricarpus

I have to say that I have never witnessed any difficulties of this sort among the large number of women whom I have known to take the remedy over the last 35 years, but it is as well to be aware of possible difficulties.

There is some evidence of the remedy's efficacy from human and veterinary studies. Ullman quotes a French double-blind trial using Caulophyllum and four other homeopathic remedies to treat pregnant women which showed that women who were given a remedy were in labour for an average of approximately 5 hours compared with 8 hours for those on placebo (Dorfman et al., 1987). In an Italian clinical study Caulophyllum 7c was given to 22 women in their first pregnancies who had gone into labour spontaneously; 17 had normal deliveries. Compared with 34 labours retrospectively selected by the same criteria, the duration of labour in Caulophyllum-treated women was reduced by a statistically significant 90 minutes (Eid et al., 1993). Christopher Day, the highly respected homeopathic vet, has carried out work on the incidence of stillbirths in a herd of 200 pigs and found that Caulophyllum reduced the rate substantially (Day, 1993).

Two or three days prior to expected delivery Arnica may also be given at the acute level, increasing to first aid level for six doses if possible on the day of delivery, then continuing post partum at the acute level for 7–10 days as necessary. The remedy will not help to reduce pain to any great extent but will help with tiredness from the effort of childbirth and speed recovery. If stitching has been necessary, Hypericum could be taken as well as the Arnica, allowing half an hour between the two remedies. If any tearing has occurred or a Caesarean was necessary, then Bellis perennis may be taken in place of the Arnica. Calendula cream may be applied to cracked nipples.

REMEDIES FOR TREATING INFANTS

The notion of a specialist homeopathic provision for children followed the trend established in early orthodox medicine (Leary, 1995). A textbook was published by Hartman (1853) dealing with infants and their management, although it covered the diseases of older children as well. Another textbook by Teste (1854) with similar content appeared 2 years later. The London Homeopathic Hospital opened a children's ward in 1895, at which time 17% of admissions were children under the age of 14 years. This percentage rose to 33% of admissions within 20 years. Glasgow enjoyed the presence of a dedicated Children's Hospital for many years. Paediatric homeopathy is similar to homeopathy in that clinical observation of symptoms and behaviour replace subjective assessments. Infants respond well to homeopathic treatment; the vital force is young and strong and environmental influences have not taken hold. In the early stages of life any of the remedies listed in the first section of this chapter can be used safely whether as crystals, granules, liquid or crushed tablets. Crushing of tablets for infants can be most easily carried out between two teaspoons.

Early stages

The most widely used of all infant remedies is Chamomilla. The indications for this remedy are colic and teething, particularly in children who are fretful and want to be carried. Another remedy for teething is a combination of three ingredients: Aconite, Belladonna and Chamomilla, known as ABC. For colic alone Colocynth is an excellent remedy. Babies who do not sleep at night may be given Coffea, or if they have suffered a fright then Aconite is effective.

Later stages

For nappy rash, Calendula cream or ointment is effective, rubbed well in at each change, and covered with white soft paraffin as a barrier against the urine. Occasionally help is requested in the control of bedwetting. A normal child can be expected to gain bladder control during the day from about 18 months old, and during the night about 6 months later. About 50% of enuretic children still wet their beds between the ages of 6 and 7 years. This presents a major problem when the child is going to scout camp or on a school trip and is likely to be embarrassed in the presence of other children. There can be a substantial element of emotional involvement, so counter-prescribing on the basis of physical symptoms alone is unsatisfactory in the long term. A distinction can be made between primary bedwetting, when a child has never been dry, and secondary bedwetting, where the child has been dry but suddenly starts to wet again. The remedy that has been found most useful in the second case is Equisetum. Sanicula may also be indicated for enuresis. The latter remedy has also been used in stubborn constipation in children when symptoms of many drugs overlap (Satti, 1997). There are many possible causes, including allergies, infection and anxiety, as well as physiological causes, so if the problem does not resolve within a fortnight then referral should be considered. Constitutional treatment can be useful.

Childhood diseases can be helped. Chickenpox, for example, responds to Rhus tox where the child is listless, has a fever and rash, or Sulphur where the child has similar symptoms but refuses to eat, despite being very thirsty and hungry.

For further information the reader is referred to the text by Neustaedter entitled *Homeopathic Paediatrics* (Neustaedter, 1991).

REMEDIES FOR TREATING TEENAGERS' PROBLEMS

The teenage years are difficult because although such children seek independence from the parental nest this is nevertheless the very time that support is needed. Childhood needs are still very much present within the teenage body. Parents can offer homeopathic remedies to their offspring with confidence, because homeopathy allows individualisation at each different adolescent stage of development without the possibility of upsetting the delicate behavioural balance that may have been established at any given time. Some suitable remedies to consider are indicated in Table 9.17.

Ruta is an excellent remedy to place in the box of provisions given to a returning student at the start of a new term. It offers a solution for the effects of late night studying (eye-strain, headache and back problems), and also for muscular strain caused by sports activities. The usual first aid remedies – Arnica (mental and physical exhaustion, bruising), Arsen alb (diarrhoea),

Table 9.17   Useful remedies for some common teenage problems (adapted from Smith, 1994)

Condition	Remedies	Indications
Acne	Antim crud	Thick, hard, painful and often infected, worse for heat (especially at night) and application of cold water
	Graphites	Dry, crusty, oozing, worse for warmth at night
	Sulphur	Dry, scaly; grey colour, itches and suppurates
Blushing	Belladonna	Shyness, anxiety in social situations
	Lycopodium	Lack of confidence
Body odour	Carbo veg	Gastric problems, distention and flatulence
	Merc sol	Skin covered with offensive perspiration
Boils	Antim crud	Recurrent pustular eruptions that itch
	Hepar sulph	Unhealthy cracked skin that becomes infected Better for heat
	Sulphur	Recurrent boils, diarrhoea, greasy skin
Concentration – poor	Lycopodium	Constant distraction, feelings of insecurity
	Pulsatilla	Concentration affected by a changeable nature
	Natrum mur	Distraction caused by anxiety and worry
Examination fears	Aconite	Terror – not likely to turn up for exam
	Argent nit	Worry about failure, anxiety; aggravated by heat
	Gelsemium	Milder types of anxiety
Eyestrain	Euphrasia	Acrid lachrymation; red – conjunctivitis
	Ruta grav	Eyestrain from reading, eyes hot and painful, headache; back pain
Home sickness	Acid phos	Anxiety, depression and home sickness
Perspiration – excess	Ipecac	Sweating associated with nausea and vomiting
	Pulsatilla	Sweating associated with shyness and anxiety
	Thuja	Sweating is offensive and associated with warts
Shyness	Arsen alb	The neat and tidy loner who avoids others
	Gelsemium	Milder shyness
	Natrum mur	Anxious and possibly depressed
	Pulsatilla	Terrified by being in the limelight

Belladonna (sore throats, headaches) and Gelsemium (colds and flu, exam nerves) – could also be components of a small kit.

Some of the Bach flower remedies have been used successfully to treat mental symptoms, particularly Rescue Remedy for examination worries (see Ch. 10).

For further information on this subject, the reader is referred to a slim volume by Dr Trevor Smith entitled *Homeopathy for Teenagers' Problems* from which the table has been adapted (Smith, 1994).

There is a German product called Traumee that can be applied topically with gentle massage. It is also available as drops for internal use and comprises no fewer than 14 different homeopathic medicines, mostly in the 1x and 3x potencies. It is occasionally requested by foreign visitors. The product has been the subject of an impressive number of clinical trials and is one of a number of complex products for sports use marketed in Europe and the USA.

Common sports-related illnesses and their treatment

Here there are two classes of problems, those contracted during sports activity (examples are scrumpox, water-related conditions, climatic problems and insect bites) and those contracted in the changing room (fungal infections and verrucae):

1. Scrumpox. This is commonly caused by the virus herpes simplex. It is highly infectious, spreading by direct contact and droplet spread. Impetigo and erysipelas are also blamed for this condition. Rhus tox or Apis might be appropriate in the latter cases, while a Herpes nosode is available for the former.
2. Water-related conditions. Swimmers are susceptible to a number of illnesses including eye conditions that may respond to Calendula or Euphrasia eyedrops. Gastrointestinal diseases may be treated with Arsen alb, or Nux vom. Jellyfish stings respond to Ledum.
3. Effects of climate. In hot weather the possibility of heat exhaustion must be considered. Together with the normal first aid activities (lying the patient down in the cool, giving plenty of fluids, etc.), Natrum carb (patient quiet, thirsty and sensitive to noise), Glonoinum (better from uncovering the head, throbbing headache and absence of thirst) or Belladonna (red hot swollen face, sudden onset of headache) should be administered. Frostbite medicines include Agaricus, Apis and Lachesis; hypothermia is treated with Camphor.
4. Effects of altitude. The symptoms of altitude sickness come on suddenly and include pounding headaches, nausea, loss of appetite, dehydration and breathlessness. Sleep is also a problem with disrupted breathing patterns. Diazepam and temazepam have been used to help sleep at altitude, but the hangover effect from these two drugs is dangerous, for climbers must be alert at all times. Mountaineers have used the diuretic effect of acetazolamide to help with acclimatisation, but this can be substituted by Coca in the 30c potency. Cactus has also been used (Kayne, 1992a).
5. Insect bites. These can be treated with Apis or Ledum. A commercial mixture of seven homeopathic tinctures is also effective.
6. Fungal infections. The most commonly occurring fungal infection is athlete's foot (tinea pedis). Generally this and other similar ringworm infections including tinea cruris are self-limiting, but athletes are unwilling to allow these conditions to linger on untreated for weeks or even months. Old-fashioned remedies like Whitfield's ointment and

potassium permanganate may be augmented with remedies such as Rhus tox, Sepia, Sulphur or Tellurium.

7. Verrucae and warts may be treated orally twice or three times daily with either Acid nitric or Thuja. If the skin is not broken Thuja may be applied topically as ointment or mother tincture. Both are usually applied sparingly once daily.

Other conditions

One of the difficulties in treating sports persons is that the WADA regulations state that athletes at elite and sub-elite levels can be dope tested during training as well as during competition. This means that an athlete complaining of a cough or cold might be sold an OTC product containing a banned substance. The range of homeopathic cough and cold remedies provides a useful means of ensuring that the athlete is not at risk. There are problems like insomnia and anxiety for which no orthodox remedies are available.

Anxiety and excitement can affect performance in competitive sport. They may also lead to diarrhoea and insomnia. In such circumstances Argent nit or Aconite is effective. Two doses of Gelsemium have also been suggested to relieve anxiety before a boxing match (Schmidt, 1988). Insomnia responds to Coffea or Passiflora, and diarrhoea to Arsenicum album. There are a number of other antidiarrhoeals including Podophyllum, Veratrum alb and Croton tig, but these drug pictures are less frequently indicated in sports persons.

Performance-enhancing preparations

There is one remarkable report in the literature of homeopathic Arsenic being administered to the members of a boxing team in the Indian Military Academy with apparent success. Two unexpected wins were subsequently recorded (Negi, 1985). In order to accelerate the oxidation rate within cells, which is important to facilitate the release of energy, it has been suggested that the remedies Vanadium and Ferrum met should be used, together with Cobalt to improve nervous reflexes. The report is recorded without further comment!

DENTAL APPLICATIONS

The use of homeopathy by dental colleagues is small in quantity at present, but growing at an impressive rate. Examples of dental uses are summarised in Table 9.18. The main advantages of using homeopathy are that the remedies do not interfere with existing medication and that there is no possibility of an overdose of analgesics or antianxiolytics.

It should be noted that some remedies should be used prophylactically. Arnica, for instance, should be given prior to dental surgery. It does not reduce pain but speeds the recovery process. The box below gives a case study of the use of Arnica here. It is fully acknowledged that the case described is hardly the stuff clinical trials are made of – but it does give cir-

Table 9.18 Remedies that can be used for dental conditions

Indication	Remedy to be considered
Anticipation, anxiety	Argent nit, Aconite, Staphysagria (after extraction)
Preoperative	Arnica (as prophylactic, start 2 days before), Calendula
Postoperative	Arnica (bruising), Belladonna (pain), Calendula (antiseptic), Staphysagria (pain and anxiety after surgery)
Bone involvement	Symphytum, Calc phos
Gum disorders	Belladonna, Merc sol
Cold sores	Hypericum and Calendula mother tincture
Mouth – soreness and ulcers	Borax, Calendula mouthwash

cumstantial evidence of the efficacy of Arnica. In a Norwegian randomised double-blind trial six homeopathic medicines were chosen in the 30x potency (Arnica, Hypericum, Staphysagria, Ledum, Phosphorus and Plantago) to study the effect of using homeopathy after dental surgery (Lökken et al., 1995). The remedies were individualised to each patient; 21 out of the 24 patients eventually ended up with Arnica. Treatment started 3 hours after completion of surgery. Not surprisingly, no positive evidence was found for the efficacy of homeopathic treatment, because for a beneficial clinical result the remedy must be given before treatment, and continued immediately after.

Case Study: Dental surgery

A 26-year-old woman attended the dental surgery for removal of her left upper wisdom tooth under local anaesthetic 'in the chair'. She experienced considerable pain and discomfort that subsided after 5 days with the help of analgesics.

Remedy: Arnica 30c
Dose: Two days prior to returning for another similar extraction she took two tablets of Arnica 30c three times a day, increasing every 15 minutes for six doses on the day of the visit. After the extraction she took two tablets four times a day for 4 days
Result: She was able to go out to a dance on the night of the day on which her extraction took place. Pain and swelling were much less than before and she recovered with only minor discomfort after 24 hours

Subsequently the patient was given Symphytum 30c (at the acute level for 7 days) to aid repair of the bone.

Arnica can also be used as a gargle; 15 ml of mother tincture in 500 ml of warm water is an effective mouthwash or gargle. It may be combined with Hypericum or Calendula.

Almeida et al. (2004) compared the preventive action of fluorine and evaluated the effect of homeopathic medicines on the teeth of 60 male rats fed a cariogenic diet. The double-blind randomised placebo controlled trial used six remedies: placebo, Calc phos, Calc fluor, Kreos, Nat fluor 6c and Fluorine (NaF 0.05%).

Calc phos and Calc fluor were indicated due to their relation with basic dental salts (particularly calcium phosphate and calcium fluoride) and based on the pathophysiology of dental caries which considers that this disease is a consequence of a lack of the balance in the calcium salts' metabolism (Schüssler's Theory, see Ch. 10). Kreosotum was included because of the similarity between signs and symptoms described in homeopathic materia medica and the signs and symptoms of dental caries (similarity principle). Fluorine, which is widely used to prevent dental caries, can cause an intoxication called 'fluorosis', which is very similar to dental caries. Sodium fluoride was included for this reason.

A swab was applied directly in the dental surface and gingival mucous membrane daily for 35 days. None of the groups included in this study developed caries. Commenting on this work, Darby and Villano Bonamin (2004) stated it is likely that the prevention of dental decay with homeopathic medicines is some way in the future.

The dental applications of homeopathy are covered comprehensively by Colin Lessell in his *Textbook of Dental Homeopathy* (Lessell, 1995).

THE TRAVELLING HOMEOPATH

Useful remedies for a traveller's kit are summarised in Table 9.19. Some case studies are illustrated below.

Case Studies: Homeopathy for travellers

Flying
Man, aged 35, terrified at the thought of flying. Had already cancelled a holiday at the last moment because it involved flying

Remedy: Aconite 30c tablets
Dose: Two tablets three times daily, starting 7 days before departure, increased to two tablets every half hour on day of departure. Similar regimen for return flight
Result: Still unhappy, but did take flights in both directions without feelings of terror

'Holiday tummy'
Teenager, returned from holiday abroad, with diarrhoea and vomiting

Remedy: Arsen alb granules
Dose: One dose of granules every 15 minutes for six doses, then three times daily
Result: Condition improved within an hour; cleared up within 24 hours

---

Use of nosodes and sarcodes as 'vaccines'

From time to time requests for 'vaccines' are received from people who are visiting areas where the risk of diseases such as malaria and cholera is high.

Table 9.19 Some suitable remedies for travellers

Indication	Remedy
Abrasions (superficial), antiseptic	Calendula (as liquid or cream)
Accidents	Arnica (as tablets or topicals)
Allergies	Euphrasia
Antiseptic; superficial abrasions	Calendula (as liquid or cream)
Anxiety about flying	Argent nit (worry), Aconite (terror)
'Blood and crush' remedy	Hypericum
Diarrhoea and vomiting	Arsen alb, Melissa Co (Weleda)
Heat stroke, sudden headache	Belladonna
Indigestion, overeating and drinking	Nux vom
Insect bites	Apis (stings), Ledum (puncture), Combudoron® (Weleda)
Insect repellent	Pyrethrum spray (A Nelson & Co)
Insomnia	Coffea, Passiflora, Noctura® (A Nelson & Co)
Jet lag	Arnica
Mouth wash	Calendula mother tincture
Motion sickness*	Cocculus (air, car), Petroleum (car, train), Sanicula (sea), Tabacum (sea)
Skin rash from the sun	Belladonna
Sunburn	Burn ointment, Urtica cream (after sun), Combudoron® (Weleda): Cantharis

* Cocculus: headache, nausea, 'weakness all over', aversion to food.
Petroleum: occipital headache with nausea, vertigo; pains in the stomach.
Sanicula: profuse sweat on occiput, constipation, nausea and vomiting; thirst.
Tabacum: cold feeling, profuse sweat and exhaustion; nausea.

The so-called vaccines are really nosodes, or in some cases sarcodes (see Ch. 8). There is no evidence that they confer any protection. Health authorities are unlikely to accept vaccination certificates on the basis of homeopathic remedies (see p. 171).

Reactions to sun

There is a remedy called Sol, in which the mother tincture is made by exposing an alcohol/water mixture to direct sunlight for 5 hours. The 6c potency can be taken prophylactically by clients who suffer from exposure to the sun, commencing 5 or 6 days prior to departure, at the acute level of dosing, rising to the first aid level immediately prior to departure and then reverting to the acute level for the remainder of the trip.

Reactions to insect bites

Pyrethrum can also be potentised and given in a similar manner to clients who are in the habit of reacting badly to insect stings and bites, although it is more usually applied topically.

Effects of X–ray exposure on remedies

It is not unusual for customers to ask if their homeopathic remedies are likely to be adversely affected by X-ray security machines at airports. The intensity of the rays used in these machines is relatively low and in my opinion remedies are unlikely to suffer any deterioration during the three or four exposures an average holiday might involve. However, if repeated exposure is likely, on an extended business trip for example, then it would be prudent to request a hand search. If this is done the traveller should be careful not to arouse suspicion – homeopathic remedies look remarkably similar to certain drugs of abuse. On more than one occasion I have been disturbed from my slumbers by an irate customs officer wanting assurance that the innocent-looking granules found in someone's case were not something more sinister. Another solution is to pack the remedies in the lead bags sold in photography shops to protect films.

Further information

If you are interested in this aspect of homeopathic practice there is a comprehensive text written by Colin Lessell that comes highly recommended (Lessell, 1993). According to a review by Richard Laing (1993), *The World Traveller's Manual of Homeopathy* gives 'a fascinating panorama of the myriad ways in which the unwary traveller may be infected, infested, stung, bitten or envenomed, quite apart from the common ailments resulting from fatigue, sprains, heat and cold. From travellers' nerves and fractious children, sore feet and back strain, to typhoid fever and the sting of the box jellyfish, no stone is left unturned'.

AGRICULTURAL AND VETERINARY HOMEOPATHY

Pharmacists with an interest in agricultural and veterinary pharmacy (or pet care) may wish to take advantage of the growing market in homeopathy in these areas.

Agricultural applications

Unfortunately there is no agricultural pharmacopoeia to which one can refer and much work remains to be done to enable suitable remedies and potencies to be chosen with confidence. Homeopathic remedies are sometimes used in organic farming, both as sprays and in ground feed. Some of these applications are outlined in the section dealing with anthroposophical medicines (see Ch. 10). An example of homeopathic medication was the treatment with Tabacum 30c of a papaya tree where the leaves were mosaic, curled and closed. The leaves began to spread open within 4 days. The medicine was selected on the basis of resemblance of tobacco leaf characters to the affected leaves of the papaya (Sinha, 1976).

Dr Marjorie Blackie, in her book *The Patient not the Cure* (1976), reports the case of two turkey oaks with oozing wounds that responded to treatment with Sulphur 6c and Mercurius 6c and 30c. McIvor (1980) has reported success in treating fruit trees, including nectarine, plum and peach, isopathically using dilutions of the fungus that causes leaf curl. A fine hole was drilled into the tree trunk about 15 cm above ground level and the 6c potency injected under pressure.

Veterinary applications

Some time between 1811 and 1829 Hahnemann expressed an interest in veterinary homeopathy. He produced 12 pages of notes for a lecture entitled 'The homeopathic science of healing domestic animals'. It is not clear for whom the lecture was prepared, nor whether it was ever delivered (Kaiser, 1991). In his final paragraph Hahnemann wrote 'they (animals) do not lie to us or deceive us, as humans do when they indulge secretly in what is harmful to them without letting the physician know it. In one word, animals can be cured homeopathically at least as safely and certainly as humans.' I have already referred to Joseph Wilhelm Lux (credited with inventing the term 'isopathy') who was appointed Professor of Veterinary Science at the University of Leipzig in 1806 at the age of 30 years. He used homeopathy in treating animals from about 1820 onwards. In 1831 he was asked for a homeopathic remedy to treat anthrax and distemper. Not knowing of an appropriate homeopathic remedy, the Professor suggested that the animals were treated respectively with either a 30c dilution of a drop of blood or nasal mucus. The favourable results of this new procedure led to a range of disease agents and body fluids being potentised for both contagious and non-contagious conditions (Bellavite and Signorini, 1995).

Veterinary homeopathy reached its greatest popularity during the final years of the last century in both the UK and the USA (Coulter, 1979). In 1889 James Moore & Son published their tenth edition of *Outlines of Veterinary Homeopathy* comprising horse, cow, pig, sheep and dog diseases and homeopathic treatments; it was aimed at both practitioners and the general public (Moore, 1889).

They claimed homeopathy to be superior to other medicines because:

- small amounts of medicine were used, giving financial savings
- the animals recovered more quickly and could return to work sooner

- the working animals were treated in a more kindly manner, resulting in less diminution of strength
- many diseases, such as 'pleuro-pneumonia' and 'milk fever' in cattle, often would not respond to the medicines of the day but could be cured by homeopathy.

Moore's text described the disease progressions listing appropriate medicines in great detail; early homeopaths believed that medicines should not be mixed, but that treatment could begin with one remedy and end with another.

Homeopathic treatment fell out of favour for many years but is now enjoying a revival. It is currently being used in the treatment of both domestic and farm animals to great effect. Homeopathy is especially useful for animals that form part of the food chain, obviating the necessity for protracted withdrawal periods after drug use.

Chris Day, currently Veterinary Dean at the UK Faculty of Homeopathy, has outlined the subtle nuances of veterinary case taking by not interfering with the animal's reality and suggests that the picture presented is like a clear reflection in a tranquil pool. Disturb the water even slightly, he says, 'and the chance to grasp the emerging drug picture is lost'. There is an obvious problem in treating animals effectively without mental or subjective symptoms. The key to successful repertorisation lies in behavioural observation, especially distant observation, and an analysis of disposition and demeanour (Day, 1993). Changes in normal routine are important; it is highly significant if a dog drinks or sits in its basket more than usual, or if its faeces change in their consistency. With information obtained from an owner, veterinarians can even use homeopathic remedies to treat aggressive or emotionally disturbed dogs, obviating the necessity for the often far more drastic orthodox treatment involving powerful sedatives. Naturally shy species, for example Shetland sheepdogs ('Shelties'), respond well to remedies such as Gelsemium.

Pharmacists are well placed to supply homeopathic remedies by counter trade, and on prescription, but the very large number of remedies available often frightens off potential stockists. At the time of writing there are no licensed homeopathic veterinary products in the UK although the necessary regulatory framework exists. Licensed human remedies may be used under an arrangement known as 'the cascade' or the remedies may be made extemporaneously by pharmacists with the necessary authorisation.

In the USA, Homeopet of Westhampton Beach, New York, has a range of small animal, equine and bovine remedies (www.homeopet.com/index.htm). Several Indian companies advertise veterinary products on the internet (www.indianindustry.com/animalhealth/5171.html).

A study has been carried out to identify the six remedies most widely used by a sample of homeopathic veterinarians and the conditions for which they were indicated (Kayne, 1992b). The main results are set out in Table 9.20. The most popular remedies were found to be similar to those used for humans, so to cater for the veterinary market no extra stock is required.

Table 9.20 Veterinary use
of homeopathic remedies

Remedy	% sample using	Main veterinary indications of remedy
Arnica	82	Pain in small animals, pre- and post-surgery, injuries
Arsen alb	41	Diarrhoea, enteritis, eczema in dogs
Hypericum	29	Nerve injuries, spinal crush injuries, damaged nails
Pulsatilla	35	Cat flu, runny noses, hormonal disturbances
Rhus tox	71	Arthritic pain, rheumatism, lameness
Sulphur	29	Skin problems, itches, rashes

There is an increasing demand from the public for homeopathic medicines to treat animals. Under the Veterinary Surgeons' Act 1966, diagnosis and treatment of animals is restricted to veterinarians and owners and this applies to homeopathy too. An illustration of the potential problems that can occur is provided by pharmacists' involvement in supplying Borax to farmers during a disastrous foot and mouth disease (FMD) epidemic in the UK in 2001 (see Box 9.1).

There are several veterinary materia medica available but since there have been no provings carried out on animals the books represent human uses translated into animal terms. A true match with a veterinary drug picture is therefore not possible. There are problems in drawing parallels. Animals have widely differing anatomies; the cow's alimentary canal is quite unlike the human's, for instance. A gerbil's morphology is different from a pig's. Yet, despite these differences, vets have had great success in treating animals on the basis of human indications.

It has already been noted that nosodes are used in veterinary medicine, both prophylactically, when they are often inaccurately called 'vaccines' (e.g. for kennel cough, parvo in dogs), and as an isopathic treatment (e.g. for mastitis in cows, sheep and goats, foot scald in goats, etc.). The Welsh Hedgehog Hospital in Llanddeiniol, Dyfed, has used miasmic nosodes and polychrests very successfully in treating its diminutive patients (Sykes and Durrant, 1995). Animals with parasitic infections, for example coughs due to lung worm, seem to benefit from Sulphur, especially if they are thin and eat a lot.

Some of the most useful homeopathic veterinary books are listed in Appendix 2.

Box 9.1   Homeopathic Borax and foot and mouth disease

In the first quarter of 2001 the UK was in the grip of a major epidemic of foot and mouth disease with hundreds of thousands of animals being slaughtered throughout the country. The disease started at a pig farm in northern England and spread quickly throughout the country. Farmers desperate to provide protection for their animals turned to homeopathy for help, placing extreme pressure on many pharmacies to supply them with the appropriate remedy. Demand for the remedy Borax 30c increased rapidly as the knowledge of its existence spread among the farming community. There was some anecdotal evidence of its beneficial use during the last foot and mouth epidemic to hit the UK in the 1960s but the Faculty of Homeopathy, the governing body for medical and veterinary homeopathy, felt that this was insufficient to claim its effectiveness in preventing the disease.

The Faculty of Homeopathy issued a statement on 2 March 2001 stating that in view of the legal status of this notifiable disease and the MAFF slaughter policy, it did not advise the use of any prophylactic (preventative) medication. The statement pointed out that an eradication scheme and slaughter policy relied on a wholly susceptible animal population, in order to be able to detect disease signs promptly. The danger of using any prophylactic medicine was that, if it is effective, it may render animals unsusceptible. This could result in animals being able to harbour the virus and to shed it, while they remain symptom-free. If they were to become 'carriers', the virus could multiply within them with potentially devastating effect for the national herd.

The statement acknowledged that while there is anecdotal evidence of the beneficial use of homeopathic Borax during the previous foot and mouth outbreak, the Faculty of Homeopathy felt that this was insufficient to claim its efficacy in preventing the spread of the disease.

REFERENCES

Aabel, S (2000) No beneficial effect of isopathic prophylactic treatment for birch pollen allergy during a low-pollen season: a double-blind, placebo-controlled clinical trial of homeopathic Betula 30c. *Br Homeopath J*, 89: 169–173.

Aabel, S (2001) Prophylactic and acute treatment with the homeopathic medicine Betula 30c for birch pollen allergy: a double-blind, randomized, placebo-controlled study of consistency of VAS responses. *Br Homeopath J*, 90: 73–78.

Aabel, S, Laerum, E, Dølvik, S and Djupesland, P (2000) Homeopathic 'immunotherapy' effective? A double-blind, placebo-controlled trial with the isopathic remedy Betula 30c for patients with birch pollen allergy. *Br Homeopath J*, 89: 161–168.

Almeida, NT, D'Almeida, V and Pustiglione, M (2004) The effect of fluorine and homeopathic medicines in rats fed a cariogenic diet. *Homeopathy*, 93: 138–143.

Anon. (1959) Homeopathic injury remedies [Discussion report]. *Br Homeopath J*, 48: 281–285.

Beattie, N and Kayne, SB (2000) Unpublished results.

Bellavite, P and Signorini, A (1995) *Homeopathy: A Frontier in Medical Science*. North Atlantic Books, Berkeley, CA, p 25.

Blackie, M (1976) *The Patient not the Cure*. Macdonald, London, p 144.

Campbell, A (1976) Two pilot controlled trials of Arnica montana. *Br Homeopath J*, 65: 154–158.

Castro, M (1992) *Homeopathy for Mother and Baby*. Macmillan, London.

Clover, A (1990) *Homeopathic First Aid*. Thorsons, Wellingborough.

Clover, A and Ratsey, D (2002) Homeopathic treatment of hot flushes: a pilot study. *Homeopathy*, 91: 75–79.

Coulter, DB (1979) Veterinary homeopathy: the implications of its history for unorthodox veterinary concepts and veterinary medical information. *J Vet Med*, 6: 117–122.

Darby, P and Villano Bonamin, L (2004) Homeopathy and dental caries: implications for dental practice and veterinary research [Editorial]. *Homeopathy*, 93: 119.

Day, CEI (1993) Diagnosis in veterinary homeopathy. *Homeopathic Links*, 6(1): 6–8.

Dorfman, P, Lasserre, M and Tetau, M (1987) Préparation à l'accouchement par homéopathie: expérimentation en double-insu versus placebo. *Cahiers de Biotherapie*, 94: 77–81. (Quoted by: Ullman, D (1988) *Homeopathy: Medicine for the 21st Century*. North Atlantic Books, Berkeley, CA, p 61.)

Eid, P, Felisi, E and Sidera, M (1993) Applicability of homeopathic Caulophyllum thalictroides during labour. *Br Homeopath J*, 82: 245–248.

English, J (1995) Homeopathic treatment of URTI in general practice. *Br Homeopath J*, 84: 207–212.

Gibson, DM (1993) *First Aid Homeopathic in Accidents and Ailments*, 16th edn. British Homeopathic Association, London.

Gray, M (1995) Dr Jean Hindmarsh [Obituary]. *Br Homeopath J*, 84: 247–248.

Hartman, F (1995) Diseases of children (trans. Mempel, New York, 1853). (In: Leary, B (1995) A century of homeopathic paediatrics. *Br Homeopath J*, 84: 238–242.)

Homeopathic Development Foundation (1991) *Homeopathy for the Family*. Wigmore, London.

Kaiser, DA (1991) Rediscovered manuscript of one of Hahnemann's basic writings. *Classical Homeopathy Quarterly*, 4: 66–71.

Kayne, SB (1992a) A mountaineer's homeopathic first aid kit. *Homeopathy*, 42: 222–223.

Kayne, SB (1992b) Homeopathic veterinary practice. *Br Homeopath J*, 81: 25–28.

Kayne, SB and Reeves, A (1994) Sports care and the pharmacist – an opportunity not to be missed. *Pharm J*, 253: 66–67.

Khan, MT (1997) How I treat. *Br Homeopath J*, 86: 92–97.

Labrecque, M, Aider, D, Latulippe, L et al. (1992) Homeopathic treatment of plantar warts. *Can Med Assoc J*, 146(10): 1749–1753.

Laing, R (1993) Book review. *Br Homeopath J*, 82(4): 279–280.

Leary, B (1986) Letter to the editor. *Br Homeopath J*, 75(1): 54.

Leary, B (1995) A century of homeopathic paediatrics. *Br Homeopath J*, 84: 238–242.

Lessell, C (1993) *The World Traveller's Manual of Homeopathy*. CW Daniel, Saffron Walden.

Lessell, C (1995) *Textbook of Dental Homeopathy*. CW Daniel, Saffron Walden.

Lockie, A (1989) *The Family Guide to Homeopathy*. Elm Tree Books, London.

Lockie, A and Geddes, N (1999) *A Woman's Guide to Homeopathy*. Hamish Hamilton, London.

Lokken, P, Straumsheim, PA, Tveiten, D et al. (1995) Effect of homeopathy on pain and other events after acute trauma: placebo controlled trial with bilateral oral surgery. *Br Med J*, 310: 1439–1442.

McIvor, G (1980) Letters to the Editor. *J Am Inst Homeopath*, 73: 43, 48.

Moore, J (Ed) (1889) *Outlines of Veterinary Homeopathy*. Leith and Ross, London.

Muscari-Tomaioli, G, Allegri, F, Miali, E et al. (2001) Observational study of quality of life in patients with headache, receiving homeopathic treatment. *Homeopathy*, 90: 189–197.

Negi, RS (1985) Homeopathy in sports medicine. *Hahnemannian Gleanings*, 52: 244–248.

Neustaedter, R (1991) *Homeopathic Paediatrics*. North Atlantic Books, Berkeley, CA.

Poitevan, B (1998) Review of experimental studies in allergy, part 1. Clinical studies. *Br Homeopath J*, 87: 89–99.

Satti, JA (1997) Sanicula aqua [Letter]. *Br Homeopath J*, 86: 60.

Savage, R (1984) Homeopathy: when no effective alternative. *Br Homeopath J*, 73: 75–83.

Schafer, T (2004) Epidemiology of complementary alternative medicine for asthma and allergy in Europe and Germany. *Ann Allergy Asthma Immunol*, 93: S5–10.

Schmidt, P (1988) Athletic injuries. *Hahnemannian Homeopathic Sandesh*, 12: 115–123.

Shepherd, D (1945) *Homeopathy for the First Aider*. Homeopathic Publishing Company, London.

Shore, J (1994) How I treat seasonal allergies. *Br Homeopath J*, 83: 68–77.

Sinha, EP (1976) Agro-homeopathy. *J Am Inst Homeopath*, 68: 37–40.

Smith, T (1994) *Homeopathy for Teenagers' Problems*. Insight Edition, Worthing.

Stass, M, Michaels, C, Peter, E, Beeutke, R and Carter, RW (2000) Prospective cohort trial of Euphrasia single-dose eye drops in conjunctivitis. *J Altern Complement Med*, 6: 499–508.

Subotnick, S (1991) *Sports and Exercise Injuries: Conventional, Homeopathic and Alternative Treatments*. North Atlantic Books, Berkeley, CA.

Sykes, L and Durrant, J (1995) *The Natural Hedgehog*. Gaia Books, London, p 103.

Taylor, MA, Reilly, D, Llewellyn-Jones, RH, McSharry, C and Aitchison, TA (2000) Randomised controlled trial of homeopathy versus placebo in perennial allergic rhinitis with overview of four trial series. *Br Med J*, 321: 471–476.

Teste, A (1854) *Diseases of Children*. Cincinnati. (In: Leary, B (1995) A century of homeopathic paediatrics. *Br Homeopath J*, 84: 238–242.)

Tveiten, D and Bruset, S (2003) Effect of Arnica D30 in marathon runners: pooled results from two double-blind placebo controlled studies. *Homeopathy*, 93: 187–189.

Ullman, D (1988) *Homeopathy: Medicine for the 21st Century*. North Atlantic Books, Berkeley, CA.

Vickers, AJ, Fisher, P, Smith, C, Wyllie, SE and Rees, R (1998) Homeopathic Arnica 30x is ineffective for muscle soreness after long-distance running: a randomized, double-blind, placebo-controlled trial. *Clin J Pain*, 14: 227–231.

Walach, H, Lowes, T, Mussbach, D et al. (2001) The long-term effects of homeopathic treatment of chronic headaches: one year follow-up and single case time series analysis. *Homeopathy*, 90: 63–72.

Webb, P and Gray, J (1994) Caullophyllum survey. *Simile*, 4: 8–10.

Chapter 10

Therapies allied to homeopathy

CHAPTER CONTENTS

Anthroposophical medicine 255
Evidence 256
Flower remedies 257
Bach flower remedies 258
   Edward Bach 258
   Preparation of Bach remedies 259

Clinical uses of the Bach flower
   remedies 259
Rescue remedy 260
   Evidence 261
Other flower remedies 262
Biochemic tissue salts ('Schüssler salts') 263

ANTHROPOSOPHICAL MEDICINE

The anthroposophic philosophy is based on the idea that the human intellect has the ability to contact spiritual worlds. It owes its popularisation to Rudolf Steiner (1861–1925), an Austrian-born scientist and artist who believed that man once participated more fully in spiritual processes of the world through a dreamlike consciousness, but had since become restricted by his attachment to material things. The name is derived from the Greek *anthropos*, meaning 'human', and *sophia*, meaning 'wisdom', and its main aim is to stimulate the natural healing forces of the patient. These healing forces comprise:

- a life force that maintains the physical body functions
- an etheric body of non-physical formative forces, particularly active in growth and nutrition
- an astral body, particularly active in the nervous system

a spritual core or ego, reflected in a person's ability to change themselves inwardly.

Anthroposophical practitioners seek to understand illness in terms of the way in which these four elements interact.

Steiner's early experiments in Switzerland finally led to the founding of the Waldorf School Movement, which by 1969 had 80 schools attended by more than 25 000 children in the USA and Europe. Many other projects grew out of Steiner's work, including centres for handicapped children, schools of art, sculpture and drama and research centres.

Great care is taken in collecting raw materials for preparing anthroposophical medicines (Evans and Rodger, 1992). Vegetable material is grown using methods of biodynamic farming, a development of organic practice where the soil is fed to improve its structure and fertility. Soil additives are restricted to homeopathic remedies only; all other hormones and chemicals are excluded. Due cognisance is taken of the natural cycles of the moon, sun and seasons. The first growth of plants is harvested and composted, and a second crop grown on the composted material. The process is repeated, and the third generation of plants is used to prepare the medicine. Manufacturers prefer to produce their own source material whenever possible. Weleda of Ilkeston, Derbyshire, one of 26 Weleda companies world-wide, grows many medicinal plants in its extensive herb gardens. Anthroposophical pharmacy uses different temperatures during the manufacturing process according to the particular remedy involved. Aconite, said to exhibit the properties of 'coolness', is prepared at a lower temperature than Crataegus, a remedy acting on heart muscle and therefore active at body temperature. Anthroposophical practitioners believe that there is a link between warmth and the ego. Paying attention to the temperature during preparation can be seen as helping to relate the remedies to human use. The remedies are extracted, diluted and used without potentisation, or prepared using the homeopathic process of serial dilution and succussion. Iscador, marketed by Weleda in the UK (see Ch. 4), is a mistletoe preparation used to treat cancer. Its complex method of extraction involves mixing winter and summer sap. Drops of one are added to a fine film of the other on a rapidly spinning disc; there is also a controlled fermentation process.

Although an anthroposophical prescription is often highly individualised, taking into account the physical and spiritual features of a patient, there are 'specifics', usually mixtures of several potentised remedies, that can be used in all patients to alleviate certain symptoms. There are treatments for bruises and sprains, burns, chilblains, constipation, indigestion and many other common ailments. Disci comp is an injection comprising potentised Formica (red ant juice) and Bambusa (bamboo nodes) combined with either silver or tin, which is indicated for a variety of acute or chronic back pain problems. Silicea comp contains potencies of Silica (quartz), Belladonna (deadly nightshade) and Argent Nit (silver nitrate) and is used to treat sinusitis.

Evidence

Evidence of anthroposophical medicine is sparse. In a German study 18 unselected patients with chronic inflammatory rheumatic conditions including

10 with confirmed rheumatoid arthritis were treated according to anthropo-sophical principles in an open prospective uncontrolled pilot study with a mean follow up period of 12 months (Simon et al., 1997). Main outcome targets were local and systemic inflammation, subjective status and functional capacity. Treatment comprised a combination of Bryonia, Rhus tox, Apis, Formica and Vespa, individualised to each patient's requirements. There appeared to be a definite reduction in local and systemic inflammatory activity and improvement in mental symptoms. These results must be considered to be of limited validity since the patients were self-selected in that they asked to be treated using anthroposophical medicine, the numbers of patients were low and there was no double blinding. After carrying out a systematic review to summarise and critically evaluate all randomised clinical trials testing the effectiveness of the whole system of anthroposophical medicine, Ernst (2004) concluded that, at present, the question whether the anthroposophical concept of healing generates more good than harm cannot be answered. As with much of complementary medicine the evidence supporting the use of anthroposophy is not robust. However, in international study of more than a thousand patients, Hamre et al. (2005) showed that anthroposophic treatment of primary care patients with acute respiratory and ear symptoms had more favourable outcomes, lower antibiotic prescription rates, fewer adverse drug reactions and higher patient satisfaction.

FLOWER REMEDIES

Over the years the flower remedies have become included under the homeopathic umbrella, and the best known variant, the Bach flower remedies, are included in the *BHomP*. However, there is considerable doubt among homeopaths as to whether they are in fact homeopathic for a number of reasons:

- flower remedies are not prepared by trituration or alcoholic extraction
- there is doubt as to whether the manufacturing process of flower remedies includes standard potentisation
- the flower remedies have not undergone provings
- prescribing is based on accurate perception of archetypes with a psyche (i.e. mental state) rather than matching symptoms to a drug picture
- flower remedies have a wide spectrum of activity and are not known to be negatively affected by aromatic agents, tea, coffee, etc.

This is reflected by the fact that the remedies have to be called 'essences' rather than 'remedies' in the United States for legal reasons. I will use the terms interchangeably. As flower remedies are becoming increasingly popular, and are stocked by many pharmacies, they are included here. Pharmacists practising in tourist areas may experience demand from German visitors particularly, for the Bach flower remedies are difficult to find and extremely expensive in their own country.

Bach flower remedies

Edward Bach

A range of flower remedies were discovered by the English bacteriologist and physician Edward Bach, born in Moseley, Birmingham, on 24 September 1886. Dr Bach (whose name is usually pronounced 'Batch' although the guttural 'ch', as in Scottish 'loch', is also used) trained in medicine and early on became a convinced homeopath, although he found the complexity of homeopathic prescribing rather difficult. He was a profoundly religious man and took up medicine from a desire to heal. Bach took his holidays in Wales and Norfolk, enjoying long walks in the countryside either alone, or latterly with his companion and assistant Nora Weeks. It is claimed that he was intuitively drawn towards certain wild flowers that he was able to associate with particular emotions. Thus, if he experienced a sudden adverse emotion and went outside to seek fresh air and exercise he would always be drawn inextricably towards a particular plant or tree. Simply being in its presence would relieve his emotional state. He believed that these were not just chance occurrences, but indications that he had been led divinely towards a new method of healing.

Initially he found 12 remedies, usually referred to as the 'original healers'. These were as follows:

- **Agimony** (*Agrimonia eupatoria*): for those not wishing to overburden others with their problems
- **Centaury** (*Centaurium umbellatum*): for those who cannot refuse and are anxious to please
- **Cerato** (*Ceratostigma willmottiana*): for those who doubt their ability to make decisions
- **Chicory** (*Cichorium intybus*): for those who are overprotective of others
- **Clematis** (*Clematis vitalba*): for lack of interest in present circumstances
- **Gentian** (*Gentiana amarella*): for those who hesitate in making decisions
- **Impatiens** (*Impatiens glandulifera*): for those who are quick thinking, but impatient
- **Mimulus** (*Mimulus gluttatus*): for timidity and shyness
- **Rock rose** (*Helianthemum nummularium*): for those suffering from terror
- **Scleranthus** (*Scleranthus annuus*): for the indecisive
- **Vervain** (*Verbena officinalis*): for those with fanatical opinions
- **Water violet** (*Hottonia palustris*): for those who prefer to be alone.

In 1934, Dr Bach established a healing centre in a small house at Mount Vernon in Oxfordshire, where many of the plants used in his remedies could be grown in the garden or were available as wild specimens close by. It was here during the final 2 years of his life that he completed his collection of flower remedies with the following:

Aspen, Beech, Cherry plum, Chestnut bud, Crab apple, Elm, Gorse, Heather, Holly, Honeysuckle, Hornbeam, Larch, Mustard, Oak, Olive, Pine, Red chestnut, Rock water, Star of Bethlehem, Sweet chestnut, Vine, Walnut, White chestnut, Wild oat, Wild rose, Willow.

He considered the final total of 38 sufficient to treat the most common negative moods that afflict mankind.

Bach interpreted the doctrine of 'like cures like' rather differently from Hahnemann. He felt that it was wrong to apply a poison to eradicate a disease. Wrong could never drive out wrong: only good could triumph over evil. Bach stated (Barnard, 1987):

> Disease is the natural consequence of disharmony between our bodies and our Souls: it is 'like cures like' because it is the very disease itself which hinders and prevents our carrying our wrong actions too far, and at the same time, is a lesson to teach us to correct our ways and harmonise our lives with the dictates of our Soul.

Dr Bach's explanation for the healing power of his medicinal herbs was quite simple: he believed they were Divinely enriched.

Preparation of Bach remedies

There are two methods of preparation detailed in the *BHomP*.

The 'Sun method' is used to prepare mother tinctures from flowers that bloom during late spring and summer, when the sun is at its strongest. The procedure is carried out where the plants or trees have been gathered, commencing around 9.00 a.m. on a calm settled day. Fifty parts of pure spring water (although the *BHomP* states just 'water', not specifically spring water) are added to a glass container until the level reaches just below the brim. One part of flower heads is floated on the surface of the water. The container is then left in the sunshine for 3 hours, after which the flowers are removed and the remaining solution strained into a glass bottle. It is mixed with an equal quantity of grape brandy, vigorously shaken and stored in a cool dark place.

The 'boiling method' is used to prepare mother tinctures from flowers and twigs of trees, bushes and plants that bloom early in the year, before there is much sunshine. The material is gathered as before, and one part added to 10 parts of water in a glass vessel. The resulting mixture is boiled for half an hour and allowed to cool before being diluted with grape brandy and vigorously shaken.

In both cases the resulting solutions are diluted to 5x using 22% ethanol. There is considerable discussion on the method being used to achieve the 5x dilution. Some authorities are of the opinion that it does not constitute proper potentisation, but it is on the basis of this process that manufacturers claim the homeopathic label for their product.

Clinical uses of the Bach flower remedies

The Bach flower remedies are the most fully described and tested, apart from being the best known, so I will deal with them in a little detail.

How often the remedies are taken depends on each individual patient. If the mood is transient then only one dose might be appropriate; if the condition persists many doses might be taken. Clients should be instructed to add two to four drops of the Bach flower remedy to a cold drink of their choice (fruit juice or still mineral water are both acceptable) and the mixture sipped every 3–5 minutes for acute problems until the feelings have subsided. The remedy should be held in the mouth for a moment before

Table 10.1 Examples of useful Bach flower remedies

Emotion	Bach flower remedy suggested
Terror	Rock rose
Uncertainty through indecision	Scleranthus
Lack of energy	Olive
Envy and jealousy	Holly
Lack of confidence	Larch
Over-enthusiasm	Vervain

swallowing. If no suitable beverage is available, four drops of the remedy may be placed under the tongue. For longer use a dose should be taken four times daily.

The remedies are not used directly for physical symptoms but for the state of mind, the rationale behind this being that this not only hinders recovery but may also be the primary cause of certain diseases. This emphasises the idea that all true healing must come from a spiritual level.

The 38 remedies can be split into six groups:

1. Fear (Aspen, Cherry plum, Mimulus, Red chestnut, Rock rose)
2. Uncertainty (Cerato, Gentian, Gorse, Hornbeam, Scleranthus, Wild oat)
3. Insufficient interest in present circumstances (Chestnut, Clematis, Heather, Honeysuckle, Impatiens, Mustard, Olive, Water violet, White chestnut, Wild rose)
4. Oversensitivity to influences and ideas (Agrimony, Centaury, Holly, Walnut)
5. Despondency or despair (Crab apple, Elm, Larch, Oak, Pine, Star of Bethlehem, Sweet chestnut, Willow)
6. Over-care for the welfare of others (Beech, Chicory, Rock water, Vervain, Vine).

A discussion on the differences within each group is beyond the scope of this book, and the reader is referred to more specialised works available from the manufacturers whose addresses are listed in Appendix 1. Some suitable books are listed in the bibliography (see Appendix 2). As a guide, the most useful remedy from each group is listed in Table 10.1. All Bach's remedies, with the exceptions of Cerato, Olive and Vine, can be found growing naturally in the British Isles.

Rescue remedy

One of the difficulties is that one is treating a mood that can change. Indeed as the patient feels better there is a likelihood that a different flower remedy will be more appropriate. In order to deal with this there is an extremely useful combination of five Bach flower remedies known as Rescue remedy. It was so named for its stabilising and calming effect on the emotions during a crisis. Other variants have similar products called simply 'five flower remedy'.

Three of the five constituents (Clematis, Impatiens and Rock rose) were first used successfully by Bach to treat an ailing crew member from a ship wrecked in a storm off Cromer, eastern England (Vlamis, 1994). The remedy comprises Cherry plum (for fear of not being able to cope mentally), Clematis (for unconsciousness or the 'detached' sensations that often accompany trauma), Impatiens (for impatience, agitation), Rock rose (for terror), and Star of Bethlehem (for the after-effects of shock). This remedy is often used in place of Arnica where the mental symptoms resulting from an accident or overwork are more evident than the physical.

Rescue remedy is also used in veterinary cases, particularly by breeders prior to mating and when showing. Four drops of the remedy can be added to the animal's drinking water. Gregory Vlamis claims that 10 drops to a bucket of water have been reported as being beneficial in the case of large animals but does not give references (Vlamis, 1994).

Plants are known to be affected by environmental stimuli as well as by interrelations with other forms of life. Thus Bach remedies can be used botanically too. When treating plants or trees 'one must put oneself in their place and try and imagine how they are feeling', according to Chancellor (1971). For example, a transplanted tree may suffer from shock, indicating Star of Bethlehem. If it seems to lack the strength to recover from the transplanting, Hornbeam or Olive would be appropriate. If a pot plant is knocked over accidentally or damaged in some other way Rescue remedy® is often useful. Infested or diseased plants may benefit from Crab apple.

Bach Rescue Cream is a skin salve that is claimed to help a wide range of skin conditions. The cream contains the same five remedies as the drops plus Crab apple (sense of uncleanliness).

Evidence

Numerous anecdotal reports exist supporting the view that Rescue remedy is of substantial benefit in stressful situations for both human and veterinary patients (Vlamis, 1994). One is attributed to a Dr Alec Forbes of Bristol. Dr Forbes said that while travelling on a ship he had been called to treat a woman who would not come out of her cabin. She was having an emotional crisis and was distressed and crying. One hour after a dose of Rescue remedy, the woman had recovered sufficiently to walk about on deck. However, a randomised double-blind clinical trial using 100 university students who had previously suffered from examination nerves in which participants took one to four doses daily of Rescue remedy or identical placebo revealed no benefit from taking the remedy (Armstrong and Ernst. 1999). However, it should be stressed that this is only one piece of evidence; users do testify to the effectiveness of the product.

Other flower remedies

The remedies that follow are included for general interest to demonstrate that other flower essences are available (Harvey and Cochrane, 1995; Mansfield, 1995). They will not normally be requested by members of the public. For many years after Edward Bach died no attempts were made to create new flower remedies. Then in 1982 essences were produced from the native plants of California according to methods of Bach, to the opposition of the Bach Centre in the UK who maintain that Bach finished the system when he died. The main themes of the Californian essences, of which there are well over 200, are sexuality, social integration, work, life and growth.

The Australian Bush essences were created by Ian and Kirstin White in the 1980s, although the practice of using essences dates back much earlier. The Australian Aborigines obtained the beneficial effects of a flower essence by eating the whole flower (White, 1993). The essence in the form of dew made potent by the sun would thus be consumed with the flower. These essences have a strong focus on the issues of healing relationships and sexuality, aiming to bring out and cultivate people's positive qualities. Like the Bach flower remedies, the descriptions are almost entirely based on emotional characteristics. However, the method used to choose the appropriate remedy is rather more complicated and may involve some diagnostic techniques, for example kinesiology. The first essence made by the Whites was Bush iris, a remedy claimed to help spiritual development and meditation. There is now a range of 50 remedies in the group, all derived from Australian plants and trees including Banksia, Bottlebrush, Jacaranda, Paw paw and Waratah. They are usually taken as a single essence but can be used in combinations of up to a maximum of seven essences for an enhanced effect if they are all addressing the same theme (www.ausflowers.com.au).

The Alaskan essences, first produced commercially in the summer of 1983 from the native plants of the state, are mainly focused on mental and spiritual ideas, considered 'abstract' by many (http://healthyherbs.about.com/od/floweressences/index_a.htm).

A group of 45 flower essences were developed over a period of 20 years by Dr Arthur Bailey at his practice in Yorkshire. Most of the Bailey flower essences are made from the flowering parts of specimens, although a few use other parts of the respective plants. Most are made by the Bach sun method using either water or alcohol. Although many of the sources are similar to homeopathic remedies, their suggested uses differ widely (www.baileyessences.com).

Another range of related essences are the Green Man group, covering 74 trees grown in the British Isles and offering separate male and female forms where the trees are sexed. The first essence made was from the flowers of the hazel tree, whose qualities encourage the growth of new skills and information (www.greenmantrees.demon.co.uk).

There is currently great interest in essences from the flowers of tropical, subtropical and equatorial regions. The Himalayan tree and flower essences, the Amazon orchid essences and the Hawaiian essences are examples. The Christchurch flower essences were assembled in New Zealand by Dr Wendy Isbell. They comprise spring, summer and blended essences. Like all the

PART 5

Research and education

PART CONTENTS

11. Homeopathic research   269

12. Education   321

Chapter 11

Homeopathic research

CHAPTER CONTENTS

Introduction 270
Classification of homeopathic research 271
Providing an evidence base for
   homeopathy 271
General difficulties 271
   Availability of resources 271
Research techniques 272
   Aims 272
   Methodology 272
   Accuracy of test materials 273
   Reproducibility of test materials 273
   Placebo error 273
   Recording measurements 273
   Quantifying the placebo response 275
Interaction with colleagues 275
   Cooperation 275
   Institutional censorship 275
Publication issues 275
   Poor presentation 275
   Biased journals 275
   Editorial censorship 276
   Value of peer review 276
   Misleading content 276
   Ongoing work 277
Designing research protocols 277

Clinical research to address the
   question: Does homeopathy work? 279
Early work 279
Measures of efficacy and effectiveness 280
Outcome measures 281
   The VAS 281
   GHHOS 282
   The OPIC 283
Randomised clinical trials 285
   Early trials 286
   Gibson's rheumatoid arthritis trials 286
   Placebo studies 288
Trials on specific remedies 291
   Arnica 291
   So, does Arnica work? 293
   Arsenicum album 293
   Rhus tox 293
Other trials 294
The meta-analysis and review of
   homeopathic trials 294
Problems with RCTs 296
   Selecting subjects 296
   Randomisation 297
   Complexity of homeopathic response 297
   Quality of evidence 298

Maybe not a gold standard?	298	The Benveniste controversy	302
Another approach	298	Benveniste – an interview	304
Examples of outcomes and		Entanglement theories	306
observational research	298	Other research	307
Case reports	299	Audit studies	307
The Delphi project	300	Attitudes and awareness studies	307
Research to address the question:		Agricultural research	308
How does homeopathy work?	300	Veterinary research	310
Local causality	300	Homeopathic research – time for a	
Non-local causality: interaction		change of emphasis?	311
with diluent	301	Summary	313

INTRODUCTION

Homeopathy is enjoying increased consumer-led demand, even though objectively convincing data to support its claims tend to be conflicting (Walach, 2000) due to difficulties in obtaining consistent results with conventional medical trials (Stevinson et al., 2003). In order to secure general acceptance for homeopathy it is crucial to secure an overall theory to explain its effects.

According to Walach (2003a), 'we face the situation that homeopathy, as a medical theory, is only weakly supported by experimental facts, and highly endorsed by circumstantial and anecdotal evidence, which is unique in the history of medicine over such a long time.'

Colleagues demand high quality evidence from RCTs yet even when this is provided it is rejected if positive (Vandenbroucke, 1997). Speaking at a conference in 1998 on integrated medicine in the UK Iain Chalmers, the director of the UK Cochrane Centre, said that critics of complementary medicine often seem to operate a double standard, being far more assiduous in their attempts to outlaw unevaluated complementary practices than unevaluated orthodox practices. He went on to say that these double standards might be acceptable if orthodox medicine was based solely on practices which had been shown to do more good than harm, and if the mechanisms through which their beneficial elements had their effects were understood, but that neither of these conditions applied (Bower, 1998). Ernst has been particularly active in questioning the evidence produced for homeopathy (and indeed other complementary disciplines), asking whether the demise of homeopathy was imminent (Ernst, 2000) and whether we should be using 'powerful placebos' (Ernst, 2004a). His views have been branded 'misleading' (Kayne and Kayne, 2000) and 'neither balanced nor penetrating' (Mathie and Kayne, 2004).

Throughout the text I have quoted research papers where appropriate. In this chapter I intend to look at homeopathic research in a broader way, discussing the problems, methodology and protocol design. Some of the more important contributions will be critically reviewed in a little more detail. Hopefully this will give a feel for the mix of positive and negative research literature; it is not the intention to offer an exhaustive critical review and make a pronouncement on the worth of using homeopathy. Readers wishing to follow up current research in greater detail may wish to contact the Glasgow Homeopathic Library and its Hom-Inform service (see Appendix 1 for address).

CLASSIFICATION OF HOMEOPATHIC RESEARCH

Essentially homeopathic research falls into two categories:

1. clinical and scientific studies to provide evidence that homeopathy works
2. research aimed at improving homeopathic practice to secure better outcomes.

In practice it is not so simple – nothing is, in homeopathy! There is a crossover between the two areas in terms of the aims of research and in some cases the techniques used to measure outcomes. For example, studies aimed at unravelling the mechanisms of homeopathic interventions might be considered to fall into the first category but could theoretically lead to improving practice as well – as they often do in allopathic medicine. Audit could also fit into either group.

PROVIDING AN EVIDENCE BASE FOR HOMEOPATHY

General difficulties

Availability of resources

Few well-designed studies have been reproduced by independent research teams. This situation exists for two major reasons: lack of sufficient funding and lack of a sufficient number of well-trained homeopaths qualified and interested to participate in research.

Funding for orthodox research by large multinational companies continues to be significant; by comparison that available for homeopathy is small. The pharmaceutical industry invests some 36% of turnover back into research and development in the UK, that is, £3.3 billion a year (ABPI, 2004). Certainly, the possible rewards from bringing a new allopathic drug to the market are huge compared with the possible turnover from homeopathy.

Availability of high quality research facilities may also be a problem. These limitations mean that industry sponsored research on own products, particularly in France and Germany, forms a larger proportion of the research activities than might be desirable.

Apart from the UK sources of funds identified in Chapter 1 for CAM as a whole, in which homeopathy shares, research grants are available from the British Homeopathic Association, the Faculty of Homeopathy and the Scottish Homeopathic Research and Education Trust (SHRET). There are other sources of funds too, including the Research Council for Complementary Medicine France, and the US has government funded research.

Research techniques

Aims

Certain scientific standards must be met in the objectives. Thus a hypothesis should be set and tested. With such uncertainty as to the mechanisms of action of homeopathy, research tends to proceed in an uncoordinated fashion, a large number of different ideas being investigated by individuals almost in isolation.

Methodology

Scofield (1984a) has stated that: 'despite the great deal of experimental and clinical work there is only little evidence to suggest that homeopathy is effective. This is because of bad design, execution, reporting or failure to repeat experimental work.'

Many of the published studies are indeed flawed, with numerous methodological problems (Merrell and Shalts, 2002). This problem is not confined to homeopathy, for it has been estimated that only 1% of the millions of scientific papers published annually may be considered sound (Anon., 1998a). It depends to some extent on the bias of those making the critique and the importance placed on individual elements of the research.

In a review by Ezzo et al. (2001) the authors conclude that both the number and quality of the primary studies on which much contemporary medical practice stands are remarkably weak. The most common statement in Cochrane reviews was the complaint of the very poor quality of many clinical trials. The number of reviews indicating that modern biomedical procedures show no effect (32/160; 20%) or insufficient evidence (34/160; 21%) seems very high, and the number indicating significant evidence of desirable effect (36/160; 23%) seems very low.

In some articles that report positive outcomes for homeopathy, numerous homeopathic remedies have been prescribed for the same diagnostic category. Critics suggest that the pooling of data from trials using different therapeutic agents to assess the overall success of homeopathic prescribing is incorrect. Research protocols that employ combination remedies, in which a medication contains several homeopathic remedies, fall into the same category.

One of the most common problems is a lack of objective validated outcome measures. Another common problem is a small sample size. In most positive and negative meta-analyses published to date, research data are pulled together artificially based on either a diagnostic category or a particular remedy. Frequently the concentration of the remedy used and the conditions to which it has been applied are different.

In a letter concerning the benefits of Arnica, Rutten (2004) suggests that the homeopathic community needs to work on the shortcomings of the methods, while colleagues in conventional medicine should acknowledge that researchers deserve some space to develop their own scientific identity. Lessons can be learnt from unsuccessful trials (Jansen et al., 1992) and it is important that failures as well as successes are published to allow a balanced view to be advanced.

Accuracy of test materials

Choice of remedy. There is virtually no evidence supporting the choice of the remedy and the potency to be used in any given therapeutic situation (Kleijnen, 2001). Hahnemann's principles have been brought into practice in innumerable ways, as is indicated by the differences among the trials presented in systematic reviews. The process of producing preparations (the percentage of alcohol in the solution, the number of times that the substance must be succussed during potentiation, etc.) and their composition (especially when herbs are used) differ greatly among manufacturers.

Reproducibility of test materials

The reproducibility of remedies across national borders and from producer to producer within domestic markets means that replication of research is often difficult. Orthodox research is used to extreme accuracy in its test material. For homeopathy, however, 'one drop plus 99' varies with the method being used to deliver the drop. In the best estimation it will approximate to 0.1 ml, but bearing in mind that the dilution process may be carried out 30, 200 or even 1000 times the variation could be substantial. Homeopaths would say that within the scale of dilution a few noughts more or less would be hardly significant, and this is probably true, but it worries orthodox researchers. If there are potential inaccuracies with the classical Hahnemannian method of potentisation, what can be said of the Korsakoffian, LM or the very high Skinner potencies (see Ch. 4)? The difficulties implicit in using remedies made in this way for research are obvious. There are other inherent problems with the potentisation process. While the most modern producers prepare their remedies in controlled environments, others do not, and the possibility of unclean laboratory air introducing contaminants exists. Finally, evaporation of alcohol from opened containers means that absolute values for potencies are not possible. None of these inaccuracies appears to affect the efficacy of remedies in a clinical sense, but are examples of the difficulties that exist in applying standard research methodologies to homeopathy. Hornung (1991a) addressed this problem by proposing guidelines for the preparation of serial dilutions used in research. So far standardisation has not been adopted.

Placebo error

A frequent source of error in placebo controlled trials is introduced by the use of unmedicated solid dose forms comprised of lactose alone. For accuracy the placebo should be medicated with alcohol potentised to the same level as the remedy.

Recording measurements

Validity of measurements. Measurements may be:

- invalid or incomplete
- taken over an insufficient length of time.

Figure 11.1   Example of a visual analogue scale (VAS)

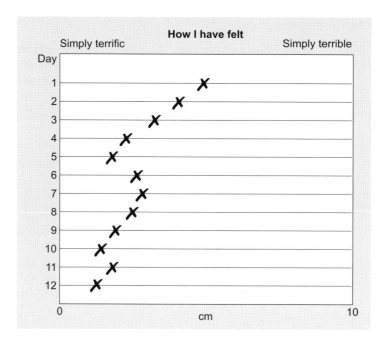

Two responses. All the usual pharmacological tests available today have been developed to investigate potent and toxic drugs of orthodox medicine. If we accept that homeopathy works by stimulating the body to heal itself, without actually disturbing the body's function, the parameters to be measured must be carefully selected and related back to an individual's control. We are interested in whether this particular patient experienced an improvement and so measurements need to be designed with this in mind. If one were to ask 'Who knows best as to whether a patient has improved?' the answer must surely be 'the patient'.

There are really two results for every homeopathic test involving patients:

1. There is a clinical result reflected in an improvement in the diseased state. This can be measured objectively in terms of smaller lesions, or less coughing in a day, or it may be a subjective assessment by the patient, scoring progress on a VAS of 1 to 10 (Fig. 11.1).
2. There is a 'well-being' result, reflected in the patient feeling better 'in themselves'; this feeling may not be directly related to the disease. Thus, a person suffering from an allergic reaction may feel better after taking a homeopathic remedy, even though their symptoms are still troublesome. This assessment has been recognised only recently in allopathic medicine. It is rather more difficult to measure than clinical improvement and often involves the subjective approach mentioned above.

The problems with RCT methodology are outlined below.

Quantifying the placebo response

Quantifying the contribution to data as a result of the placebo response may be difficult. The influence of a prescriber in taking the case, explaining homeopathic principles and the act of taking the remedy may all influence results. A good example of this is the 1978 Gibson et al. study (see p. 286).

Interaction with colleagues

Cooperation

In organising homeopathic research it is often necessary to enlist the assistance of non-homeopathic colleagues in referring patients, handing out questionnaires and allowing access to medical records. Although time is taken to give the necessary explanations, cooperation is often denied; worse still, cooperation may be implied only to be withdrawn half-way through an investigation. Certainly things are improving with time, with good collaborative studies now ongoing in both the UK and US.

Institutional censorship

On the other side of the fence is institutional censorship, a term that refers to explicit or implied intimidation: isolating the so-called heretic from his or her colleagues or threatening sanctions if certain work is pursued. It may result from a researcher's belligerent manner as well as from his or her scientific views. Benveniste, for example, was ostracised from the scientific community following his 'memory of water' experiments (see below, p. 304).

Publication issues

Poor presentation

There may be incomplete statistical evaluation: too few patients to be meaningful and/or poor presentation of results and inappropriate conclusions.

Biased journals

Kleijnen et al. (1991) identified a possible problem in searching the literature. Many homeopathic trials with positive results are accepted for publication only by so-called 'alternative' journals with limited exposure, whereas those with more negative results are likely to be published by orthodox journals, leading to reinforcement of the ideas already held by readers of these journals. Those members of the scientific community who are interested in homeopathic research often find accessibility to homeopathic journals difficult.

Vickers (2000) has examined the scientific debate on whether homeopathy could have effects greater than placebo in humans. He identified five rigorous clinical studies published in high impact journals that favoured homeopathy. Letters and other articles written in response to these papers were then retrieved and analysed. Much of the content of responses to positive homeopathic research was rhetorical in nature and antagonistic; researchers were accused of bias. Vickers concluded that investigators undertaking clinical research need to be responsive to the dangers of publication bias and to the requirement for stronger than usual levels of evidence.

As the editorial points out, meta-analyses of results of trials of homeopathic treatments suggest benefit greater than placebo in some cases, but this can easily be discounted by publication bias. Statistically, some trials of homeopathic treatments will show some benefit even when the real effect of the treatment is zero, and these are the trials that are most likely to be published.

Editorial censorship

The use of 'editorial censorship' to reject unwanted papers has been addressed by Schiff (1995), citing the difficulties experienced by Dr Benveniste in publishing his work on the memory of water (see below). Schiff claims that editors may reject work on the basis of dubious technical arguments that form a smokescreen for the real reason – a bias against the new concepts being put forward.

Value of peer review

Although applied widely, peer review is by no means a secure discipline (Horton, 1995). For instance, Altman (1990) is critical of the entire notion of peer review, a term that he believes is jargon with no agreed meaning. He has described good peer review as the equivalent of effective technical editing. Horton suggests that emotional investment in particular ideas and personal interest in academic success may lead investigators to overemphasise the importance of their findings and the quality of their work. Even more serious conflicts arise when for profit organisations, including pharmaceutical companies, provide funds for research and consulting, conduct data management and analyses, and write reports on behalf of the investigators.

Misleading content

When important outcomes occur infrequently, clinicians should focus on individual outcomes rather than on composite end points. Under these circumstances, inferences about the effect of treatment on the more important end points (which, because they occur infrequently will have very wide confidence intervals) will be weak.

Guides to help recognise methodological weaknesses that may introduce bias are available (Goodman et al., 1993; Montori et al., 2004) but these criteria do not protect readers against misleading interpretations of methodologically sound studies.

Ongoing work

Publishing information about an ongoing trial is useful for it lets the research community, potential funders and the lay public know that the trial exists (Ezzo, 2003). For researchers conducting systematic reviews of the evidence, knowledge of in-progress work is vital. There are few examples in the literature (Walach and Guthlin, 2000). One example of reporting ongoing work is the paper by Steinsbekk et al. (2004) reporting a study that was investigating whether treatment by homeopathy was more efficacious than self-selected conventional health care and whether self-treatment with self-selected homeopathic medicines was more efficacious than placebo in preventing upper respiratory tract infection in children. It was predicted that the results would be available within a few months.

DESIGNING RESEARCH PROTOCOLS

A series of articles that provides an outline of the main methods for researching CAM-related issues, including clinical trials, cross-sectional studies and qualitative methodologies, is now available. Drawing on the experiences of a range of experts in CAM research, each article in this series addresses the scope and strengths of a particular methodological approach (Broom et al., 2004).

The first stage in any research project is the protocol design, drawn up after a period of reflection and discussion. A clear concise protocol is the first requisite for funding. It should comprise a number of headings and, in the first instance, run to no more than about 1000 words:

1. title of project
2. names, qualifications and affiliations of researchers
3. a brief introduction, giving background and previous related work obtained by carrying out a comprehensive literature search. The Glasgow Homeopathic Library may well be able to help in this task (address in Appendix 1)
4. an indication of the project's importance or relevance and timescale
5. an outline of the project methodology, including subjects (numbers, nature, selection criteria, exclusion and arrangements for consent), sampling and measurement techniques, and data handling
6. a realistic financial budget that covers equipment, materials, researchers' time, locums, etc., and makes allowance for time spent analysing data. Most researchers are offered only one bite of the grant allocation cherry, so it is important to ensure that everything is covered
7. if the project involves treatment of patients (either human or veterinary), as opposed to audit, then a member of that profession must be involved. It may be necessary to seek approval from the ethical committees covering the geographic location where the trial is to be carried out. Input from these colleagues will be required. The protocol should record whether ethical approval is necessary and the mechanism for securing patients' agreement to participate
8. appropriate references should be included.

Table 11.1 Internal validity of trials

Item	Parameter	Example
Subjects	Adequacy and comparability Eligibility Sample size Randomisation Control group	Subjects from same source of population? Appropriate exclusion criteria Adequate? Procedures adequate? Is a control group required?
Measurement of outcome	Valid measurements taken Blinding of participants and observers where necessary	Measurements appropriate to type of study Subjects and researchers blind to treatment allocations?
Data	Compliance Withdrawals recorded	Compliance with instructions by patients and researchers? Withdrawals at acceptable level?
Statistics	Presentation Limits of confidence	Results sufficient? Limits stated
Conclusions	Clear conclusions stated Limitations of method	Do results support conclusions? Ways to improve procedures?

Help with drawing up a protocol is available from the Research Officer at the Faculty of Homeopathy, Luton. There are also a number of experienced researchers among the Faculty members who will be pleased to offer advice on protocols and suggest possible sources of financial support. They will know what research is going on elsewhere and be in a position to refine any ideas you may have.

In formulating a research procedure, two important areas of control must be addressed (Vickers, 1995). The issues are broadly the same whether a full scale clinical trial or an attitudes and awareness survey is being contemplated:

1. internal validity is concerned with matters such as control of confounding and bias, sample size and statistical interpretation. It is related to accuracy within the studied group
2. external validity involves two separate questions: that concerning the population chosen and that concerning the validity of the experimental model. It is related to the validity of extrapolating results from the research groups to the general population and the precise nature of the questions (Anon., 1998).

The various issues to be considered in organising a piece of research work are outlined in Tables 11.1 and 11.2.

The more variables a study attempts to control – i.e. the greater the internal validity – the less likely it is to reflect common daily practices – i.e. the less external validity can be achieved. Against this, however, the less a study attempts to change everyday practices the more likely it is to be invalidated by uncontrolled variables. A trade-off between the two is necessary.

Table 11.2 External validity of trials

Item	Parameter	Example
Subjects	Applicability of results	Features of population chosen Number of withdrawals or refusals to take part
Validity of experimental model	'Quality' of researchers Realism of procedures	Experience, qualifications and number Procedures are common practice

Methodology and presentation checklists have been suggested as useful tools to ensure that procedures are standardised, not only in research (Linde et al., 1994), but also in complementary medicine (Reit et al., 1990) and mainstream pharmacy (Hayes et al., 1992; Kayne et al., 1994). Checklists and scoring systems using predefined criteria have become standard methods in systematic reviews for assessing the quality of randomised clinical trials (Kleijnen et al., 1991), so it would seem appropriate to adopt these techniques in setting up the research procedures themselves. A checklist based on the information in Tables 11.1 and 11.2, or on the extensive example provided by Linde in the article referenced above, is recommended.

Mathie (2003a) notes that there are two principal categories of research design: experimental and observational. Each of these forms of research with its particular strengths and weaknesses has importance in homeopathy (Walach et al., 2002).

In a typical experimental study, the researcher investigates the effect of an intervention in comparison with the responses of a randomised control group. Any difference between the groups may be associated with the efficacy of the intervention (see below) . The randomised clinical trial is generally considered to be the gold standard for prospective experimental clinical research.

In an observational study, the researcher does not seek to influence the outcome; rather, he or she merely describes what happens. Observational research can be both prospective and retrospective and includes clinical outcomes and case studies. It measures effectiveness (see below).

CLINICAL RESEARCH TO ADDRESS THE QUESTION: DOES HOMEOPATHY WORK?

Early work

Dean (2004) uncovered 45 studies and trials from 1821 to 1953. Essentially the designs of this research fall into three categories:

1. observational studies of classical homeopathy in mixed conditions (1821–35)
2. pragmatic open label comparisons of classical homeopathy with allopathy or no treatment for mixed or specific conditions (1844–86).

This group includes the cholera trials at the Royal London Homeopathic Hospital in 1854 (see Ch. 1)
3. controlled trials of clinical homeopathy (1914–53).

At the turn of the 20th century, a book was published containing numerous charts that compared scarlet fever, yellow fever, typhoid disease and death rates in homeopathic and allopathic hospitals (Bradford, 1900). The homeopathic hospitals usually had between 50 and 80% less deaths per 100 people, depending on the disease compared.

Measures of efficacy and effectiveness

Studies can be designed to be either *explanatory* or *pragmatic* (Schwartz and Lellouch, 1967). Explanatory trials are designed to find out whether a treatment has any efficacy (usually compared with placebo) under ideal, experimental conditions. Pragmatic trials are designed to find out about how effective a treatment actually is in routine, everyday practice (MacPhaerson, 2004).

Efficacy is a term of medical evaluation. It tends to be clinically oriented. An assessment is made of the effects actually observed, in relation to the desired or expected therapeutic goals. The results are therefore evaluated according to the perceived therapeutic success. Examples are randomised trials of homeopathy against standard care or no intervention, and long-term audit studies using validated measures that can answer such questions as 'What is the efficacy of homeopathy in practice?' and 'Which patients and conditions respond to homeopathy?' The outcome is usually measured by the researcher.

Effectiveness is represented by any influence on a biological system that is not specifically directed towards a certain therapeutic goal, the tangible results of which can be observed and measured after a drug has been administered. Outcomes tend to be patient oriented and refer to a clinical result measured (or perceived) under 'field' or 'real-world' conditions. Thus, if a homeopathic medicine is given to a patient who is then seen to improve, one would say the remedy was effective rather than efficacious. Theoretical justification is not usually an issue. There is no doubt that what is perceived as being 'effective' differs widely between patients, and in many cases between patient and prescriber too.

Part of this divergence may be due to the fact that it is possible to identify two treatment outcomes. The first, an improvement in the clinical characteristics of the condition being treated, can be assessed in terms of any or all the following:

- resolution of symptoms
- less discomfort
- a need to take less medication.

The second outcome concerns the patient's overall feeling of wellness. This is largely subjective and may vary from day to day. Patients differ in their ability to deal with disease and this may be reflected in the success or otherwise of treatment.

Table 11.3 Basic homeopathic research

Research on effect	Research on efficacy
Aim: gathering scientific proof	Aim: improvement of techniques
Limited patient input	Patient's attitudes and awareness and their perceptions of efficacy important
Experiments carried out mainly in vitro	Clinical trials and audit studies
Investigations and evaluation by *scientists* to find out *what* happens	Evaluation of results by *statisticians* to find out if the results are significant
Investigations by scientists to find out *how* it happens: crucial to acceptance of the discipline of homeopathy	Mechanisms of action are less important
Verification of homeopathic laws: experiments to test the Law of Similars	Clinical observations; patient based studies on interactions and posology
Result: academic scientific evidence (may result in improved procedures)	**Result:** clinical: improved procedures

In fact, some research overlaps, and it is not always possible to place studies in one group or the other. Table 11.3 sums up the features of the two approaches.

Outcome measures

There is a range of outcome measures routinely used for pragmatic studies:

- Simple yes/no/don't know
- A Visual Analogue Scale (VAS)
- Glasgow Homeopathic Hospital Outcome Scale (GHHOS)
- Overall progress interaction chart (OPIC)
- Yes/no.

The simple yes/no response to a question 'Do you feel better?' or 'Did the medicine help you?' has obvious limitations both in amount of information given and the uncertainty it may create. Adding two further options, 'Too soon to say' or the infamous 'Don't know', may offer some refinement. When applied to homeopathy it is often found that women appear to be more positive than men, whose score for 'Too soon to say' is higher than female respondents (Kayne et al., 1999).

The VAS

An example of a VAS is shown above in Figure 11.1. It comprises a number of parallel 10 cm lines corresponding to days of the month on which patients may be invited to place a cross signifying the severity of symptoms or

---

Box 11.1   Glasgow Homeopathic Hospital Outcome Scale

+ 4 Cured or 'back to normal'
+ 3 Major improvement
+ 2 Moderate improvement
+ 1 Slight improvement
0 No change or 'don't know'
− 1 Slight deterioration
− 2 Moderate deterioration
− 3 Major deterioration
− 4 Disastrous deterioration

---

quality of life on the appropriate day. If a run-in period of no medication is not used to establish a base score patients should consider the first day score to be half way down the line so they have sufficient room to go in either direction.

GHHOS

The Glasgow Homeopathic Hospital Outcome Scale is an attempt at turning subjective observations into a more structured subjective score. It measures both clinical symptoms and quality of life or 'well-being'. Patients (and practitioners) are required to self-assess their progress from + 4 to − 4 according to the scale illustrated in Box 11.1. The practitioner generally also scores the situation for comparison.

The GHHOS may be used on a case-by-case basis but it is also possible to pool the results from large numbers of patients using a particular remedy and gain some insight into the degree of help a patient might expect. Figure 11.2 shows how pooled results can be displayed. In this example some interesting trends emerge:

- Arnica: 95% of all cases treated with Arnica responded positively with 43% of cases scoring + 2 or + 3 and a further 18% scoring + 4
- Belladonna: 87% of cases responded to Belladonna; 55% of all cases scored + 2 or + 3 and a further 12% scored + 4. More Belladonna cases showed no improvement or deterioration than the other two remedies
- Chamomilla: 95% of all cases responded to Chamomilla; 61% of all cases scored + 2 or + 3 and a further 17% scored + 4.

It should theoretically be possible to record the pooled results against time and determine the faster acting common remedies. The possibility exists to be able to indicate to patients the degree of healing and speed with which improvement may be expected, thus aiding concordance.

Richardson (2001) reported an outcome survey carried out at Liverpool Regional Department of Homeopathic Medicine over a 12-month period between 1 June 1999 and 31 May 2000, using self-assessment by the GHHOS.

Figure 11.2 Illustration of how pooled results from GHHOS assessments may be shown

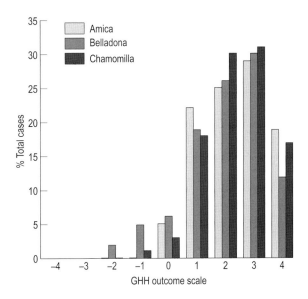

Overall, 76.6% of patients reported an improvement in their condition since starting homeopathic treatment, while 60.3% scored + 2, + 3 or + 4 on the GHHOS; 52% of patients reduced their conventional medication.

The GHHOS was used in many countries but has now been superseded internationally by the Integrative Medicine Outcomes Scale (IMOS) promoted by the Integrative Medicine Data Collection Network (IMDCN) (Heger and Haidvog, 2000).

A hybrid version of the VAS and GHHOS is provided by the cards illustrated in Figure 11.3. These cards are handed out by some British pharmacies to monitor progress following the supply of a homeopathic medicine. Clients are asked to place a tick in the appropriate box on the grid having assessed their condition using the GHHOS. An assessment is made by viewing the slope of a best fit line through the ticks to identify whether the trend is positive or negative.

The OPIC

A method of recording patients' subjective assessment of their clinical or wellness states has been developed by Dr David Reilly and Dr Neil Beattie working at Glasgow Homeopathic Hospital, from an idea described by George Vithoulkas (Vithoulkas, 1980).

It is known as an Overall Progress Interactive Chart or an Observer Patient Interaction Chart and a version is illustrated in Figure 11.4. The abbreviation for both terms is the same – OPIC.

After an initial 4-week 'run-in' period (week – 4 to week 0) during which no remedy is given, patients are asked to draw a purely subjective curve to represent their own assessment of how their symptoms and well-being have

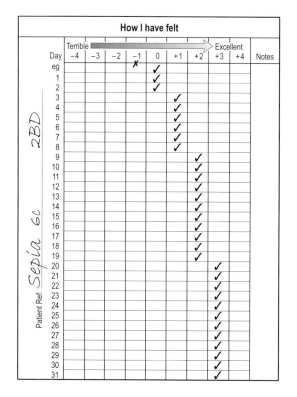
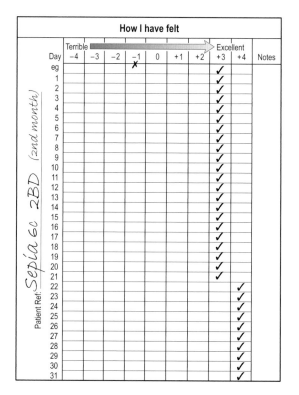

Figure 11.3 Hybrid GHHOS/VAS card (result over 2 months)

Figure 11.4 Example of an OPIC

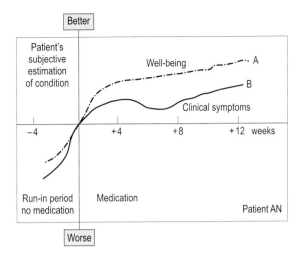

changed. These values are plotted on the diagram as shown in Figure 11.4 and give individual baseline controls for each patient. A remedy is then administered and the patients asked to record their assessments again after a further 4 weeks, by extending the existing lines as appropriate. An estimation of the perceived degree of change can be obtained by measuring the area between the curves and the baseline. An interesting difference between the shapes of the two curves often occurs, assessments of well-being often being quite different from patients' assessments of changes in the symptom pattern. In another variant of the OPIC, the baseline is set at the patients' estimation of well-being and symptoms at – 4 weeks.

Randomised clinical trials

RCTs have been used both to test homeopathy as a therapy against placebo and to assess the response to individual remedies. Most studies in this category refer to the former.

The place of the blinded, randomized, controlled trial (RCT) in assessing forms of homeopathy has been widely questioned, some authors even apparently advocating the view that the time for RCTs in homeopathy is past (Walach, 2003b) and that energy, time and money spent on this form of investigation is bound to be wasted in the long run, as single RCTs of single conventionally diagnosed medical conditions will, at most, sway opinion very slightly in favour for the use of homeopathy in that particular condition, but are very unlikely to change perceptions about homeopathy as a method of helping a large number of people suffering from a very wide range of diagnoses. Supporters of the continued relevance of performing RCTs in homeopathy point to the fact that this is the best and most accepted method yet devised for looking in detail at the efficacy of a particular medical intervention. If homeopathy is to be accepted by the wider medical community, it must expect to use the standard methods of assessment (Oberbaum et al., 2003).

Early trials

According to a review of early homeopathic work by King (1995), the first double-blind cross-over study ever performed was carried out in 1906 by homeopaths (Bellows, 1906). This impressive study was carried out concurrently in 11 different cities on 51 subjects and involved Belladonna.

Gibson's rheumatoid arthritis trials

The first controlled clinical trials are generally ascribed to Gibson et al., working in Glasgow in the 1970s. Their first paper reported the results of a pilot study in which 41 patients with rheumatoid arthritis were treated with 3.9 g per day of aspirin (group 1) and the results compared with a further 54 similar patients treated with homeopathy (group 2). Both groups were compared with a control group of 100 patients who received placebo (Gibson et al., 1978).

All 95 patients admitted to the trial had clinically well diagnosed rheumatoid arthritis and had been under therapy before the trial for a period of at least 4 months up to 6 years, mostly without success. They were assigned alternately to the two therapeutic groups by clinic nursing staff, after having first been seen by the consultant, and were scheduled to maintain their therapy for 1 year. A further 100 rheumatoid patients from the clinic list were placed in the placebo group. The conditions of treatment are summarised in Table 11.4 (adapted from Hornung, 1991b).

A total of 200 different remedies were used in the individualised homeopathic treatment; the most commonly used were Bryonia, Calc carb, Lycopodium, Natrum mur, Pulsatilla and Rhus tox.

The results showed that within the aspirin group (group 1) only six of the 41 patients maintained their medication for the year; these patients showed an improvement in their symptoms. Results for the homeopathic group were more encouraging; 74% of the group maintained their treatment throughout the year and only four patients achieved no improvement in their symptoms. However, there are a number of problems in accepting this apparently positive result:

- The homeopathic physicians may have influenced their group by a comprehensive and sympathetic case-taking technique that could have enhanced a placebo response. The authors stated that the design of the trial was such that it was not possible to distinguish between the effects due to the influence of the physicians' actions and those due to the drugs alone.
- A positive response may have been generated by the fact that patients on homeopathy were allowed free access to the drugs they took prior to entering the trial and therefore enjoyed a substantial advantage. The patients' own responsibility to fight their disease might have been strengthened in contrast to the inflexible protocol for group 1. One of the most interesting results of this preliminary study was that none of the homeopathic group experienced toxic effects, whereas over a third of the aspirin group dropped out the trial for this reason.

ation could be identified between the action of homeopathy and placebo. On average, over the last 2 weeks after randomisation, patients who received homeopathy had a 28% improvement compared with 3% among those in the placebo group. There was a mean reduction of the visual analogue scale score of 10.9 mm in the homeopathy group compared with 1.1 mm in the placebo group (95% confidence interval for difference 4.2 to 15.4, $P = 0.0007$; two sided, two sample t test).

Taylor and colleagues (2000) found that homeopathy and placebo had different effects.

Compared with placebo, homeopathy provoked a clear, significant, and clinically relevant improvement in nasal inspiratory peak flow, similar to that found with topical steroids. However, the subjective improvement was less clear. The primary outcome used to calculate the sample size was a visual analogue score measuring patients' perceived improvement in symptoms. In contrast to the earlier studies, the researchers detected no effect of homeopathic treatment on the visual analogue score.

In a commentary on the fourth paper in the series, Lancaster and Vickers acknowledge the rigorous nature of the work but call for much larger trials (Lancaster and Vickers, 2000).

Unfortunately Lewith et al. (2002) were unable to validate the procedure of homeopathic immunotherapy. They carried out a double blind randomised trial to evaluate the efficacy of homeopathic immunotherapy on lung function and respiratory symptoms in asthmatic people allergic to house dust mite. They found there was no difference in most outcomes between placebo and homeopathic remedy and concluded that homeopathic immunotherapy is not effective in the treatment of patients with asthma.

Trials on specific remedies

Evidence based medicine seeks to establish proof of efficacy of treatments for specific diagnoses. In homeopathy it is based on clinical verification of symptoms used in homeopathic practice within the framework of the homeopathic concept of similarity.

The organisation of such verification is not simple because homeopaths use different methodologies and strategies varying according to their training, expertise and clinical experience Robust evidence of positive outcome from a particular remedy chosen from its drug picture is scant. Presented below are examples of studies on individual remedies.

Arnica

Arnica is the homeopathic remedy most frequently studied in placebo-controlled clinical trials and demonstrates the difficulty of applying strict measures of efficacy to homeopathic remedies.

Ernst and Pittler (1998) systematically reviewed the clinical efficacy of homeopathic Arnica. Most of the trials related to conditions associated with tissue trauma and were burdened with severe methodological flaws. They suggested that that homeopathic Arnica was not more efficacious than placebo.

Three randomised double-blind, placebo-controlled clinical trials evaluated the efficacy of homeopathic Arnica after knee surgery (Ludtke and Wilkins, 1998). The indications were simple knee arthroscopy for diagnostic purposes, implantation of artificial knee joints and rupture of cruciate ligaments. The primary outcome parameter was swelling; secondary outcome criteria: pain, drainage fluid. The authors concluded that Arnica is not as efficacious in pain control as in swelling. They recommended that combining Arnica with other homeopathic remedies, e.g. Hypericum, was more efficacious in reducing pain.

Researchers from Exeter University and the Royal Devon and Exeter Hospital carried out a double-blind, placebo-controlled, randomised trial on Arnica with three parallel arms using 64 adults undergoing elective surgery for carpal tunnel syndrome (Stevinson et al., 2003). The group were randomised to take three tablets daily of Arnica 30c or 6c or placebo for 7 days before surgery and 14 days after surgery. Primary outcome measures were pain (short form McGill Pain Questionnaire) and bruising (colour separation analysis) at 4 days after surgery. Secondary outcome measures were swelling (wrist circumference) and use of analgesic medication (patient diary). Sixty-two patients could be included in the intention-to-treat analysis. There were no group differences on the primary outcome measures of pain ($P = 0.79$) and bruising ($P = 0.45$) at day 4. Swelling and use of analgesic medication also did not differ between Arnica and placebo groups. The authors stated that the results do not support the routine use of homeopathic Arnica for preventing or reducing postoperative bruising, swelling or pain. As a caveat they do not rule out the possibility that individual patients could benefit. These sweeping conclusions attracted critical comment, for although the remedy appeared not to work at the doses and in the context studied, it might have had positive effects at other doses, in other forms and in different applications (Hutton, 2003; Needleman, 2003; Simmons, 2003). These possibilities were actually acknowledged by Ernst in 1995 in a critique of work carried out by others (Ernst, 1995). Commenting on the negative outcome of a trial, Professor Ernst wrote:

> Homeopaths might well have doubts about this conclusion, arguing that the RCT protocol does not allow for the necessary freedom of homeopathic prescription: the doses are usually fixed and so was the treatment schedule, yet homeopathy requires these to be flexible and fully individualised. Thus homeopaths might think that the results would be different if true homeopathy was practised.

In addition, the use of Arnica in pain control was suspect since it had already been demonstrated 3 years earlier that Arnica alone is not generally indicated in pain control (Ludtke and Wilkins, 1998).

Following publication of the trial one of the authors published a collection of 16 case studies apparently showing the beneficial use of Arnica (Ernst, 2003). He made the following comments:

Topical Arnica preparations are often wrongly equated with homeopathic Arnica; the former are herbal preparations (i.e. not homeopathically diluted), which have undisputed pharmacological activity. Taken orally they would even be toxic. Thus all Arnica for oral administration must be highly diluted and is therefore less likely to have pharmacological effects.

The case reports show that many lay people seem to be unclear about the difference between herbal and homeopathic Arnica.

The anti-inflammatory effect of Arnica 6c was evaluated using acute and chronic inflammation models (Macêdo et al., 2004). Wistar male rats (*Rattus norvegicus*), weighing between 180 and 200 g, were used in the experiments. In the acute model, carrageenin-induced rat paw oedema, the group treated with Arnica 6c showed 30% inhibition compared to control ($P < 0.05$). Treatment with Arnica 6cH 30 min prior to carrageenin did not produce any inhibition of the inflammatory process. In the chronic model, nystatin-induced oedema, the group treated 3 days previously with Arnica 6c had reduced inflammation 6 h after the inflammatory agent was applied ($P < 0.05$). When treatment was given 6 h after nystatin treatment, there was no significant inhibitory effect. In a model based on histamine-induced increase of vascular permeability, pretreatment with Arnica 6c blocked the action of histamine in increasing vascular permeability.

So, does Arnica work?

There is much contradictory information about Arnica in the literature. However, many of the Arnica studies have been designed with either an inappropriately chosen procedure or an inappropriate dosing regimen. Apparently positive responses could be due to other factors including the use of herbal (non-diluted) Arnica, placebo response and the natural course of disease. Robust evidence of efficacy has not been proven to accepted scientific standards. Edzard Ernst (2004a) has claimed that the results of rigorous clinical trials collectively show that Arnica is no better than placebo. In a tortuous argument he points out that as both placebo and Arnica are associated with respectable clinical improvements, depending on one's point of view one could conclude that Arnica is ineffective (i.e. it is no better than placebo) or effective (same effect as placebo).

Arsenicun album

It has been demonstrated in various animal models that ultra-high homeopathic dilutions of Arsenicum alb seem to have significant biological effect (Datta et al., 1999) (see also Ch. 8 – Tautodes).

Rhus tox

In a double-blind crossover trial, Fisher et al. (1989) showed that Rhus tox 6c was twice as effective as placebo in treating a selected subgroup of patients suffering from fibrositis.

Other trials

A Dutch/Belgian trial (Klerk et al., 1994) investigated the effect of homeopathic medicines on the daily burden of symptoms in children with recurrent upper respiratory tract infections. A total of 175 children were included in the study (five dropped out after 26 weeks) and the trial ran for nearly 5 years. The results were inconclusive; individually prescribed homeopathic remedies seemed to be of little assistance in complementing counselling and antibiotic therapy although when combined with dietary advice there was an excellent response.

Jennifer Jacobs and colleagues carried out a randomised double-blind clinical trial in Nicaragua, comparing homeopathic medicine with placebo in the treatment of acute childhood diarrhoea (Jacobs et al., 1994). A sample of 81 children aged from 6 months to 5 years were studied. Individualised treatment was prescribed together with oral rehydration therapy. There was a statistically significant decrease in the duration of diarrhoea in the treatment group.

There is also evidence from randomised, controlled trials that homeopathy may be effective for the treatment of influenza, allergies, postoperative ileus and childhood diarrhoea (Jonas et al., 2003). Evidence suggests that homeopathy is ineffective for migraine, delayed-onset muscle soreness and influenza prevention. There is a lack of conclusive evidence on the effectiveness of homeopathy for most conditions. Homeopathy deserves an open-minded opportunity to demonstrate its value by using evidence based principles, but it should not be substituted for proven therapies.

The meta-analysis and review of homeopathic trials

One of the most frequently cited papers in the literature is by Jos Kleijnen and his colleagues (1991) working at the Department of Epidemiology in the University of Limburg in Maastricht. The objective of their work was to establish whether there was any firm evidence of the efficacy of homeopathy from all the many controlled trials that have been carried out since Gibson started the ball rolling in 1978. They used the technique of meta-analysis to assess the methodological quality of 107 controlled trials, published in 96 journals world-wide. The trials were scored using a list of predefined criteria of good methodology (e.g. number of patients in the trial, randomisation methods, double blinding, presentation of results) and the outcome of the trials interpreted according to their quality. All the trials were scored by at least two of the researchers, and any differences in opinion resolved by discussion.

The top two trials, scoring 90 points out of 100, were those by the French government-sponsored research group known as GRECO (1989) and Reilly et al. (1986). The former reported the effect of two homeopathic preparations (Opium 15c and Raphanus 5c) on the resumption of intestinal peristalsis after operations on the digestive tract. The authors failed to identify any effect. Reilly's pollen trials were discussed above; they appeared to report a positive effect.

Table 11.5 Success rates of homeopathic trials studied by Kleijnen et al. (1991)

Indication	No. of trials assessed	Percentage positive
Vascular diseases (0)*	9	44
Respiratory infections (2)	19	68
Other infections (1)	7	86
Digestive diseases	7	71
Allergic reactions (3)	5	100
Recovery of bowel movement after surgery (3)	7	71
Rheumatic disease (0)	6	67
Trauma or pain (1)	20	90
Mental or psychological problems (0)	10	80
Other conditions (1)	15	87

*(The numbers in parentheses indicate studies within the therapeutic group that scored 70 or above.)

Overall, of the 105 trials with interpretable results, 81 positive trials were recorded. In 24 trials no positive effects of homeopathy were found. The results, summarised by condition treated, are given in Table 11.5. Of the 11 trials scoring 70 and above, spread over six therapeutic groups, nine showed positive results and two, relating to post-surgical ileus and postoperative infection respectively, showed negative results.

Kleijnen acknowledged that the weight of presented evidence was probably not sufficient for most people to decide whether homeopathy works or not but that there would probably be sufficient evidence to support a number of day-to-day applications if it were an orthodox therapy. It was concluded that additional evidence is required, and that it must consist of a few well-performed human trials with large numbers, performed under rigorous double-blind conditions.

Meta-analyses of RCTs of homeopathy against placebo showing positive results in favour of homeopathy have been seized upon by the homeopathic community as 'manna from heaven' (Linde et al., 1997). Cucherat et al. (2000) concluded from a meta-analysis of 16 trials that there was some evidence that homeopathic treatments were more effective than placebo, but that the strength of this evidence was low because of the low methodological quality of the trials. Studies of high methodological quality were more likely to be negative than the lower quality studies. These less positive results and criticisms are often conveniently bypassed (Linde et al., 1999).

Ernst searched electronic databases for homeopathic systematic reviews/ meta-analysis (Ernst, 2002). Seventeen articles fulfilled the inclusion/ exclusion criteria. Six of them related to re-analyses of one landmark meta-analysis. Collectively they implied that the overall positive result of this meta-analysis is not supported by a critical analysis of the data. Eleven independent systematic reviews were located. Collectively they failed to provide strong evidence in favour of homeopathy. In particular, there was no condition which responds convincingly better to homeopathic treatment than to placebo or other control interventions. Similarly, there was no homeopathic remedy that was demonstrated to yield clinical effects that are convincingly different from placebo. It is concluded that the best clinical evidence for homeopathy available to date does not warrant positive recommendations for its use in clinical practice.

Mathie (2003b) conducted an analysis of the 93 substantive RCTs that compare homeopathy either with placebo or another treatment. He found 50 papers that reported a significant benefit of homeopathy in at least one clinical outcome measure, 41 that failed to discern any inter-group differences, and two that described an inferior response with homeopathy. Considering the relative number of research articles on the 35 different medical conditions in which such research has been carried out, the weight of evidence currently favours a positive treatment effect in eight: childhood diarrhoea, fibrositis, hayfever, influenza, pain (miscellaneous), side-effects of radio- or chemotherapy, sprains and upper respiratory tract infection. Based on published research to date, it seems unlikely that homeopathy is efficacious for headache, stroke or warts. Insufficient research prevents conclusions from being drawn about any other medical conditions. Mathie concluded that available research evidence emphasises the need for much more and better-directed research in homeopathy. A fresh agenda of enquiry should consider beyond (but include) the placebo-controlled trial. Each study should adopt research methods and outcome measurements linked to a question addressing the *clinical* significance of homeopathy's effects.

Shang et al. (2005) compared the treatment effects in homeopathy and conventional medicine. They initially identified 110 placebo-controlled trials of both to study but once they had excluded small and low quality trials only eight homeopathic and six orthodox trials remained to be analysed. The Swiss researchers concluded that the clinical effect of homeopathy was a placebo effect. Protagonists of homeopathy questioned the findings but the *Lancet* thought them to be of such quality as to signify the end of homeopathy (Anon., 2005).

Problems with RCTs

Selecting subjects

The double-blind clinical trial requires two groups of similar patients, one to act as a control and the other to receive active ingredients. Normally, in day-to-day medical research, groups will be compared for age, sex, racial origin, social status or occupation. There may be other special factors including number of cigarettes smoked or alcohol consumption; if the two groups are comparable on four or five main parameters, then it is assumed that they are statistically comparable in every other way. If one considers the diversity of human personality and physical type, it can be appreciated that this is an assumption that cannot be made from a homeopathic viewpoint. It is necessary to use either a very big group, where there is a fair chance of a genuine sample of the community, or to control for some other important homeopathic factors summarised under the general heading of 'constitutional'. In homeopathy several aspects of different levels of the human being are analysed leading to the comparison of the patient's symptoms with a drug picture. The requirement to individualise homeopathic treatment means that it is not possible to assemble two groups of people all with exactly the same remedy requirements unless limited to specific prescriptions, complexes or isopathic remedies. It was pointed out within the first few pages of this book that remedies indicated for one patient may be totally different from another, even though the symptoms appear very similar. For clinical trials of homeopathy to be accurate representations of practice, we need modified designs that take into account the complexity of the homeopathic intervention. There are methods available to enable double-blind trials to take place with homeopathic remedies (Vithoulkas, 1985), but once changes are made to standard research techniques suspicions are expressed by the orthodox research community.

Assembling a homogeneous group of patients is an important factor (Wiegant et al., 1991). Indeed, attracting sufficient participants of any type to arrive at statistically significant conclusions may prove difficult for a variety of reasons (Jansen et al., 1992). However, only with such trials will the results be generalisable to homeopathic practice in the real world.

Randomisation

Randomisation and blinding of participants substantially distorts the context of homeopathic prescribing, potentially weakening its effect. It is not uncommon for the positive outcomes experienced in day-to-day homeopathic practice not to be confirmed by RCTs (Baas, 2004). The selection of homeopathic medicines is often simplified in such studies. This makes it easier to design a methodologically robust clinical trial. However, the selection process of homeopathic remedies in practice is different. Thus RCTs do not always study the same thing as observational outcome studies.

Complexity of homeopathic response

There is another fundamental problem with the interpretation of results from placebo-controlled trials in homeopathy (Weatherley-Jones et al., 2004). It is not reasonable to assume that the specific effects of homeopathic medicine and the non-specific effects of consultations are independent of each other – specific effects of the medicine (as manifested by patients' reactions) may influence the nature of subsequent consultations and the non-specific effects of the consultation may enhance or diminish the effects of the medicine.

Quality of evidence

The question as to why one should bother to read about a trial comparing homeopathic treatment to placebo has been posed by Feder and Katz (2002). After all, if one is comfortable using homeopathic medicines a trial will probably not influence prescribing decisions, mainly because, as stated above, most trials of homeopathic medicines do not reflect individualised treatment, the hallmark of homeopathic practice. If they do and a homeopathic effect over placebo can be shown (Linde and Melchart, 1998) it is difficult to apply the results to individual treatment decisions in practice.

Maybe not a gold standard?

There are other more general problems with the RCT. Even after a drug has been subjected to rigorous RCTs it may have to be withdrawn because of concerns about adverse reactions. Some chemotherapeutic agents have been made available on the basis of evidence from trials with limited patient numbers and for obvious reasons no RCTs are carried out on children or indeed animals (although the latter may be implicated in human research). For these reasons the RCT may not be considered to be an absolute gold standard for gathering evidence of efficacy and safety.

Another approach

Dean (2000) has advanced the argument that randomised placebo-controlled trials of homeopathy might usefully be replaced by observational studies, audit and quality-of-life assessment. Randomised equivalence and patient-preference trials are proposed as more informative alternatives. They have the merit of providing hard information for health services on the comparative value of treatments, and can facilitate internal comparisons of competing homeopathic methods. Dean suggests that this pragmatic approach also allows clinical change during the homeopathic treatment of chronic disease to be assessed without the time constraints usually imposed by placebo controls.

Examples of outcomes and observational research

There have been a number of effectiveness studies which have looked at groups of patients treated with homeopathic remedies in real-world settings:

- for a small number of well-defined diagnoses (Riley et al., 2001)
- for the treatment of a specific condition with a remedy chosen on the basis of repertorisation (Gerhard and Wallis, 2002; Schlappak, 2004)
- for many diagnoses in a tightly defined patient social group (Walach and Guthlin, 2000)
- for chronic headache, Muscari-Tomaioli et al. (2001) reported very positive results for homeopathy evaluated using real-world outcome studies contrasting with RCT results, which have been generally unimpressive with the homeopathic treatment of headache (Whitmarsh, 2002).

A Norwegian study investigated whether the homeopathic medicine Betula 30c was more effective than placebo in reducing symptoms of pollen allergy in patients sensitive to birch pollen (Aabel, 2000). It was a double-blind, randomised, placebo-controlled trial. Tablets were given both as a prophylactic agent, once a week 4 weeks before the pollen season, and as an acute remedy during the pollen season. The study was carried out in Oslo, and involved 73 children, adolescents and young adults from 7 to 25 years of age. Allergy symptoms were assessed on a VAS by patients or parents. Surprisingly, the verum treated patients fared worse than the placebo group; they used more rescue medication and had higher symptom scores during these 3 days. Homeopaths might attribute the findings to a putative aggravation response, but the results certainly do not lend support to the usefulness of the tested prophylactic approach, under conditions of low allergen exposure.

Further examples of observational studies in other areas of homeopathic practice are provided by the following:

A study to evaluate the effect of a GP-led practice-based homeopathy service was carried out in Coventry observing symptoms, activity, well-being, general practice consultation rate and the use of conventional medications (Slade et al., 2004). Data were collected for 97 consecutive patients referred to a homeopathy service over a 6-month period. Following homeopathy, symptoms and well-being improved. Following use of the homeopathy service, the mean 6-month general practice consultation rate decreased by 1.18 consultations per patient (95% CI 0.40–1.99; $P = 0.004$). A total of 57% of patients reduced or stopped taking their conventional medication, saving £2807.30 per year. The main limitation of this study is the absence of a control group.

In a prospective uncontrolled observational multicentre outcome study, patients visiting 80 homeopaths all over Norway for the first time in eight different time periods from 1996 to 1998 were approached (Steinsbekk and Lüdtke, 2005). Patients wrote down their main complaint and scored its impact on daily living on a 100 mm VAS at the first consultation. Six months later they were asked to score again. Seven out of 10 patients visiting a Norwegian homeopath reported a meaningful improvement in their main complaint 6 months after the initial consultation ($n = 654$).

Case reports

Detailed anecdotal information is usually called a 'case report'. To be acceptable these reports must be rigorously structured and not subject to journalistic 'hype' (Ernst, 2004b). There is a requirement for information on the disease and its extent, and information about any other patients who did not recover after being administered similar treatment. From an orthodox point of view such observations are interesting but do not necessarily mean that the next patient will respond in the same manner. Despite this, several orthodox medicines, especially in the field of psychiatry, are administered on the basis of case studies, although the acceptability of such justification is often challenged by more orthodox colleagues.

The case report is one of the chief sources of clinical knowledge for the homeopath. In teaching seminars the world over, most established teachers will only present cases that fulfill stringent quality criteria (see www. mangialavori.org). A good case brings the different parts together into a coherent narrative whereas in materia medicas and provings the information can feel jumbled and unconnected. Cases demonstrate the practical application of the principles of homeopathy direction of cure, prescribing strategies, potency choices, etc. By supplying cases, without details of medicines given, teachers of homeopathy have the perfect tool for modern 'problem-based learning'. There is a growing momentum in conventional medicine to recognise the value of patients' narratives (Greenhalgh and Hurwitz, 1999). The sophisticated methodology of homeopathic case taking, developed over many years of reflective work, has much to offer this process (Swayne, 1998).

The Delphi project

The Delphi project was started in 1997 with the aim of gathering homeopathic case reports and making them available for comparison and study. Most attention was given to identifying criteria for the quality of case descriptions and to ways of prompting homeopathic prescribers to participate and submit cases to the Delphi library. The basic criterion was that the case be described in such a way that the readers could make their own decision about the quality and usefulness of the case.

Several years of work on the development of the Delphi project have brought to the surface many of the challenges and pitfalls of clinical case research in homeopathy (Baas, 2004). The legal and ethical aspects have taken up the most time and energy, but it seems these can be overcome by a more formal description and organisation of the project. The variability in case reports and peer reviews, however, are ongoing problems. The Delphi brochure is available electronically from delphi.project@hccnet.nl.

RESEARCH TO ADDRESS THE QUESTION: HOW DOES HOMEOPATHY WORK?

Modern trends lean towards systematic investigation of the basic mechanisms of an observed effect before proof of efficacy is accepted by the scientific establishment. Any effects must be fully explainable using accepted paradigms. Pressure from legislators who demand proof of pharmacodynamic and therapeutic efficacy of all pharmaceuticals on the market has made this area important.

The debate on possible mechanisms of action for homeopathy centres around whether the effects of homeopathy are due to local or non-local causes. The 'local causality hypothesis' is the traditional explanation; the action of homeopathic medicines is pharmacological (or at least quasi-pharmacological), due to some specific factor contained in the medicine. Current thinking appears to favour the non-local option, considering the mechanism to involve some form of information storage in the physical substrate.

Local causality

Among homeopaths the common idea about a working hypothesis for homeopathic effects seems to be that, during the potentisation process, 'information' or 'energy' is being preserved or even enhanced in homeopathic remedies. The organism is said to be able to pick up this information, which in turn will stimulate the organism into a self-healing response. According to this view the decisive element of homeopathic therapy is the remedy which locally contains and conveys this information (Walach, 2000).

The pharmacological view was given enhanced credibility by Belon et al. (2004) who performed a series of experiments using ultramolecular dilutions of Histamine 10^{-30}–10^{-38}M (15–19c), prepared in steps of 1:100 with vortexing (instead of succussion). The methodology was based on inhibition of basophil activation. The overall result, including all stimulatory concentrations of anti-IgE and all dilutions of Histamine, showed statistically highly significant inhibition from ultramolecular dilutions of Histamine. The researchers were unable to explain their results but suggested that it may involve biological information from the solvent. Although not much used in the UK, Histamine (often in the form of lung Histamine) is widely used in homeopathic dilution elsewhere in the world, in the treatment of allergy.

Non-local causality: interaction with diluent

A literature search will reveal numerous hypotheses on the theory of minimal doses and a review of these is beyond the scope of this book. The subject is well covered in a book by Bellavite and Signorini (1995). Only a very brief overview is given here of the so-called 'biophysical paradigm' that reflects a need to seek explanations beyond the biochemical interpretations of orthodox drug action.

There are three basic diluents utilised in homeopathic pharmacy, namely water, alcohol and lactose, all of which play an important part in the mode of action (Singh and Chhabra, 1993). Of these, the first has received the most attention. Numerous hypotheses based on an ability of water to retain molecular imprints have been advanced to try and explain the apparent therapeutic efficacy of high dilutions. Endler (1989) suggested in a report on a symposium entitled 'Water and information' that the concept of information transfer leads us to change our understanding of the nature of substance itself from the old static conception to one in which substance is understood in terms of processes. Antonchenko and Ilyin (1992) argue that the stability of various dissipative structures in water systems is explained by their presence in the earth's electromagnetic field, and by the stabilising processes of proton transfer along hydrogen-bonded chains in these structures. A possible connection between the processes occurring in dissipative water structures and the radiation characteristics of homeopathic preparations is possible. In a BBC television programme entitled 'Medicine or Magic' in 1993, Dr David Reilly referred to the many different physical forms of water in trying to explain how homeopathic dilutions might work using snowflakes as examples of biochemically identical, but biophysically different forms. Others have followed a similar track. Cohen (1993) pointed out that this approach is especially appropriate because the most popular disparaging comments about homeopathy refer to there being 'nothing present but a molecule or two in an ocean of water'. However, little is known about the complex microscopic behaviour of the liquid state: in fact it is often

Figure 11.5   Water
molecules forming an
hydration shell around a
positive remedy ion (Lessell,
1995)

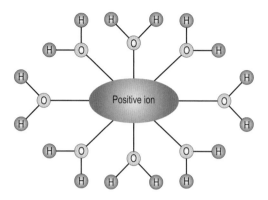

viewed as being one of a class of 'chaotic systems' whose behaviour is highly unpredictable. Cohen says that water is 10 times more complex and enigmatic than other liquids, therefore this vehicle is thought to play an important part in homeopathic activity. Chemical bonding always requires an exchange of electrons, and it is impossible to describe such reactions involving water at a molecular level without accepting that the solvent plays more of a role than just supporting dissolved material. Knowledge of water/ice structures and semiconductor theory can in fact be used to develop a further argument that shows molecular and subatomic structures of aqueous and solid state solutions to be analogous.

In his book entitled *The Infinitesimal Dose*, Lessell (1995) points out that the 'molecular imprint' theories of water involvement are fraught with difficulties. There are other possible explanations based on molecular geometries or shapes; a concept of hydration shells formed by the close association of water molecules with ions of remedy molecules is one that I favour (Fig. 11.5). However, while this may be an acceptable explanation for demonstrable quantities of molecules, it still does not really explain activity beyond Avogadro's number.

It is possible to construct a mathematical model for the potentisation process, identifying a relationship between the dilution factor, the number of succussions and the oscillatory function that is said to contribute to a biological effect. Lessell's book is a good place to start to try and unravel the mystery of how medicines can possibly become stronger the weaker chemically they become. Despite the plethora of hypotheses, little has changed in the time that has elapsed since George Vithoulkas (1985) wrote: 'as far as is yet known there is no available explanation in modern physics or chemistry for the phenomenon of potentisation'. We are still very much in the dark.

The Benveniste controversy

Of all the attempts to unravel the mystery of homeopathic mechanisms of action, undoubtedly the most controversial in modern times was contained in a paper published after a 3-year delay in the prestigious British journal *Nature* on June 30 1988 (Davenas et al., 1988). The paper was authored by 13 scientists working at INSDERM U 200, a research institute at the

University of South Paris, and was hailed as a breakthrough by many supporters of complementary medicine in providing the elusive scientific explanations for the mechanisms of action of homeopathic remedies. The team was led by an immunologist called Jacques Benveniste, arguably the most controversial scientist of the last 50 years (Edwards, 2005). At its height, 'l'affaire Benveniste' involved some of the cream of the scientific establishment on both sides of the English Channel, but their treatment of the man sometimes smacked more of a Papal Inquisition than of sober scientific appraisal.

The so-called 'ghost molecule' or 'memory of water' studies were based on a hypothesis that water had the ability to 'remember' the pattern or imprint of biologically active material with which it had been in contact. The phenomenon was investigated using human basophils, a type of white blood cell, with antibodies of the E-type immunoglobulin, IgE, on its surface, which when exposed to the large anti-IgE antibodies release histamine from their intracellular granules and change their staining properties. Solutions of anti-IgE antibodies were repeatedly diluted, with succussion, until well beyond the Avogadro number. Although there were then theoretically no molecules left, the solution still apparently evoked a response from immune cells at concentrations down to 10^{-120}, which is equivalent to a 60c potency. Since the dilutions were accompanied by vigorous shaking for the effects to be observed, Benveniste and his colleagues concluded that transmission of the biological information could be related to the molecular organisation of water in the solvent. For a more detailed commentary on the methodology and Benveniste's problems, the reader is referred to Michel Schiff's book *The Memory of Water* (1995).

Although Benveniste's findings seemed to provide experimental support for homeopathic observations, the journal nevertheless concurrently published a disclaimer (Anon., 1988a), stating: 'readers of this article may share the incredulity of many referees who have commented on several versions of it during the past several months'.

The journal subsequently sent a team to investigate the results. It was an ill-assorted bunch who descended upon Professor Benveniste's laboratory: John Maddox, Editor of *Nature*, James 'The Amazing' Randi, a magician (the same man whose jibe directed at me on his website was reported in Ch. 2) and Walter W. Stewart, an American scientist with special interest in scientific fraud. The investigators were surprised to find that the experiments did not always work. There were several months at a time during which solutions of a high dilution had not degranulated the basophils; these results were discarded. Further, the experiments seemed to work more often when carried out by one particular investigator, described as being 'exceptionally devoted to her work' (Smith, 1988). After a week-long inspection the work was condemned as being seriously flawed, a delusion, and 'not to be believed' (Madox et al., 1988). Randi told a reporter from the *New Scientist*: 'As a conjuror I could see 15 ways to bias the results without sleight of hand.' Not surprisingly, Benveniste, convinced that he was the subject of a witch hunt, struck back at his critics, asking why his paper was published one week, only to be destroyed a fortnight later. He claimed that the investigation was 'a mockery of scientific enquiry' and gave details of disturbing behaviour by the *Nature* investigators (Benveniste, 1988). The episode received wide coverage in the press. For example, *The Guardian*, in a piece entitled 'Nature's call dampens hopes of homeopathic breakthrough', stated 'The scientific journal *Nature* admits that it does not believe one of its own learned articles' (Anon., 1988b).

Three years after these events, Benveniste published new evidence in the journal of the French Academy of Sciences, having had the paper rejected by *Nature* and the American journal *Science* on the grounds of alleged 'statistical errors' (Benveniste et al., 1991). There were two series of experiments in this later research. The first was essentially a repetition of the studies reported in *Nature*, except that this time the effect of human anti-IgE serum was compared with goat anti-human IgG antiserum and distilled water at dilutions down to 10^{-30}. The second series looked at the inhibitory effects of the homeopathic remedy Apis on basophil 'achromasia', the new term for granulation. Specific basophils were incubated with an anti-IgE anti-serum after treatment with either potencies of Natrum mur or Apis mellifica. A statistically significant inhibition of the anti-IgE antibody-induced achromasia was observed when cells were treated with some potencies of Apis. No such effect was seen with the Natrum mur. This work was greeted with further widespread scepticism (Concar, 1991). Similar experiments carried out in Utrecht by van Wijk and Ovelgönne in 1991 and reviewed by Bol (1991) did not appear to support the French results. Dr Benveniste's funding was subsequently withdrawn and the research team disbanded.

Fraud or fact? Benveniste's papers have been the subject of much animated discussion over the years. A literature search will reveal that a number of groups have achieved varying degrees of success in replicating aspects of these high dilution experiments. John Maddox, though held in high regard by the scientific community, was well known to be opposed to research that conflicted with accepted scientific paradigms. It has been suggested that his 'editorial censorship' (see p. 276) was the real reason for rejecting the validity of Benveniste's work, rather than scientific incompetency as claimed (Walker, 1995). Criticism also came from quarters other than Maddox. For instance, the deputy editor of *Nature*, Peter Newark, called Benveniste's work 'bizarre and . . . a piece of outrageous research' (MacEoin, 1988), while an article in *The Guardian* referred to 'invalid biological research' (Anon., 1988c). Debate still continues (Fisher, 2004a). A television programme made by the BBC (*Horizon*) and broadcast in the UK in November 2002 and subsequently in many other countries alleged that experiments related to Benveniste's were irreproducible. Similar claims were broadcast by ABC Network's *20/20* programme in the USA in early 2004.

Benveniste – an interview

I met with Jacques Benveniste (Fig. 11.6) in Moscow, for the opening of the second annual Russian Homeopathic Congress. With colleagues I was sitting at a large round table waiting to start lunch. As the first of our nine courses arrived 'M. le Français' swept in. Jacques Benveniste, researcher extraordinaire, made his entrance in style. He was wearing an expensive suit

Figure 11.6 Jacques Benveniste (12 March 1935–4 October 2004)

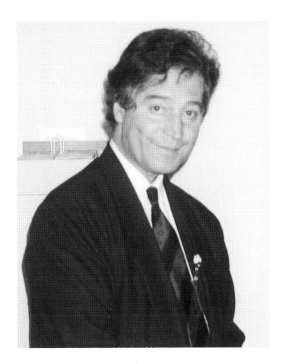

complete with designer creases. He introduced himself, apologising profusely for his late arrival and explaining that he had been held up at some government agency. His infectious laugh and sympathetic personality soon prompted freely flowing conversation. Jacques Benveniste said that he was deeply hurt by this criticism of his work, especially the personal nature of some of the comments. He was a man with over 300 scientific papers, a respected researcher, whose credibility was being questioned.

'I saw the results with my own eyes', he said. 'To sit back and say nothing would have betrayed my colleagues and implied acceptance of the criticism, some of which I considered childish. OK, we made mistakes, but the basic thrust of our work was based on hard facts.' Here he thumped his left fist into the palm of his right hand to emphasise his statement and repeated the words 'hard facts'. He continued, 'They also said I was arrogant. Peter Medawar, the British Nobel Laureate researcher, said that "humility is not a state of mind conducive to the advancement of learning" and I agree with him to some extent. Those people will apologise to me some time.'

Dr Benveniste leaned forward, as if to tell me a secret: 'In 1982, I thought homeopathy was a new sexual disease', he joked, eyes sparkling impishly.

> *I knew nothing – in fact I still know little of the discipline, except in the context of considering its mechanisms as a branch of nature's general transmission of messages through electro-magnetic forces. That year I took on a new member of staff, Bernard Poitevin, a young medical doctor with a side-interest in homeopathy. He asked me if he could try out some homeopathic preparations 'on my allergy test' for his MD thesis and I gave permission, providing that he did not waste time. His results were interesting and I became involved in my present work from 1983.*

I asked Benveniste why homeopathy appeared to suffer in English speaking countries.

> *That's interesting; I had not thought of that. Ah, oui, I know why. It is because you are more concerned with scientific evidence than with empirical results. There is also a publication bias in English language journals against positive results – especially ones that cannot easily be explained.*

Dr Benveniste delivered an excellent paper on his work on the following day, despite being kept waiting for 2 hours, suffering slide projection problems and speaking in short phrases that were then translated into Russian. As he left the Congress on his way to visit the Institute for Medical Problems he generously invited me to his laboratory in Paris.

> *We will set up the experiments for you and you can prepare your own potencies. You will see for your own eyes. The results will be reproducible, I promise you.*

Unfortunately I did not manage to take up the invitation before he lost his funding, so for me at least, the mystery is still a mystery. That is not to say that I ever doubted Jacques' integrity, but it would have been good to see it with my own eyes. Dr Jacques Benveniste died during the evening of 3 October 2004 at the Pitié-Salpétrière Hospital in Paris.

Entanglement theories

In the last few years, the most radical challenge in the entire history of homeopathy has emerged: the non-local causality hypothesis, based on 'entanglement' (Fisher, 2004b). This theory was first proposed by Walach (2000) who concluded that the database is too weak and contradictory to substantiate a local interpretation of homeopathy, in which the remedy is endowed with causal-informational content irrespective of the circumstances and proposed a non-local interpretation. Subsequently other versions and interpretations have emerged, including those of Hyland (2003), Weingärtner (2003) and a series of papers by Milgrom (2004a,b). These hypotheses all share the idea of quantum entanglement.

The extended network generalised entanglement theory (entanglement theory for short) combines two theories based on complexity theory and quantum mechanics. According to Hyland (2003) the theory's assumptions are: the body is a complex, self-organising system (the extended network) that self-organises so as to achieve genetically defined patterns (where patterns include morphologic as well as lifestyle patterns). These pattern-specifying genes require feedback that is provided by generalised quantum entanglement. Additionally, generalised entanglement has evolved as a form of communication between people (and animals) and can be used in healing. Entanglement theory suggests that several processes are involved in CAM. Direct subtle therapy creates network change through lifestyle management, some manual therapies, and psychologically mediated effects of therapy. Indirect subtle therapy is a process of entanglement with other people or physical entities (e.g. remedies, healing sites).

OTHER RESEARCH

Audit studies

This is the systematic evaluation of clinical activity – the effectiveness of a particular intervention. It involves the identification of a problem and its resolution as part of an audit cycle. Audit is about ultimately improving a procedure. Rarely is this work carried out as part of an audit cycle. Practitioners often conduct an uncontrolled observational study by recording an outcome in isolation without any recommendations or a commitment to improving clinical practice.

There are two sorts of audit studies:

- those concerned with recording what has been prescribed
- those concerned with measuring clinical outcomes.

Although homeopathic medicine has been available under the UK National Health Service since 1948, there have been few comprehensive audits in either category.

Jeremy Swayne (1989) carried out two 'usage' studies. In his first, he analysed some 7218 consultations among medical practitioners who used homeopathy, and found that 35% of them were managed using the discipline, 8.5% of the total in conjunction with allopathic medicines. Over 3000 prescriptions were recorded, involving 278 different remedies. Respiratory disorders accounted for most of the homeopathic treatments. In his second study Swayne showed the cost advantages and effectiveness of homeopathy (Swayne, 1992).

Haselen and Fisher (1994) have presented a proposal to establish common basic data collection methodology for homeopaths throughout Europe, together with a systematic study of the results of homeopathic treatment of patients with arthritis using quality of life and objective assessments. These attempts at standardisation will make audit studies easier to compare across different countries. Their paper also presents a set of homeopathic prescribing features for Rhus tox.

An audit was conducted of 829 consecutive patients presenting for homeopathic treatment of a chronic illness; conventional treatment had failed, plateaued in effect, or was contraindicated by adverse effects, age or condition of the patient (Sevar, 2000). Of the 829 patients, 503 (61%) had a sustained improvement from homeopathic treatment.

Researchers at Bristol Homeopathic Hospital carried out an audit to investigate the incidence of adverse reactions among 116 patients attending the outpatients department (Thompson et al., 2004). They concluded that remedy reactions are common in clinical practice; some patients experience them as adverse events (see also Ch. 8).

Attitudes and awareness studies

In this category several papers are of general interest, especially with respect to the methods used. Such studies are useful in establishing where people obtain their information about homeopathy and how they perceive its efficacy. Not only do the results have educational and marketing implications but also it is known that high expectations of success can affect the outcome of a therapy. A positive attitude to homeopathy may assist treatment.

Furnham and Smith (1988) have been concerned with the different health and illness beliefs of patients choosing traditional versus complementary medicine. Two similar groups of patients, one visiting a GP and the other a homeopath, were asked to complete questionnaires that included questions on the efficacy of the two types of medicine. The major differences between the groups were that the homeopathic group was much more critical and sceptical about the efficacy of traditional medicine. The results suggested that people who chose homeopathy did so from disenchantment with, and bad experiences of, traditional medicine.

Finnegan (1991) has documented a scale for examining the attitudes and expectations of complementary medicine. Alton and Kayne (1992), Davies and Kayne (1992) and Kayne and McGuire (1993) have provided models for 'attitudes and awareness' studies among pharmacy customers, pharmacy staff and veterinary surgeons respectively. An example of such a study questionnaire is illustrated in Figure 11.7.

AGRICULTURAL RESEARCH

A number of well-controlled botanical experiments have been performed by homeopathic investigators, the reason perhaps being that a placebo effect in plants may be discounted. Numerous experiments were performed to demonstrate the effect of homeopathic dilutions, mostly on wheat, by Kolisko (1959). It was found that growth was promoted by lower dilutions, then inhibited with higher dilutions and finally stimulated at even higher dilutions, results that are rather different from what might have been expected by Ardnt's Law.

Wannamaker (1966, 1968) conducted experiments over a period of years to test the effect of Sulphur and Boron potencies on the growth of onion plants and found significant improvements in weight and dimensions. Pelikan and Unger (1971) reproduced a small amount of Kolisko's work during the late 1960s, but with experimental methods more adapted to laboratory conditions. They provided statistically significant evidence that potentised substances do have an effect on plant growth. Unfortunately some of the requirements of their method were impossible to duplicate, and alternative methods were developed by Jones and Jenkins (1981, 1983).

The techniques of these and many other workers have been discussed by Scofield (1984b) in an extensive critical review of the potential role of homeopathy in agriculture. He concludes that, despite a great deal of investigation, because of poor experimental technique there is little firm evidence to support the efficacy of homeopathic remedies. However, much circumstantial evidence exists.

The inhibitory and stimulatory effects of potencies of certain homeopathic remedies on normal growth, respiration and growth rhythms of wheat has been reviewed by Poitevin (1967), but references to fieldwork are sparse. In a study of the effects of Sulphur on plots of rye grass at Harper Adams

Short research project
We are trying to assess the efficacy of homeopathic remedies bought over the counter in community pharmacies.   We should be grateful if you would complete this card and post it back to us.

No stamp is required.

About Yourself
Age: Under 25 ☐   Sex: Male ☐   Female ☐
             26–35 ☐
             36–45 ☐   Occupation:
             46–60 ☐   Is it the first time you have used
             Over 60 ☐   homeopathic medicine: Yes ☐   No ☐

About the Remedy
For whom did you buy the remedy: Self ☐   Child ☐   Family ☐
                                                            Friend ☐   Other ☐
What was if for?
What was the remedy called?
What form was it: Tablets ☐   Pills ☐   Granules ☐
                                            Liquid ☐   Ointment ☐   Cream ☐

How often was the remedy taken: And for how long:

About buying the Remedy
What prompted you to buy a homeopathic remedy: How did you know which remedy to select:

        I always use homeopathy ☐   Information from or   Family ☐
        I saw advertisement ☐   article in   Friend ☐
        The Pharmacy staff ☐   Media ☐
        Media coverage ☐   Pharmacist ☐
        Told by someone else ☐   Doctor ☐
                                                                  Own knowledge ☐
                                                               Told by someone else ☐

Did you ask the Pharmacy staff any questions: Yes ☐   No ☐
Were the Pharmacy staff able to answer your questions: Yes ☐   No ☐

How did it work
Did the remedy help the problem: Yes ☐   No ☐
Did you (or the patient) feel generally better after taking the remedy: Yes ☐   No ☐
Did you (or the patient) take the remedy on its own: Yes ☐   No ☐
                    with another homeopathic medicine   Yes ☐   No ☐
                    with another medicine   Yes ☐   No ☐
Will you (or the patient) use homeopathy again: Yes ☐   No ☐

About other Complementary Medicines
Have you tried other complementary therapies? (Tick any that apply)
    Acupuncture ☐   Herbalism ☐   Osteopathy ☐   Hypnosis ☐
    Reflexology ☐   Aromatherapy ☐   Other ☐

Of all the complementary therapies, which do you use most often? (Tick any that apply)
    Homeopathy ☐   Acupuncture ☐   Herbalism ☐   Osteopathy ☐
    Hypnosis ☐   Reflexology ☐   Aromatherapy ☐   Other ☐

Do you think availability of complementary therapies under the NHS is:
    Too little ☐   About right ☐   Too much ☐

Have you ever received an NHS prescription for homeopathy from your Doctor?
    Yes ☐   No ☐   Thank you very much

Figure 11.7   Example of an 'attitudes and awareness'-type questionnaire

Agricultural College, I was unable to demonstrate a significant result at the potency levels chosen (Kayne, 1991).

A randomised blind trial was carried out to evaluate the effects of 5 and 45 centesimal and decimal potencies of arsenic trioxide (As_2O_3) on tobacco plants subjected to tobacco mosaic virus (TMV) inoculation as biotic stress (Betti et al., 2003). Homeopathic treatments of arsenic appeared to increase resistance to TMV with decimal potencies inducing significantly increased resistance. The researchers claimed that the findings could indicate that decimal potencies are more suited to plants than centesimal potencies.

VETERINARY RESEARCH

In the veterinary discipline homeopathic treatment fell out of favour for many years, but is now enjoying a revival. Biddis (1979) has posed the question: 'How does homeopathy fit in with twentieth century veterinary medicine?' He suggests that homeopathy provides a wider range of medicaments on which to treat, for example, fright symptoms or awkward nervous conditions. Macleod (1981) expounded the principles and practice of homeopathy with relation to cattle, as did Day (1985). Day has also demonstrated the control of stillbirths in pigs using homeopathy (Day, 1984).

Work has been reported on the effects of some homeopathic remedies on the growth and feeding efficiency in broilers (Trehan et al., 1985). A paper by Taylor et al. (1989) describes a trial using the same scientific criteria as those required for the evaluation of conventional medicines; it examines the effect of a homeopathic prophylactic against artificial infection of *Dictyocaulus viviparus* and compares the results in untreated control calves. There were no discernible differences between the treated and untreated groups.

A study by Mackie et al. (1990) was more successful in appearing to demonstrate a difference in effect between a Sepia-treated group and a control group. It has been suggested that veterinarians should carry out their own homeopathic clinical trials (Morton, 1988). Neo-natal scouring in calves has been shown to respond to a nosode prepared from *E. coli*, the causative organism, by McLeod (1974) and also to Arsenicum album, which was tested in conjunction with orthodox methods (Kayne & Rafferty, 1994) and shown to be effective in reducing recovery time in a small sample of animals.

In an interesting study by Maria Bowler, an MSc student at Stirling University Institute of Aquaculture, the efficacy of a homeopathic treatment of *Aeromonas salmonicida* infection (furunculosis) in Atlantic salmon parr was investigated (Fig. 11.8; Bowler, 1993). The condition is one that affects many fish farms on the west coast of Scotland. I prepared one nosode for Maria using furuncle material obtained from experimentally infected fish, and a second using a pure culture of *A. salmonicida*.

The efficacy of the two nosodes was assessed through a pre-trial, a therapeutic trial and two prophylactic trials. The study showed that the nosodes, though not effective against acute furunculosis, appeared to act as immuno-stimulants of non-specific defence, conferring some degree of protection against the disease (Bowler, 1993).

The use of a variety of homeopathic remedies to treat mastitis has been reported for many years. Day (1986) prescribed nosodes while other

Figure 11.8 Salmon with furunculosis. Courtesy of Professor Roland Smith, University of Stirling Institute of Aquaculture

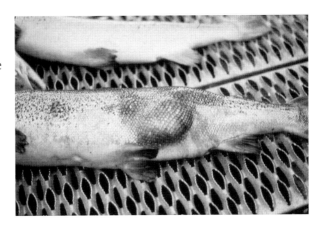

veterinarians have relied on single or complex remedies. Fifty cows with acute mastitis were used in the study. The initial treatment comprised Aconitum D 4, Phytolacca D 1 and Bryonia D 4 (Merck et al., 1989). In subsequent treatments Phytolacca D 1, Bryonia D 4 and Lachesis D 8 either singly or in combination were used; Mercurius solubilis D 4 was also used. Encouraging results, especially in the treatment of cases of *E. coli* mastitis, were achieved. A three-armed, stratified, semi-crossover design comparing homeopathy, placebo and a standardised antibiotic treatment involving 57 dairy cows was carried out in Norway (Hektoen et al., 2004). The antibiotic treatment was significantly better than placebo. Two-thirds of the cases both in the homeopathy and placebo groups responded clinically within 7 days. Evidence of efficacy of homeopathic treatment beyond placebo was not found in this study. An uncontrolled observational study of the treatment of udder diseases of buffalo showed that a homeopathic complex comprising Phytolacca 200c, Calcarea fluorica 200c, Silicea 30c, Belladona 30c, Bryonia 30c, Arnica 30c, Conium 30c and Ipecacuanha 30c could be effective and economical in the management of udder health problems of buffaloes (Varshney and Naresh, 2004). A total of 102 mastitic quarters (40 fibrosed, 62 non-fibrosed) and five cases each of blood in milk and udder oedema in lactating buffaloes were treated. Treatment was 80 and 96.72% effective in cases of fibrotic mastitis and non-fibrosed mastitis respectively. Recovery period was 21–42 days (fibrosed) and 4–15 days (non-fibrosed). In other work on mastitis, Varshney and Naresh (2005) concluded that a combination of homeopathic Phytolacca, Calcarea fluorica, Silica, Belladonna, Bryonia, Arnica, Conium and Ipecacuanha was effective and economical in the management of mastitis in lactating dairy cows.

A review of early veterinary research may be found at www. chiroweb.com/archives/13/19/19.html.

HOMEOPATHIC RESEARCH – TIME FOR A CHANGE OF EMPHASIS?

There is still a need to establish the validity of homeopathy as a credible therapy and speak loudly to the audiences who need to be convinced, namely the medical establishment and funders of health care (Whitmarsh, 2004).

Homeopathy has developed over the last 200 years as a patient-orientated discipline, with empirical case studies being the source of most prescribers' skills. The list of medicines available remained static for many years but within the last decade or so a limited number of new preparations have appeared, and there has been an increased interest in isopathy. Few other 'patient comforts' can be recorded. Most research has centred on refuting the suggestion that homeopathy acts solely by way of a placebo effect or on trying to discover a credible mechanism of action. It is certainly true that homeopathy suffers from an inability to explain how it works. It is also true that licensing authorities consider such information important and if homeopathy is to be accepted fully we must respond to these demands. Thus, we need to continue these lines of research. Undoubtedly it would help homeopathy if a mechanism of action was discovered and homeopathy would no longer be a prime example of implausibility. The definitive answer might come from a series of rigorous trials with protocols agreed by both camps beforehand. The trials themselves ought to be carried out by fully independent investigators who have no axe to grind. I would argue that, in the interest of science, truth and our patients, this would be an exercise well worth doing (Ernst, 2000).

There is one piece of evidence that cannot be dismissed by truly caring governments. If an ill patient can be shown to have recovered, or even improved, beyond any reasonable doubt, as the result of administering a safe preparation, then universal acceptance of the technique must follow eventually. Should we not direct more of our research to what is happening at the 'sharp end' of medical practice and seek to produce more of this evidence? What is the point of dressing our homeopathic shop window with exciting 'goodies' to entice new customers if the knowledge of our product and the method of its use leave much to be desired?

Effectiveness research is pragmatic and requires different methodological strategies than those used for research into efficacy, which are explanatory in nature (Jacobs, 2000). Most recent homeopathic clinical trials have focused on efficacy – does homeopathy have a significant effect above and beyond that of placebo? While this information is vital in establishing the scientific validity of homeopathy, a different strategy may be necessary to increase the use of homeopathy in clinical practice. If the goal in homeopathic research is to demonstrate the practical usefulness of homeopathy, appropriate experimental methods must be used.

Jacobs (2000) suggests that effectiveness research in homeopathy should involve interventions that are feasible for use in widespread real-world practice, compare homeopathy to usual care, involve a broad segment of the population, have sample sizes adequate to detect clinical as well as statistical significance, and have clinically and economically significant outcomes. They should be designed to guide practical decision making, rather than to answer a specific scientific question.

Homeopathy is more likely to be integrated into the prevailing healthcare system if there is clear evidence of its clinical utility for common illnesses and prescribing strategies are simplified. Homeopathic research protocols should be designed to reflect these priorities in the coming years.

A small amount of research has been carried out to determine what are the most important rubrics to be considered in matching a drug picture. More of this work is needed to improve prescribing techniques, especially for newly qualified colleagues. The 'three-legged stool' approach and the decision processes followed in the OTC environment should be investigated further.

We know little about remedy interactions, except on a purely anecdotal level. No worker has set out to investigate properly in what order remedies should be administered, or whether the 'half an hour after tea/coffee' (or is it 2 hours?) has a basis in fact. The interactions between homeopathic and allopathic medicines might yield a whole new area of treatment possibilities. Many practitioners state that steroids inactivate homeopathic remedies. A project to determine the necessary 'withdrawal period' prior to homeopathic treatment would probably improve efficacy.

How should we store our remedies? If remedies are affected by sunlight, or heat, or X-rays at airports, we should be able to tell our patients with confidence, and have evidence to back up our statements. Patients are constantly asking about shelf-life. We place arbitrary expiry dates on remedies to satisfy EU regulations; this is totally unacceptable. We should be able to determine exact expiry dates from simple experiments. It is generally accepted that the form of the carrier in solid dose forms is unimportant; pills are as good as tablets and granules. Do we have evidence for this statement? Perhaps some remedies work better in liquid form.

Which over-the-counter remedies are the most effective? It would be interesting to test all the OTC products and see whether they are effective against the range of ailments claimed. Do anti-cold and flu tablets actually protect against cold and flu? There is some evidence that they do. Does Bryonia linctus really soothe a dry, troublesome cough? The possibility of OTC trials is often dismissed as impossible to conduct, but there are techniques available. It might improve the effectiveness of these remedies if the degree of necessary counselling was determined. Are supermarkets, cash and carry premises and grocers the right places for health advice? Some research would be useful to determine the support prospective patients need. A code of practice would be appropriate.

All the disciplines involved in homeopathy, including non-medically qualified registered homeopaths, have a part to play, and this should be encouraged by interdisciplinary cooperation. The temptation of trying to fit practice to theory, as the only aim of research, must be avoided by all. Improving our existing techniques would undoubtedly improve our therapeutic success rate, and we all have the means and, perhaps with a little help, the expertise.

Research is not just for the elite of our professions; we should all do our bit and ensure that our patients get better – quicker! Then, armed with the evidence we require, the balance might well swing in our favour.

SUMMARY

Dean (2004) has summarised the current position with regard to homeopathy.

The most enthusiastic proponents of homeopathy would claim that:

- it is totally safe and free from adverse reactions
- it can be used for almost every condition at any time in any patient
- it treats the whole patient as well as the local symptoms of disease.

Evidence currently available would seem to suggest that:

- homeopathy is generally as safe as is claimed and can be used in some situations where allopathy is inappropriate but more rigorous collection of data on suspected adverse reactions is necessary
- more evidence is necessary to support the use of homeopathy in complex conditions and problem and treatment modelling is necessary
- there is evidence that in some circumstances homeopathy appears to be capable of influencing well-being and local disease
- there are economic benefits to accrue from using homeopathy.

REFERENCES

Aabel, S (2000) No beneficial effect of isopathic prophylactic treatment for birch pollen allergy during a low-pollen season: a double-blind, placebo-controlled clinical trial of homeopathic Betula 30c. *Br Homeopath J*, 89: 169–173.

ABPI (2004) [Press release] Pharmaceutical R&D remains vital to Britain. http://www.abpi.org.uk/press/press_releases_04/041025.asp (Accessed 21 January 2005.)

Altman, LK (1990) The myth of 'passing peer review.' In: CBE Editorial Policy Committee *Ethics and Policy in Scientific Publication*. Council of Biology Editors, Chicago, pp 257–268. (Cited in: Horton, R (1995) The rhetoric of research. *Br Med J*, 310: 985–987.)

Alton, S and Kayne, SB (1992) A pilot study of the attitudes and awareness of homeopathy shown by patients in three Manchester pharmacies. *Br Homeopath J*, 81: 189–193.

Anon. (1988a) Editorial reservation. *Nature*, 333: 818.

Anon. (1988b) Nature's call dampens hopes of homeopathic breakthrough. *Guardian*, 27 July 1988, p 2, col 4.

Anon. (1988c) Ghosts in a pipette: invalid biological research recently reported in Nature magazine. *Guardian*, 2 August 1988, p 30, col 7.

Anon. (1998) Ethical experiments answering precisely framed questions. Report on Science Symposium on Clinical Trials, British Pharmaceutical Conference, 1998. *Pharm J*, 261: 670.

Anon. (2005) The end of homeopathy [Editorial]. *Lancet*, 336: 699.

Antonchenko, VY and Ilyin, VV (1992) Points at issue in the physics of water and homeopathy. *Br Homeopath J*, 81: 91–93.

Baas, C (2004) The pitfalls of clinical case research: lessons from the Delphi project. *Homeopathy*, 93: 21–26.

Bellavite, P and Signorini, A (1995) *Homeopathy: A Frontier in Medical Science*. North Atlantic Books, Berkeley, CA, pp 242–301.

Bellows, HP (1906) *The Test Drug Proving of the O.O. and L. Society: A Reproving of Belladonna*. American Homeopathic Ophthalmological, Otological, and Laryngological Society, Boston.

Belon, P, Cumps, J, Ennis, M et al. (2004) Histamine dilutions modulate basophil activity. *Inflamm Res*, 53: 181–188.

Benveniste, J (1988) Reply. *Nature*, 334: 291.

Benveniste, J, Davenas, E, Ducot, B et al. (1991) L'agitation de solutions hautement diluées n'induit pas d'activité biologique spécifique. *Comptes Rendus de l'Académie des Sciences Paris*, 312(Série II): 461–466.

Betti, L, Lazzarato, L, Trebbi, G et al. (2003) Effects of homeopathic arsenic on tobacco plant resistance to tobacco mosaic virus: theoretical suggestions about system variability, based on a large experimental data set. *Homeopathy*, 92: 195–202.

Biddis, J (1979) Homeopathy. *Vet Rev*, 25: 82–85.

Bol, A (1991) Basic research in homeopathy. *HomInt Research and Development Newsletter*, 2(2): 3.

Bower, H (1998) Double standards exist in judging traditional and alternative medicine. *Br Med J*, 316: 1694.

Bowler, MT (1993) A study on the efficacy of homeopathic treatment of *Aeromonas salmonicida* infection in Atlantic salmon parr. MSc Thesis, University of Stirling, Scotland.

Bradford, TL (1900) *The Logic of Figures or Comparative Results of Homeopathic and Other Treatments*. Boericke and Tafel, Philadelphia.

Broom, A, Barnes, J and Tovey, P (2004) Introduction to the research methods in CAM series. *Complement Ther Med*, 12: 126–130.

Cohen, H (1993) Homeopathic dilutions and the crystalline nature of water. *Resonance*, 15(6): 5–11, 34.

Concar, D (1991) Ghost molecules theory back from the dead. *New Scientist*, 129: 10.

Cucherat, M, Haugh, MC, Gooch, M and Boissel, JP (2000) Evidence of clinical efficacy of homeopathy: a meta-analysis of clinical trials. *Eur J Clin Pharmacol*, 56: 27–33.

Datta, S, Mallick, P and Khuda Bukhsh, AR (1999) Efficacy of a potentized homeopathic drug (Arsenicum Album-30) in reducing genotoxic effects produced by arsenic trioxide in mice: comparative studies of pre-, post- and combined pre- and post-oral administration and comparative efficacy of two microdoses. *Complement Ther Med*, 7: 62–75.

Davenas, E, Beauvais, J, Amara, J, Belon, P and Benveniste, J (1988) Human basophil degranulation triggered by very dilute antiserum against IgE. *Nature*, 333: 816–818.

Davies, M and Kayne, SB (1992) Homeopathy – a pilot study of the attitudes and awareness of pharmacy staff in the Stoke-on-Trent area. *Br Homeopath J*, 81: 194–198.

Day, CEL (1984) Control of stillbirths in pigs using homeopathy. *Vet Record*, 114: 216.

Day, CEL (1985) Homeopathy in cattle practice – some food for thought. British Cattle Veterinary Association Proceedings, 1983–1984, pp 217–220. Beecham Animal Health.

Day, CEL (1986) Clinical trials in bovine mastitis: use of nosodes for prevention. *Br Homeopath J*, 75: 11–15.

Dean, ME (2000) More trials, fewer placebos please. *Homeopathy*, 89: 178–187.

Dean, ME (2004) *The Trials of Homeopathy*. KVC Verlag, Stuttgart, pp 245–246.

Edwards, T (2005) Obituary. Jacques Benveniste, 12 March 1935–4 October 2004. *Homeopathy*, 94: 76–77.

Endler, P (1989) Aspects of information storage in water. *Br Homeopath J*, 78: 253–254.

Ernst, E (1995) Effects of homoeopathy [Letter]. *BMJ*, 311: 510–511.

Ernst, E (2000) The demise of homoeopathy? *Pharm J*, 264: 66.

Ernst, E (2002) A systematic review of systematic reviews of homeopathy. *Br J Clin Pharmacol*, 54: 577–582.

Ernst, E (2003) The benefits of Arnica: 16 case reports. *Homeopathy*, 92: 217–219.

Ernst, E (2004a) Should we use 'powerful placebos'? *Pharm J*, 273: 795.

Ernst, E (2004b) Anecdotal obsessions? a comment on the use of anecdotes by the general media to support claims in CAM. *Complement Ther Nurs Midwifery*, 10: 254–255.

Ernst, E and Pittler, MH (1998) Efficacy of homeopathic arnica: a systematic review of placebo-controlled clinical trials. *Arch Surg*, 133: 1187–1990.

Ezzo, J (2003) Should journals devote space to trials with no results? *J Altern Complement Med*, 9: 611–612.

Ezzo, J, Bausell, B, Moerman, DE, Berman, B and Hadhazy, V (2001) CAM in the USA – reviewing the reviews. How strong is the evidence? How clear are the conclusions? *Int J Technol Assess Health Care*, 17: 457–466.

Feder, G and Katz, T (2002) Randomised controlled trials for homeopathy. *Br Med J*, 324: 498–499.

Finnegan, M (1991) Complementary medicine; attitudes and expectations, a scale for evaluation. *Complement Med Res*, 5: 79–81.

Fisher, P (2004a) A landmark for basic research in homeopathy. *Homeopathy*, 93: 162–163.

Fisher, P (2004b) Entangled, or tied in knots [Editorial]? *Homeopathy*, 93: 171–172.

Fisher, P, Greenwood, A, Huskisson, EC, Turner, P and Belon, P (1989) Effect of homeopathic treatment on fibrositis. *Br Med J*, 299: 365–366.

Furnham, A and Smith, C (1988) Choosing alternative medicine: a comparison of the beliefs of patients visiting a general practitioner and a homoeopath. *Soc Sci Med*, 26(7): 685–689.

Gerhard, I and Wallis, E (2002) Individualized homeopathic therapy for male infertility. *Homeopathy*, 91: 133–144.

Gibson, RG, Gibson, SL, MacNeill, AD et al. (1978) Salicylates and homeopathy in rheumatoid arthritis. *Br J Clin Pharmacol*, 6: 391–395.

Gibson, RG, Gibson, SL, MacNeill, AD and Watson-Buchanan, W (1980) Homeopathic therapy in arthritis – evaluation by double blind clinical therapeutic trial. *Br J Clin Pharmacol*, 9: 453–459.

Goodman, SN, Berlin, JA, Fletcher, SW and Fletcher, RH (1993) Effect of peer review and editorial changes on the quality of manuscripts published in the Annals of Internal Medicine. Proceedings of Second International Congress on Peer Review in Biomedical Publications, Chicago, September, 1993. (Cited in: Horton, R (1995) The rhetoric of research. *Br Med J*, 310: 985–987).

GRECO (1989) Evaluation de deux produits homéopathiques sur la reprise du transit après chirurgie digestive. *La Presse Médicale*, 18(2): 59–62.

Greenhalgh, T and Hurwitz, B (1999) Why study narrative? *Br Med J*, 318: 48–50.

Haselen, R, van and Fisher, P (1994) Describing and improving homeopathy. *Br Homeopath J*, 83: 135–141.

Hayes, P, Kayne, SB and Martin, T (1992) Use of professional self audit in pharmacy practice. *Pharm J*, 249: 650–652.

Heger, M and Haidvog, DSM (2000) International integrative primary care outcomes study (IIPCOS-2): an international research project of homeopathy in primary care. *Homeopathy*, 89(Suppl. 1): S10–S13.

Hektoen, L, Larsen, S, Odegaard, SA and Loken, T (2004) Comparison of homeopathy, placebo and antibiotic treatment of clinical mastitis in dairy cows – methodological issues and results from a randomized-clinical trial. *J Vet Med A Physiol Pathol Clin Med*, 51(9–10): 439–446.

HMRG (1996) Report to the European Commission Directorate General XII: science, research and development. Vol 1 (short version). Homeopathic Medicine Research Group, Brussels: European Commission, 16–17. (Cited in: Taylor, MA, Reilly, D, Llewellyn-Jones, RH, McSharry, C and Aitchison, TA (2000) Randomised controlled trial of homeopathy versus placebo in perennial allergic rhinitis with overview of four trial series *Br Med J*, 321: 471–476.)

Hornung, J (1990) Misconception or guidepost – the 1978 study by Gibson et al. on rheumatoid arthritis reviewed. *Berlin J Res Homeopathy*, 1(1): 77–84.

Hornung, J (1991a) Guidelines for the exact description of the preparation and mode of application of serial dilutions and potencies in publications on ultra low dose effects and homeopathic research: a proposal. *Berlin J Res Homeopathy*, 1(2): 121–123.

Hornung, J (1991b) Was it the better way? The 1980 study by Gibson et al. – reviewed. *Berlin J Res Homeopathy*, 1(2): 124–128.

Horton, R (1995) The rhetoric of research. *Br Med J*, 310: 985–987.

Hutton, H (2003) Arnica works if used properly. BMJ Rapid Response, 9th February. Available at http://bmj.bmjjournals.com/cgi/eletters/326/7384/303/c#29493.

Hyland, M (2003) Extended network generalized entanglement theory therapeutic mechanisms, empirical predictions, and investigations. *J Altern Comp Med*, 9: 919–936.

Jacobs, J (2000) Effectiveness research in homeopathy methodology and practical considerations. *Br Homeopath J*, 89(Suppl. 1): S47.

Jacobs, J, Jimenez, LM, Gloyd, S, Gale, J and Crothers, D (1994) Treatment of acute childhood diarrhea with homeopathic medicine: a randomised clinical trial in Nicaragua. *Paediatrics*, 93(5): 719–725.

Jansen, GRHJ, v.d. Veer, ALJ, Hagenaars, J and v.d. Kuy, A (1992) Lessons learnt from an unsuccessful clinical trial of homeopathy. *Br Homeopath J*, 81: 132–138.

Jonas, W, Kaptchuk, T and Linde, K (2003) Critical overview of homeopathy. *Ann Intern Med*, 138: 393–399.

Jones, RL and Jenkins, MD (1981) Plant responses to homeopathic medicines. *Br Homeopath J*, 70: 120–128.

Jones, RL and Jenkins, MD (1983) Comparison of wheat and yeast as in vitro models for investigating homeopathic medicines. *Br Homeopath J*, 72: 143–147.

Kayne, SB (1991) An agricultural application of homeopathy. *Br Homeopath J*, 80: 157–160.

Kayne, SB and Kayne, LR (2000) Misleading [Letter]. *Pharm J*, 264: 94.

Kayne, SB and McGuire, A (1993) Attitudes to homeopathy in a sample of veterinarians. *Complement Ther Med*, 1: 185–188.

Kayne, S and Rafferty, A (1994) The use of Arsenicum album 30c to complement conventional treatment of neonatal diarrhoea ('scours') in calves. *Br Homeopath J*, 83: 202–204.

Kayne, SB, McGovern, EM and Taylor, A (1994) Professional self-audit in Greater Glasgow community pharmacies. *Pharm J*, 252: 261–262.

Kayne, SB, Beattie, N and Reeves, A (1999) Survey of buyers of over-the-counter homoeopathic medicines. *Pharm J*, 263: 210–212.

King, D (1995) Homeopathy Dynamic Chiropractic; 13. Available at http://www.chiroweb.com/archives/13/19/19.html. (Accessed 10 January 2004.)

Kleijnen, J (2001) What research is needed to show the effectiveness of homeopathy? *Br Homeopath J*, 89(Suppl. 1): 51–52.

Kleijnen, J, Knipschild, P and ter Riet, G (1991) Clinical trials of homeopathy. *Br Med J*, 302: 316–323.

Klerk, ESM de Lange de, Blommers, J, Kuik, DJ et al. (1994) Effect of homeopathic medicines on daily burden of symptoms in children with recurrent upper respiratory infections. *Br Med J*, 309: 1329–1332.

Kolisko, L (1959) *Physiologischer und physikalischer Nachweis der Wirksamkeit kleinster Entitaeten, 1923–1959*. Arbgmschaft anthroposophie Aerzte, Stuttgart.

Lancaster, T and Vickers, A (2000) Commentary. Larger trials necessary. *Br Med J*, 321: 476.

Langman, MJS (1997) Homoeopathy trials, reasons for good ones but are they warranted? *Lancet*, 350: 825.

Lessell, CB (1995) *The Infinitesimal Dose*. CW Daniel, Saffron Walden.

Lewith, GT, Watkins, AD, Hyland, ME et al. (2002) Use of ultramolecular potencies of allergen to treat asthmatic people allergic to house dust mite: double blind randomised controlled clinical trial. *Br Med J*, 324: 520.

Linde, K and Melchart, D (1998) Randomized controlled trials of individualized homeopathy: a state-of-the-art review. *J Altern Complement Med*, 4: 371–388.

Linde, K, Melchart, D, Jonas, WB et al. (1994) Ways to enhance the quality and acceptance of clinical and laboratory studies in homeopathy. *Br Homeopath J*, 83: 3–7.

Linde, K, Clausius, N, Ramirez, G et al. (1997) Are the clinical effects of homeopathy placebo effects? A meta-analysis of placebo-controlled trials. *Lancet*, 350: 834–843.

Linde, K, Scholz, M, Ramirez, G et al. (1999) Impact of study quality on outcome in placebo-controlled trials of homeopathy. *J Clin Epidemiol*, 52: 631–636.

Ludtke, R and Wilkens, J (1998) Arnica 30DH after knee surgery: three randomised double-blind clinical trials. Presented at the 5th Annual Symposium on Complementary Healthcare, 10–12 December 1998, Exeter.

Macêdo, SB, Ferreira, LR, Perazzo, FF et al. (2004) Anti-inflammatory activity of *Arnica montana* 6cH: preclinical study in animals. *Homeopathy*, 93: 84–87.

MacEoin, D (1988) The Benveniste affair and the denaturing of science. *J Altern Complement Med*, (Sept): 14, 16, 30, 38.

Mackie, WL, Williamson, AV, Crawford, WJ et al. (1990) A study model with initial findings using Sepia 200 given prophylactically to prevent anoestrus problems in the dairy cow. *Br Homeopath J*, 79: 132–134.

Macleod, G (1974) Coli-bacillosis of calves, or scour in calves and the rational approach to treatment and prevention. *Homeopathy*, 20: 30–31.

Macleod, G (1981) *The Treatment of Cattle by Homeopathy*. Health Science Press, Saffron Walden.

MacPhaerson, H (2004) Pragmatic clinical trials. *Complement Ther Med*, 12: 136–140.

Madox, J, Randi, J and Stewart, WW (1988) High dilution experiments a delusion. *Nature*, 334: 287–290.

Mathie, RT (2003a) Clinical outcomes research: contributions to the evidence base for homeopathy. *Homeopathy*, 92: 56–57.

Mathie, RT (2003b) The research evidence base for homeopathy: a fresh assessment of the literature. *Homeopathy*, 92: 84–91.

Mathie, RT and Kayne, LR (2004) Unbalanced opinion [Letter]. *Pharm J*, 273: 815.

Merck, CC, Sonnenwald, B and Rollwage, H (1989) The administration of homeopathic drugs for the treatment of acute mastitis in cattle. *Berl Munch Tierarztl Wochenschr*, 102(8): 266–272.

Merrell, WC and Shalts, E (2002) Homeopathy. *Med Clin North Am*, 86(1): 47–62.

Milgrom, R (2004a) Patient practitioner entanglement, part 5. Can homeopathic remedy reactions be outcomes of PPR entanglement? *Homeopathy*, 93: 94–98.

Milgrom, R (2004b) Patient practitioner entanglement, part 6. Miasms revisited, non-linear quantum theory as a model for the homeopathic process. *Homeopathy*, 93: 154–158.

Montori, VM, Jaeschke, R, Schünemann, HJ et al. (2004) Users' guide to detecting misleading claims in clinical research reports. *Br Med J*, 329: 1093–1096.

Morton, DB (1988) Homeopathy [Letter]. *Vet Record*, 12 May: 448.

Muscari-Tomaioli, G, Allegri, F, Miali, E et al. (2001) Observational study of quality of life in patients with headache receiving homeopathic treatment. *Br Homeopath J*, 90: 189–197.

Needleman, DB (2003) Would not use arnica for pain relief [Letter]. *Pharm J*, 270: 268.

Oberbaum, M, Vithoulkas, G, van Haselen, R and Singer, S (2003) Reinventing the wheel? Or the emperor's new clothes. *J Altern Complement Med*, 9: 613–617.

Pelikan, W and Unger, G (1971) The activity of potentised substances. *Br Homeopath J*, 60: 232–266.

Poitevin, B (1967) *Le Devenir de l'homéopathie: Elements de théorie et de recherche*. Doin Editeurs, Paris.

Reilly, DT and Taylor, MA (1985) Potent placebo or potency? A proposed study model with initial findings using homeopathically prepared pollens in hayfever. *Br Homeopath J*, 74: 65–75.

Reilly, DT, Taylor, MA, McSharry, C and Aitchison, TC (1986) Is homeopathy a placebo response? Controlled trial of homeopathic potency with pollen in hayfever as model. *Lancet*, ii: 881–886.

Reilly, DT, Taylor, MA, Beattie, NGM et al. (1994) Is evidence for homeopathy reproducible? *Lancet*, 344: 1601–1606.

Richardson, WR (2001) Patient benefit survey: Liverpool Regional Department of Homeopathic Medicine. *Br Homeopath J*, 90(3): 158–162.

Riet, G ter, Kleijnen, J and Knipschild, P (1990) A meta-analysis of studies into the effect of acupuncture in addiction. *Br J Gen Pract*, 40: 379–382.

Riley, D, Fischer, M, Singh, B et al. (2001) Homeopathy and conventional medicine: an outcomes study comparing effectiveness in a primary care setting. *J Altern Complement Med*, 7: 149–159.

Rutten, L (2004) The benefits of Arnica [Letter]. *Homeopathy*, 93: 63.

Schiff, M (1995) *The Memory of Water*. Thorsons, London, pp 78–82.

Schlappack, O (2004) Homeopathic treatment of radiation-induced itching in breast cancer patients: a prospective observational study. *Homeopathy*, 93: 210–215.

Schwartz, D and Lellouch, J (1967) Explanatory and pragmatic attitudes in therapeutic trials. *J Chronic Dis*, 20: 637–648. (Cited in: MacPhaerson, H (2004) Pragmatic clinical trials. *Complement Ther Med*, 12: 136–140.)

Scofield, AM (1984a) Experimental research in homeopathy – a critical review. *Br Homeopath J*, 73: 50.

Scofield, AM (1984b) Homeopathy and its potential role in agriculture – a critical review. *Biol Agriculture Horticulture*, 2: 1–50.

Sevar, R (2000) Audit of outcome in 829 consecutive patients treated with homeopathic medicines. *Br Homeopath J*, 89: 178–187.

Shang, A, Huwiler-Mütener, K, Nartey, L et al. (2005) Are the clinical effects of homeopathy placebo effects? Comparative study of homeopathy and allopathy. *Lancet*, 336: 726–732.

Simmons, AG (2003) Arnica can be of benefit at appropriate dose [Letter]. *Pharm J*, 270: 268.

Singh, PP and Chhabra, HL (1993) Topological investigation of the ethanol/water system and its implications for the mode of action of homeopathic medicines. *Br Homeopath J*, 82: 164–171.

Slade, K, Chohan, BPS and Barker, PJ (2004) Evaluation of a GP practice based homeopathy service. *Homeopathy*, 93: 67–70.

Smith, T (1988) Drop of the weak stuff. *Br Med J*, 297: 377–378.

Steinsbekk, A and Lüdtke, R (2005) Patients' assessments of the effectiveness of homeopathic care in Norway: a prospective observational multicentre outcome study. *Homeopathy*, 94: 10–16.

Steinsbekk, A, Bentzen, N, Honnebo, V and Lewith, GT (2004) Randomised clinical trials on treatment by homeopaths and self-treatment with homeopathic medicines: design and protocol. *J Altern Complement Med*, 10: 1027–1032.

Stevinson, C, Devaraj, VS, Fountain-Barber, A, Hawkins, S and Ernst, E (2003) Homeopathic arnica for prevention of pain and bruising: randomized placebo-controlled trial in hand surgery. *J R Soc Med*, 96: 60–65.

Swayne, J (1989) Survey of the use of homeopathic medicine in the UK health system. *J R Coll Gen Pract*, 39: 503–506.

Swayne, J (1992) The cost and effectiveness of homeopathy. *Br Homeopath J*, 81: 148–150.

Swayne, J (1998) Editorial. *Homeopathic Method. Implications for Clinical Practice and Medical Science*. Churchill Livingstone, London.

Taylor, SM, Mallon, TR and Green, WP (1989) Efficacy of homeopathic prophylaxis against experimental infection of calves by bovine lungworm. *Vet Record*, 124: 15–17.

Taylor, MA, Reilly, D, Llewellyn-Jones, RH, McSharry, C and Aitchison, TA (2000) Randomised controlled trial of homeopathy versus placebo in perennial allergic rhinitis with overview of four trial series. *Br Med J*, 321: 471–476.

Thompson, E, Barron, S and Spence, D (2004) Preliminary audit investigating remedy reactions including adverse events in routine homeopathic practice. *Homeopathy*, 93: 203–209.

Trehan, PK, Singh, B and Dhir, DS (1985) Effects of some homeopathic and allopathic preparations on the growth and feed efficiency in broilers. *Indian J Poultry Sci*, 20: 61–62.

Vandenbroucke, JP (1997) Homeopathic trials going nowhere. *Lancet*, 350: 824.

Varshney, JP and Naresh, R (2004) Evaluation of a homeopathic complex in the clinical management of udder diseases of riverine buffaloes. *Homeopathy*, 93: 17–20.

Varshney, JP and Naresh, R (2005) Comparative efficacy of homeopathic and allopathic systems of medicine in the management of clinical mastitis of Indian dairy cows. *Homeopathy*, 94: 81–85.

Vickers, A (1995) What conclusions should we draw from the data? *Br Homeopath J*, 84: 95–101.

Vickers, A (2000) Clinical trials of homeopathy and placebo: analysis of a scientific debate. *J Altern Complement Med*, 6: 49–56.

Vithoulkas, G (1980) *The Science of Homeopathy*. Grove Press, New York, p 103.

Vithoulkas, G (1985) Homeopathic experimentation: the problem of double blind trials and some suggestions. *J Complement Med*, 1: 10–15.

Walach, H (2000) Magic of signs: a non-local interpretation of homeopathy. *Br Homeopath J*, 89: 127–140.

Walach, H (2003a) Entanglement model of homeopathy as an example of generalised entanglement predicted by weak quantum theory. *Forsch Komp Klass Natur*, 10: 192–200. (Cited in: Milgrom, R (2004) Patient practitioner entanglement, part 5. Can homeopathic remedy reactions be outcomes of PPR entanglement? *Homeopathy*, 93: 94–98.)

Walach, H (2003b) Reinventing the wheel will not make it rounder: controlled trials of homeopathy reconsidered. *J Altern Complement Med*, 9: 7–13.

Walach, H and Guthlin, C (2000) Effects of acupuncture and homeopathy: prospective documentation. Interim results. *Br Homeopath J*, 89(Suppl. 1): S31–S34.

Walach, H, Jonas, WB and Lewith, GT (2002) The role of outcomes research in evaluating complementary and alternative medicine. *Altern Ther Health Med*, 8: 88–95.

Walker, MJ (1994) *Dirty Medicine*, revised edn. Slingshot Publications, London, p 69.

Wannamaker, AK (1966) Effects of sulphur dynamisations on onions. *J Am Inst Homeopathy*, 59: 287–295.

Wannamaker, AK (1968) Further work with boron dilutions. *J Am Inst Homeopathy*, 61: 28–29.

Weatherley-Jones, E, Thompson, EA and Thomas, KJ (2004) The placebo-controlled trial as a test of complementary and alternative medicine: observations from research experience of individualised homeopathic treatment. *Homeopathy*, 83: 186–189.

Weingärtner, O (2003) What is the therapeutically active ingredient of homeopathic potencies? *Homeopathy*, 92: 145–151.

Whitmarsh, T (2002) Editorial commentary. *Cephalalgia*, 22: 331–332.

Whitmarsh, T (2004) Clinical research in homeopathy: randomised, controlled or outcome studies? *Homeopathy*, 93: 1–2.

Wiegant, FAC, Kramers, CW and Wijk, R van (1991) Clinical research in complementary medicine: the importance of patient selection. *Complement Med Res*, 5: 110–115.

Chapter 12

Education

CHAPTER CONTENTS

Training courses	321	Gaining knowledge	329
Giving talks	324	Online sources of information	330
Deciding content	324	Setting up your stocks	330
Example of an address to an		Joining an organisation	332
unqualified audience	325	Stock control	332
A few tips ...	328	Publicising your interest	333
Getting started	329	A final word to pharmacists	333

TRAINING COURSES

Training in homeopathy has developed along two clear pathways in the UK. Medical practitioners and members of the professions allied to medicine have chosen one route, augmenting their qualification by studying at postgraduate level and, in most cases, using homeopathy as another string to their orthodox therapeutic bow. The other route is taken by professional homeopaths, whose course at a School or College of Homeopathy may be as long, or even longer, than the combined medical and postgraduate homeopathic training. It leads to qualification as a registered homeopath, differentiating these practitioners from lay or amateur homeopaths who have not received any formal training. Traditionally the two camps have not communicated, the medically qualified believing that their superior knowledge of anatomy, physiology and clinical practice set them apart. The professional homeopaths have an important contribution to make, however, and discussions are ongoing to find some common ground for cooperation.

Nurses, pharmacists, physiotherapists, podiatrists or any other similarly qualified persons from a profession allied to medicine cannot become homeopaths merely by taking a course orientated towards their own particular discipline. Any colleagues with this aim in mind should seek more comprehensive training.

The Faculty of Homeopathy was responsible for organising the training of medically qualified practitioners for over 40 years after its creation by Act of Parliament in 1950, and for veterinary surgeons too in later years. Courses were run in the main centres of Bristol, Glasgow and London. The format varied slightly, but study was usually either part-time, extending over a total of 3 years, or full-time over 6 months; both formats led to the award of Membership of the Faculty of Homeopathy (MFHom). To obtain membership, students must have been qualified in medicine for at least 3 years, and this requirement still exists. The Faculty acted as a Teaching, Examining and Accrediting body all rolled into one. The course was very comprehensive, required much application of effort and produced a handful of graduates each year.

At this time the Faculty was not involved in specialised training for members of professions other than medicine and veterinary medicine. Nelson's and Weleda both ran short pharmacy courses over the years, as did the British Homeopathic Association. They all did a good job in providing basic training for pharmacists. Unfortunately the standard and content varied greatly.

Under the guidance of Hamish Boyd and David Reilly in Glasgow, the format of the medical courses began to evolve along multidisciplinary lines in the 1980s. New, more attractive teaching methods were introduced and much of the course content was reorganised. Other centres, including Bristol, London and Oxford, followed Glasgow's lead. These changes proved popular and it was not long before the homeopathic medical course became the most popular postgraduate course in the UK. A 25-hour course was designed for pharmacists to run in parallel with the postgraduate medical course in Glasgow during the period September to November each year, starting in 1985. There were joint interdisciplinary sessions with colleagues from other professions and specialist pharmacy sessions. After 4 years, an assessment phase was introduced comprising a project, a short written paper (mainly multiple choice) and an oral examination. On successful completion the candidates were awarded a Faculty Certificate in Basic Homeopathic Pharmacy. By 1990 the course was enjoying considerable success and was 'exported' to London where numbers of candidates reached 40–50 each year. Course content and the final examination were common to both centres, assuring a measure of standardisation. The BHA then discontinued their pharmacy courses, leaving the Glasgow and London Faculty courses as the only source of education. There was considerable strain on teaching resources with courses running at both ends of the country, and although three intermediate courses were held in London, the projected advanced pharmacy course did not materialise as planned.

In 1994–5 the Faculty relinquished its teaching function to newly constituted academic departments based at the hospitals in the three main teaching centres, and assumed an examining role (which was initially given to Glasgow to administer) and an accreditation function. Concurrently, the pharmacy model was adopted by the medical courses as the basis for developing a new qualification – the Primary Care Certificate (PCC). During this time progress was made with dental, nursing and podiatry training. Veterinary training took a slightly different pathway as the NHS oriented PCC was inappropriate for the profession's needs.

The Primary Care Certificate was offered after a 1-year introductory course for those physicians who wished to understand homeopathy and achieve some proficiency in using the discipline, but without necessarily becoming medical homeopaths. The Glasgow Primary Care Certificate was then offered to pharmacists, with variants following for other disciplines. Further developments led to the establishment of a formalised system of education.

Accredited postgraduate courses are now delivered at four locations in England and two in Scotland as well as five overseas. Course provision differs by location so it is important for the would-be student to choose a curriculum that meets his or her particular needs. Faculty training is open to healthcare professionals who hold a qualification that is statutorily registerable in the UK. All Faculty-accredited courses are extensive in the depth and breadth of subject matter covered, and practitioners are expected to gain an understanding of the areas outlined below:

- core principles and concepts of homeopathy
- the historical and philosophical background to the development of homeopathy
- current scientific evidence
- homeopathic pharmacy and materia medica
- consultation and case analysis skills.

Once their training is complete, practitioners will have gained an appreciation of the scope and limits of homeopathy within contemporary medicine, and how this knowledge can be applied within their particular discipline and level of practice.

Foundation training is offered for healthcare practitioners who wish to understand the basic principles of homeopathy. The curriculum specifies the core knowledge required for the Primary Health Care Examination (PHCE) and the Preliminary Certificate in Veterinary Homeopathy (PCVH) examination. Successful candidates are eligible to become Licenced Associates of the Faculty and may use the qualification LFHom followed by a suffix denoting the practitioner's profession.

Diploma level training is available for dentists and pharmacists. It equips practitioners to use homeopathy extensively in conditions appropriate to, and within, the accepted bounds of competence of their particular profession, and prepares students to sit the Diploma examinations. Successful candidates are eligible to become Diplomate members and dentists may use the letters DFHom (Dent), and pharmacists DFHom (Pharm).

MFHom training expands substantially on introductory training and prepares doctors, nurses, vets and pharmacists who satisfy the entry criteria for the membership examination. Successful candidates are eligible to become full members of the Faculty and may use the qualification MFHom, MFHom (Nurse), MFHom (Pharm) or VetMFHom.

The Faculty awards Fellowships and Honorary Fellowships to healthcare professionals who have made a special contribution to homeopathy.

The Education Development Officer at the Faculty of Homeopathy in Luton and the Faculty Office in Glasgow will supply further details (see Appendix 1 for addresses). The Centre for Continuing Pharmacy Education for England in Manchester has produced a distance learning course in complementary medicine.

The UK is unique in having an independent body such as the Faculty to accredit training without any commercial bias. This is recognised abroad, resulting in numerous enquiries for help in designing and delivering courses. Training has been organised in countries such as Ireland, Russia, India, New Zealand and Australia with the assistance of local colleagues. In foreign countries, the training is often provided by the manufacturers; in New Zealand, Naturo Pharm and Weleda run both seminars and distance learning courses, while Brauer are active in Australia. The French producer Boiron has always been extremely active in training pharmacists and doctors.

With all the courses, emphasis is on ensuring that participants can understand the main features of homeopathy and be in a position to advise customers. This enables them to make informed decisions as to the suitability of using homeopathy in given sets of circumstances. The course will also give the student plenty of opportunities for making up his or her own mind whether or not homeopathy has a part to play in modern medicine. An important advance in gaining wider acceptance for homeopathy was the decision by the Boots Company in 1993 to train a large number of its pharmacists in preparation for a new range of own-label homeopathic remedies. The company also produced some excellent self-help material and is to be congratulated on its initiative.

The University of Exeter has the first UK Chair of Complementary Medicine (currently occupied by Professor Edzard Ernst). The Department for Complementary Medicine is part of the Peninsula Medical School and offers taught postgraduate degree courses in complementary health studies on a full-time and part-time basis; the courses are designed to provide advanced education for health professionals and cover a wide range of complementary topics (see www.pms.ac.uk/compmed).

GIVING TALKS
Deciding content

If you become known as having an interest in homeopathy or any of the other complementary disciplines you will undoubtedly be asked to talk to local groups, colleagues, or both. Putting together a talk is not easy, however, especially if you are not used to public speaking. The audience may vary from three people in a cold church hall in the middle of absolutely nowhere on a cold, snowy winter's night to 250 people in a hotel with a disco in the next room (I speak with some experience!).

The following factors influence what you might say:

- **How long do you have to speak?** About 30–40 minutes is probably about right, followed by 15 minutes of questions
- **Who is your audience?** If they are professional colleagues, you might adopt a different approach to a talk given to an unqualified audience
- **Does your audience have any special affinity?** If they are young mothers, or sports persons, you could use this fact to illustrate various points
- **Does the audience have any knowledge of the subject?** This will tell you at what level to pitch your talk.

The following section is an abstract of a talk I gave to a Ladies' Guild. It could be used to provide a starting point for a talk or article (getting started is often the most troublesome aspect of producing a script).

Example of an address to an unqualified audience

A fashionable painter in Leipzig in the late 1700s once complained that he felt unwell. He was suffering from that 'one degree under' feeling so well known today under the title of 'stress' or even 'depression'. A doctor visiting his studio noticed that he was working with sepia, a colour made by extracting the ink of the squid, and that the painter frequently sucked the tip of his brush to bring it to a sharp point. The doctor took a sample of the sepia ink away with him, and returned the next day with a homeopathic medicine made from the sample. The painter, being an extremely trusting sort of chap, took the remedy, and shortly after pronounced himself fit.

What made this treatment unusual at the time was that in the eighteenth century the idea grew up that disease was an intruder to be fought with whatever weapons were available – the battleground being the unfortunate patient's body! The poor patient would be given enormous doses of whatever remedy happened to be in vogue at the time; emetics and purgatives were frequently used and of course there were the leeches and blood-letting techniques. This was what might be called 'competitive medicine' ... if the patient recovered then all the physicians – especially the last one – would claim credit. If, as often happened, the patient died then they all blamed each other – especially the last one! The doctor I mentioned earlier was also an apothecary, and worked as a translator of medical works from English, Hebrew, Greek and French into his native German. While translating a famous textbook by the great Scottish physician William Cullen, he found himself in disagreement with the great man regarding the action of the drug quinine, a recently introduced remedy for a condition then called 'marsh fever' but now known as malaria. Testing the drug on himself, he found that it produced symptoms very similar to the condition it was being used to cure. Further, the symptoms of belladonna poisoning were similar to the symptoms of scarlet fever for which the remedy was prescribed. It seemed that there might be a law of drug action, whereby drugs that produced certain symptoms in healthy volunteers might cure sick patients presenting similar symptoms.

The doctor was Christian Samuel Hahnemann. He was born in Meissen, Saxony, in 1755, the son of a pottery painter in the famous china factory. The medical discipline he pioneered he called 'homeopathy', from the Greek *Homoeos* ('like') and *Pathos* ('suffering'). With this word we meet the first great characteristic of homeopathy: 'like cures like'.

This idea is often totally opposite to the ideas of other medical disciplines. Take, for example, the use of a laxative to treat constipation; in homeopathy we would instead use a very small dose of a remedy that in much greater concentration might well cause the symptom of constipation. Thus a remedy for insomnia comes from the green coffee bean. I can still remember the words of my dear old grandma saying 'You keep away from these new-fangled drinks like coffee; you will never get a good night's sleep again if you drink them!' A remedy to treat alcoholism comes from the very same succulent used to make tequila. Lactrodectus is a spider whose venom causes symptoms similar to angina. All the remedies we use have a 'drug picture'. This is a written survey of the symptoms noted when the drug was given to healthy volunteers, and compiled in books known as materia medica and repertories.

The second great 'rule' of homeopathy is the use of a 'minimal dose'. When Hahnemann did his original work he gave substantial doses of medicine to his patients, not always with good results! He experimented by diluting out his remedies and shaking them in a special manner. We do not know why he suddenly decided to shake or 'succuss' the remedies, but to his great amazement he found that as the remedies became more dilute they became stronger in their therapeutic effect. A teaspoonful of salt would be unpleasant to take, yet it would have little effect other than to make you very thirsty. However, when diluted down to one part in a million it becomes extremely active in the treatment of many conditions including violent and prolonged sneezing. The preparation procedure is very specialised, and because the remedy becomes stronger acting the process is known as 'potentisation'. For very acute conditions we might well use remedies diluted down to one part in 10 followed by 30 noughts! In this area, not unnaturally, we find it extremely difficult to explain how the remedy works. The idea of the minute dose is not unknown in allopathic medicine, where for example heart drugs are used in micro doses.

The third important idea is that qualified homeopaths generally treat patients with only one remedy rather than with a selection, as is often the case with orthodox medicine. Perhaps the most important idea of homeopathy, and one that is shared with many other associated therapies including herbalism and aromatherapy, is that conditions are not treated in isolation – we treat the whole person. To a homeopath there is, broadly speaking, no one remedy to treat a condition. The remedy will vary with the patient. A remedy indicated for one patient might well be totally inappropriate to another, even though the symptoms appear similar. Conversely one remedy might be used to treat very different conditions in different patients. A first consultation would involve an investigation into a patient's personality, nutritional likes and dislikes (sweet, sour or spicy food, salt, mustard), atmospheric preferences, (cold, hot, wet, dry, windy) and many other seemingly obscure investigations. In this way, it is possible to build up a total picture of the person presenting for treatment. The next stage is to catalogue the symptoms prompting the consultation, and then to match these with the 'drug picture' of all the remedies, so that the 'like treats like' philosophy may be satisfied. There are several thousand such drug pictures; to cover them all one would certainly need a computer, and the necessary software now exists. Most prescribers, however, carry the 'drug pictures' of several hundred remedies in their heads, and rely on textbooks for the rest. So don't be put out if your physician or pharmacist flicks through the pages of a book in front of you. They are ensuring that you are offered the most appropriate remedy.

Now I have to break my own rules, for there are a few remedies, known as polychrests, that do have a very wide spectrum of activity and these are the ones that you often see on pharmacy shelves or in health food shops. Arnica is a great remedy taken for bruising; it can also be taken prior to surgery to help reduce postoperative bleeding. Aconite is good for the first signs of flu. Argent nit is excellent prior to a big function – or a driving test! Calendula – from the marigold – is an agent that promotes healing. There are many more. Unfortunately the remedies have rather unfamiliar names and some are difficult to pronounce; most are abbreviations from the Latin.

Some 70% of the remedies we use come from plant tissue; that is one reason why homeopathic medicines and herbal medicines are confused. The rest of our source materials have their origins in naturally occurring minerals like sulphur, gold and iron, in biological sources such as the honey bee (Apis), spiders and snakes, and in pathological (or diseased) specimens. We do have problems in collecting raw materials, although we prefer fresh specimens whenever possible. Arnica for example grows above 3000 metres altitude and is often a protected plant by law. The source of Hawthorn (Crataegus) is important; just as wine can vary according to the growing conditions so can plants such as Crataegus. Chalk must come from the interspaces of oyster shells along with inherent impurities, and is not made pure in the laboratory.

Plant raw material is chopped up and extracted with alcohol and water, after which it is strained and the resulting tincture serially diluted with an all-important fierce burst of agitation at each dilution stage. This process is called 'succussion' and is thought to impart a special energy to the remedy. This might be the reason why more dilute solutions are more powerful – they have had more bursts of energy. These potentised solutions are then used in the preparation of tablets, pills, powders, ointments, creams and other dose forms.

Homeopathy is often referred to as 'alternative medicine'. The word 'alternative' has been defined as 'a proposition or situation offering a choice between two things, wherein if one thing is chosen, the other is rejected'. Is my task, therefore, to present the case for homeopathy, while others may champion their own alternative forms of medicine? I think not. You see, there are areas in which homeopathic medicine is inappropriate; replacement therapy and vitamin deficiencies are but two examples. In these cases it is necessary to rely on orthodox medicine along with homeopathic medicine. The two are therefore complementary – not alternatives – as, I believe, are all forms of medicine. Choosing the right 'mix' of techniques constitutes the art of healing as opposed to the 'science' of healing as practised by general practitioners. When the body is lacking important elements, homeopathic remedies are used in too great dilution to be physiologically active. In a bacterial infection, again the dose of remedy used is far too low to kill the bug. In these cases a patient might be given the best of the two disciplines: an antibiotic to kill the bug and a homeopathic remedy to help clear inflammation or other allied symptoms. Excluding these conditions, there is a very wide range of conditions that respond to homeopathic treatment.

Traditionally, the list of remedies available has not grown for many years. Within the last decade, however, a limited number of new preparations have appeared, these being mainly homeopathic dilutions of conventional medicines, and a wide range of desensitising anti-allergic preparations, including homeopathic dilutions of pollens, cat fur, house dust, etc., together with homeopathic dilutions of certain vaccines including whooping cough and measles. This is not strictly speaking homeopathy, because there is no comparison of drug pictures, but homeopathic techniques are involved. After all, it does not matter what label you put on the healing method available, so long as it does heal!

There are some theories of how homeopathic remedies work, but not unnaturally it is in this area where we find our greatest vulnerability, especially when the remedies are diluted to such great extents. Standard double-blind trials as used in drug trials are not appropriate in homeopathy because every patient is treated differently. However, slowly but surely more suitable research techniques are being devised.

The main parameters of discontent with conventional medicine concern fears of side-effects, damage to unborn children, and suitability in pregnancy and intolerance. Centuries of use have proved that homeopathy is not subject to these dangers, but provides a safe, effective method, using gentle techniques, tailored to the particular needs of every patient.

There are many books and leaflets about homeopathy; I have brought some with me tonight. More people ask their pharmacist about homeopathic remedies than ask all other health professionals together, so don't be afraid to seek advice from your local pharmacy. In Britain you can get more information from the British Homeopathic Association (see Appendix 1 for address). They also have lists of medically qualified homeopathic physicians. The Society of Homeopaths in Northampton will also be pleased to supply lists of registered homeopaths.

I hope I have given you a brief insight into the subject of homeopathy. I should be delighted to try and answer your questions, but please do not ask me to prescribe for you in public. Please restrict your questions to a general nature. Thank you.

A few tips ...

1. Do not allow yourself to become drawn into a 'prescribing session', for two reasons. First, the questioner will end up hogging your attention if you are not careful. Second, you may not be able to help anyway, especially in the early stages when you will be familiar with just a few

simple remedies. Set the ground rules for questions at the start. (People will probably approach you at the end anyway so you can pursue individual problems on a one-to-one basis, rather than involving the whole audience.)

2. People often ask about the Bach flower remedies. You might like to include a few words on these or at least be prepared to answer questions.

3. Admit openly that we do not know how the remedies work, and that all our information is based on clinical observations.

4. Have a few samples. If you write to your suppliers in plenty of time they might give you some samples and brochures etc. to leave behind. The BHA has a book list that you could photocopy. If you are a community pharmacist do not forget to leave your own promotional material.

5. In the UK Nelson's and Weleda have excellent videos that you can borrow or hire. Elsewhere approach your local suppliers or Associations. Make sure you watch them before the night. I have been in the embarrassing situation more than once of giving a comprehensive introduction to the wrong video!

GETTING STARTED

Whether it be in a community pharmacy or in a professional practice the principles of starting up are the same. If you are starting on a new venture you might consider the following, though not necessarily in this order.

Gaining knowledge

It is most important that you do know what you are talking about. Lack of knowledge means lack of confidence and this will quickly be transmitted to the customer. You might also choose the wrong remedy, and lack of progress will also upset the patient. As I said in Chapter 5 in the section 'Instructing the patient', you will be asked for information on homeopathy in general, for instance:

- Is it safe?
- What is it?
- How does it work?

and for more specific advice such as:

- Which remedy should I buy?
- How often do I take the tablets?
- How do I take them?

This book will provide most of the information you will initially need, including details of all the common remedies. If you wish for a more detailed knowledge of homeopathy you will need to purchase a materia medica and repertory (see Appendix 2). You can get this from many of the homeopathic suppliers, or from the British Homeopathic Association Book Service in Glasgow. A list of suggested starter books is given in Appendix 2.

Online sources of information

Increasingly there are electronic sources of information becoming available. An investigation on the Internet using one of the search utilities will reveal a number of sites including the Homeo-Web home page and the Homeopathy home page (see Appendix 1). Both of these have links to other areas of homeopathic interest.

HomeoNet provides a bulletin board service for exchanging messages and information. It is available by subscription through different providers according to the country of access (see Appendix 1).

Setting up your stocks

There are two good ways of introducing homeopathy into daily practice.

1. You can pick six remedies, for example: Arnica, Arsen alb, Belladonna, Chamomilla, Gelsemium, Ruta, and learn their abbreviated drug pictures off by heart – or at the very least have their applications written down on a card, so that you can consult it quickly while speaking to the customer. You will find the drug pictures of these remedies in Chapter 9 or in Chapter 13. Whenever your advice is sought on a condition that appears in the drug picture of your 'hot six' you can think about offering homeopathy. For the moment, you can remain with allopathic medicines for other conditions. As you become more proficient, you can add one or two at a time until you have a reasonable list that covers most of the common conditions that customers self-treat.

2. You can pick three or four common illnesses, for example: bruising, colds, coughs, diarrhoea, and learn the main remedies that are usually considered as being appropriate. Again, when advice is sought on these particular conditions you can offer homeopathy proactively if you think it is appropriate. You will find several tables forming a repertory section in Chapter 9, from which cards can be drawn up as an aide-mémoire.

Do not be afraid to use cards or textbooks in front of the patient. Experience shows that they quite like to join in the consultative processes and be actively involved in choosing a remedy. Whichever method you choose, do start slowly with just a handful of remedies and increase your armamentarium slowly as you gain confidence. Try to record your prescribed remedies whenever possible, so that you can build up your own source of reference.

When you are ready you can move on to a more comprehensive list. An example of a collection of 24 remedies, sometimes called the 'Glasgow Acute Kit', was developed for use by participants during the academic department courses at Glasgow Homeopathic Hospital. The remedies, with their abbreviated uses, are set out in Table 12.1.

The second example is a group of remedies, known as a 'GP kit' or 'Dr Jack's Kit' that was briefly discussed in Chapter 5:

Table 12.1 The Glasgow
Acute Kit

Remedy	Indication
Aconite	Anxiety, distress, fear; also first signs of flu
Apis	Bee stings, oedematous tissues, histamine reactions
Argent nit	Feelings of nervousness and fear (but not terror)
Arnica	Mental and physical exhaustion, trauma, bruises
Arsen alb	Diarrhoea and vomiting
Belladonna	Sudden onset, flushed appearance, throbbing headache, fever
Bryonia	Joint pains worse for movement, warmth; hacking coughs
Cantharis	Burns, scalds, sunburn; cystitis with burning sensation
Chamomilla	'Angry' children with pain from colic and/or teething
Colocynth	Severe colic, better with bending double
Euphrasia	Hayfever; streaming eyes and burning tears
Gelsemium	Influenza; pre-exam nerves
Hypericum	Blood and crush remedy; painful injuries involving nerve endings
Ignatia	Same and next day effects of grief
Ipecac	Constant nausea not relieved by vomiting; unproductive cough
Ledum	Puncture wounds that feel cold
Nux vom	Ill-effects of overeating and drinking; indigestion
Pulsatilla	Non-corrosive thick-coloured catarrh
Rhus tox	Joint pain, better for heat and gentle movement; chickenpox
Ruta	Soft tissue injuries – strains and sprains

Aconite, Antim crud, Antim tart, Arnica, Arsen alb, Belladonna, Bryonia, Camphor, Cantharis, Carbo veg, Chamomilla, Colocynth, Euphrasia, Gelsemium, Ipecac, Merc sol, Natrum mur, Nux vom, Phosphorus, Pulsatilla, Rhus tox, Sulphur.

Either list would be a suitable basis for assembling an opening stock. It is suggested that both 6c and 30c potencies of each remedy are kept to allow both acute and chronic cases to be treated.

The most important aspect of being proactive is not to be afraid to practise. Remember you can do no harm if you stick to the guidelines set out in this book.

Joining an organisation

Joining one (or more) of the following will help you keep up to date. (See Appendix 1 for addresses.) The various journals often contain helpful articles on how remedies can be used. The following organisations were dealt with in more detail in Chapter 3.

Faculty of Homeopathy. Membership of the Faculty is available to health professionals in several categories (see above). Students and colleagues at the first stage of training may apply for Associateship. Applicants for Associateship have to be proposed and seconded by a Member and may be dealt with by the Faculty Office.

The main advantages of joining the Faculty as an Associate are the quarterly journal *Homeopathy* (formerly called *British Homeopathic Journal*) and its supplement *Similima*, and access to the main British Homeopathic Library based at the Glasgow Homeopathic Hospital and the smaller library in Luton. The Glasgow librarian, who is also responsible for the Hom-Inform Homeopathic Information Centre, will be delighted to respond to requests for help in finding material. This service is available to both members and non-members of the Faculty, and has developed from a computer index of the *British Homeopathic Journal*. The result of literature searches may be sent by electronic mail. The address of the library and Hom-Inform is given in Appendix 1.

British Homeopathic Association (BHA). The BHA produces a quarterly journal called *Health and Homeopathy* aimed mainly at knowledgeable amateur homeopaths and consumers. They keep a range of brochures and leaflets and can supply lists of homeopathic practitioners and pharmacists. The BHA shares premises with the Faculty of Homeopathy in Luton. BHA Book Service can provide a wide range of consumer and professional books.

Society of Homeopaths. The Society has different classes of membership, including Fellows, Members, Subscribers and Friends. It also produces a journal dealing with topics of interest to homeopaths. The Society supports professional homeopaths.

Stock control

A list of suppliers will be found in Appendix 1. Most will be delighted to help you build your opening stock, supplying a range of the most frequently used remedies. Some have counter stands. It is best to stick to one or two potencies to start – 6c and 30c are the best options in the UK. As far as pharmacies are concerned, it does not seem to matter how many remedies you keep in stock – a prescription or OTC request will always arrive for something you have not got! If your local GP has been on a course recently he or she is very likely to prescribe all sorts of different potencies. Resist the temptation to keep adding to your stocks until a pattern has been established.

The suppliers will usually supply by return post. Some full-line wholesalers keep stock too.

Publicising your interest

It is important to let people (including local sympathetic GPs) know of your ability to supply and prescribe remedies. If you are proactive the word will get round quickly – but remember to stay within the bounds of your confidence and competence. Offer to give talks locally and perhaps write an article or two for the local newspaper. All this will serve to raise your profile and establish a new client base.

A FINAL WORD TO PHARMACISTS

Traditionally pharmacists have been involved 'behind the scenes' for many years, supporting colleagues in other homeopathic disciplines. The time has now come for a more visible role to be taken within the healthcare team. With a firm expanding educational infrastructure, a growing research base and robust licensing regulations for our manufacturers, the foundations of a higher profile for homeopathic pharmacy have been set. Homeopathy as a whole should be proud of what pharmacy has achieved. The market opportunities are there; the potential for an expansion in demand is waiting to be exploited. The future may indeed be viewed with considerable optimism.

PART 6

Reference section

PART CONTENTS

13. Materia medica   337

Chapter 13

Materia medica

CHAPTER CONTENTS

Aconite	338	Gelsemium	346
Allium cepa	338	Graphites	346
Antimonium crudum	338	Hamamelis	346
Antimonium tartaricum	339	Hepar sulphuris	346
Apis mellifica	339	Hypericum	347
Argentum nitricum	339	Ignatia	347
Arnica montana	339	Ipecacuanha	347
Arsenicum album	340	Kali bichromicum	348
Belladonna	340	Kali carbonicum	348
Bryonia	340	Ledum	348
Calcarea carbonicum	341	Lycopodium	348
Calcarea phosphoricum	341	Magnesium phosphoricum	349
Calendula	341	Mercurius solubilis	349
Camphora	341	Natrum muriaticum	349
Cantharis	342	Natrum sulphuricum	350
Caulophyllum	342	Nux vomica	350
Causticum	342	Phosphoric acid (Acid phosphoricum)	350
Chamomilla	343	Phosphorus	350
Chelidonium	343	Pulsatilla	351
China (Cinchona officinalis)	343	Rhus tox	351
Cocculus	343	Ruta grav	351
Coffea	344	Sepia	352
Colocynth	344	Silicea	352
Conium	344	Staphysagria	352
Crataegus	345	Sulphur	353
Drosera	345	Symphytum	353
Euphrasia	345	Thuja	353
Ferrum phosphoricum	345	Urtica	353

The mini materia medica in this chapter will allow you to expand your knowledge about 60 individual remedies, and to enhance your skills in differentiating between them. The drug pictures have been abbreviated so as to include only those features that are likely to be appropriate in the OTC environment. For more extensive drug pictures the reader is referred to one of the materia medicas included in Appendix 2.

Aconite

Trivial name: Blue monkshood or wolfbane
Source: Aconitum napellus, member of Ranunculaceae; lives on moist pastures and wasteland. Fresh aerial parts and tubers are used in preparing the remedy, collected at the start of the flowering season
Constitutional: Strong, healthy looking individuals with nervous disposition
Mental: Terror, distress. Fears – agoraphobia. Great tension. (cf. Argent nit and Gelsemium)
Physical: Inflammation of the eye; fever with hot dry skin; great thirst. First stages of flu (short acting)
Modalities: Worse in warm rooms and at night; better in open air

Allium cepa

Trivial name: Red onion
Source: Allium cepa – whole fresh bulbs, gathered in July–August
Constitutional: None clearly seen
Mental: Fear of pain
Physical: Acute localised conjunctivitis with bland watery discharge (cf. Euphrasia). Nasal catarrh and headache. Hacking irritating cough. Sneezing
Modalities: Worse in warm rooms, cold or damp. Better for fresh air

Antimonium crudum

Trivial name: Black sulphide of antimony (Ant crud)
Source: Comprises 29 parts Sulphur and 100 parts Antimonium
Constitutional: Most useful in the young and the elderly. Fat, sluggish people. Tendency to fall madly in love. Sensitive to the sun. Greediness. Sore corners to the mouth
Mental: Aversion to being touched. Irritable, sentimental, sulky, cross and peevish
Physical: Disturbed respiration; in the old – alternate constipation and diarrhoea. Loss of appetite
Modalities: Worse in the evening; worse in the sunshine. Better in the open air

Antimonium tartaricum

Trivial name: Tartar emetic (Ant tart)
Source: Potassium tartrate of antimony
Constitutional: Most beneficial in the young and old. Pale, sickly people who seem to be suffering and who are susceptible to chest and gastric problems
Mental: Fear of being alone
Physical: Headache (like tight band around the head), drowsiness. Indigestion. Nausea, vomiting. Inability to cough up phlegm
Modalities: Worse in the evening and from lying down at night. Better from sitting up

Apis mellifica

Trivial name: Honey bee
Source: Derived from the whole honey bee, *Apis mellifica*, killed by immersion in alcohol, minced and extracted in alcohol
Constitutional: None clearly seen
Mental: Indifference, depression, jealousy, suspicion
Physical: Oedema, especially at extremities, histamine-type reactions, stings
Modalities: Worse with application of heat or pressure. Better in cold

Argentum nitricum

Trivial name: The Devil's stone, Hellstone (Argent nit)
Source: Silver nitrate, containing not less than 99.5% of $AgNO_3$
Constitutional: Ability to think and respond quickly; extroverts. People with desire for sweets. Lack of coordination
Mental: Anticipatory anxiety; rooted to the spot. Nervous. Weak memory (cf. Aconite and Gelsemium)
Physical: Eye problems, photophobia. Headaches that come on slowly but disappear quickly. Loss of smell. Back pain. Diarrhoea from anxiety or before an ordeal
Modalities: Worse for warmth, eating, and at night. Better for fresh air and cold

Arnica montana

Trivial name: Leopard's bane or Fallkraut; Mountain tobacco
Source: Small alpine plant *Arnica montana*, with yellow flowers; grows best above 3000 m. Dried underground parts are generally used to make the homeopathic remedy
Constitutional: Tend to deny anything wrong, shy away from being comforted. Morose
Mental: Mental exhaustion or shock; forgetful following injury
Physical: Physical exhaustion, trauma, bruising. Fetid breath, angina
Modalities: Worse from touch, motion. Better lying down

Arsenicum album

Trivial name: Arsenic, White arsenic

Source: Arsenic trioxide

Constitutional: Insecure people with need of comforting. Fearful. Children are highly strung; adults emotionally sensitive, neat, tidy and fussy. Restless and anxious

Mental: General anguish and restlessness. Fear of being alone, fear of the dark. Desire to be orderly

Physical: Headaches with nausea and vomiting. Stinging, watering eyes (cf. Allium cepa and Euphrasia). Thin, watery, stinging nasal discharge. Thirsty for large quantities of water sipped slowly. Bleeding gums, mouth ulcers. Disturbed restless sleep. Fevers involving sepsis

Modalities: Worse in wet weather and after midnight. Better from heat and warm drinks

Belladonna

Trivial name: Deadly nightshade, Devil's cherries

Source: Atropa belladonna; grows luxuriantly forming bushy plant about 1 m or more high; native to Central and Southern Europe; tincture made from whole plant when it starts to flower

Constitutional: Belladonna is seldom used as a constitutional remedy but may be of value in fair skinned excitable and quarrelsome patients who are prone to flushing of face and have a vivid imagination

Mental: Changeable moods; fear of imaginary things

Physical: Burning hot flushed appearance. Tonsillitis, sore throat, earache, bursting headache, cramp and colic. Especially when symptoms come on suddenly. Effects of sunstroke

Modalities: Worse with heat of the sun, during afternoon and at night; better from bending backwards and in bed with light covering

Bryonia

Trivial name: Wild hops

Source: The remedy is made from either the whole fresh plant or the roots of *Bryonia alba*, the white bryony

Constitutional: Irritable person, 'robust' stature, with dark complexion and dark hair. Tendency towards frequent 'stitching' pains

Mental: Tiredness, sensitivity to movement of all types. Angry, anxious, irritable

Physical: Bursting headaches. Soreness in larynx and trachea. Joints red, swollen and painful (especially knees)

Modalities: Worse for warmth, movement (cf. Rhus tox). Better for pressure and application of cold

Calcarea carbonicum

Trivial name: Chalk or Calcium carbonate (Calc carb)
Source: Interspaces of broken oyster shells (mussel shells also)
Constitutional: Subjects are usually fair, flabby and overweight, with a clammy handshake. Children tend to be rather slow-moving and clumsy, with a chalky white complexion. They sweat a lot, especially at night on their heads and at the back of their neck, resulting in a wet pillow
Mental: Depression. Anxiety about health. Generally fearful. Affected badly by emotional upsets. Averse to work or exertion
Physical: Headache with cold hands and feet. Heartburn and loud belching. Tickling cough. Unhealthy, ulcerating skin. Sour smelling, sweaty feet. Lower back pain
Modalities: Worse in draughts and cold winds and for exertion. Better for constipation

Calcarea phosphoricum

Trivial name: Phosphate of lime (Calc phos)
Source: Prepared from calcium hydrogen phosphate
Constitutional: Discontented, slim (emaciated?) subjects with dark hair and long legs. Anaemic children who are 'peevish', flabby and have cold extremities
Mental: Nervousness, restlessness and dislike of routine (especially in teenage girls)
Physical: Poor weight gain in babies. Poor digestion with colicky pain in abdomen. Stiffness and pain in extremities
Modalities: Worse in damp changeable weather and for exertion. Better in the summer

Calendula

Trivial name: Marigold
Source: Prepared from the fresh flowering parts of *Calendula officinalis*
Constitutional: Tendency towards erysipelas; also likely to suffer from colds
Mental: Said to be useful in the emotional results of injury
Physical: Useful for painful and suppurating wounds; said to promote formation of granulation tissue. Topical application for superficial abrasions. Can be used to complement other treatments
Modalities: Worse in damp weather

Camphora

Trivial name: Camphor
Source: Camphor crystals obtained from the young bark of *Cinnamonium camphora*

Constitutional: Patient's body cold, yet does not cover up
Mental: None apparent
Physical: First stages of cold, with chilliness and sneezing. Shock
Modalities: Worse with motion and at night. Better with warmth
NB *Should not be given with any other homeopathic remedy (see Ch. 8)*

Cantharis

Trivial name: Spanish fly
Source: *Cantharis vesicatoria*, a species of beetle
Constitutional: Anxious restlessness with crying. Fiery sexual desire
Mental: Wild rage and loudness, screaming and insolence
Physical: Burning sensation in mouth and throat. Erysipelas. Burns. Cystitis with burning on passage of urine; urine hot and scanty
Modalities: Worse for touch, movement and cold water. Better for gentle massage of affected parts

Caulophyllum

Trivial name: Blue cohosh or squaw root (also known as blue and yellow ginseng)
Source: Roots and rhizomes of *Caulophyllum thalictroides*
Constitutional: None apparent
Mental: None apparent – though fear of unknown often associated with need for remedy
Physical: Spasmodic pains in different areas of body. Main use to establish contractions in labour; said to act on uterine muscle. Labour pains
Modalities: Worse from cold, open air and coffee
NB *See warning Chapter 8.*

Causticum

Trivial name: Potassium hydrate
Source: This remedy, potassium hydrate, is made from quicklime (calcium oxide) and potassium bisulphate
Constitutional: Sallow complexion, dark hair, dark eyes. Melancholy moods, tearful. Elderly obese subjects seem to benefit from this remedy too
Mental: Anxiety, depression, pessimism. Sudden floods of emotion. Poor concentration
Physical: Bell's palsy, dizziness when bending forward. Cracked and sore nipples; serious burns. Cystitis: frequent urge to urinate; pain and burning during flow. Incontinence in pregnancy
Modalities: Worse with cold dry winds. Better in wet weather

Chamomilla

Trivial name: Chamomile

Source: Dried roots of *Chamomilla recutita* (*BhomP*). The *GerHomP* uses fresh whole flowering plant

Constitutional: Subjects with excessive sensibility to pain; bad tempered and complaining

Mental: Angry babies that desire to be carried. Persons who are spiteful, with 'uncivil irritability'; difficult to please and cross

Physical: Especially useful for teething babies (with colic). Where slightest pain causes sweating and great discomfort. Earache, with blocked dull sensation; tinnitus

Modalities: Worse with movement, heat and touch, early morning, late afternoon. Better with milk, hot drinks and firm pressure

Chelidonium

Trivial name: Greater celandine

Source: Whole fresh flowers or the rhizomes and roots of *Chelidonium majus*

Constitutional: Thin, fair and lethargy are the constitutional features of this remedy. Anxiety and easy distraction are also indicated

Mental: Anxiety, depression

Physical: Jaundice, liver problems, distension of upper abdomen, colic; constipation

Modalities: Worse with movement, heat and touch. Better with hot drinks and firm pressure

China (Cinchona officinalis)

Trivial name: Peruvian bark, cinchona

Source: Prepared from the dried yellow bark of *Cinchona calisaya*, a South American evergreen shrub

Constitutional: Depressed anxious people, especially with artistic qualities, respond well

Mental: Apathy, indifference, nervous exhaustion. Sudden crying

Physical: Headaches; fevers with sweating and shivering; jaundice in newborn babies. Flatulence, colic; pains in limbs and joints

Modalities: Worse at night, with touch. Better with sleep, warmth and firm pressure

Cocculus

Trivial name: Indian cockle; Indian berry

Source: *Cocculus indicus* berries

Constitutional: Fair haired females, especially during pregnancy when suffering from backache and sickness. Sensitive girls

Mental: Mental exhaustion, sad and anxious about the health of others

Physical: Distended abdomen with wind, nausea and vomiting, drowsiness. Travel sickness, morning sickness

Modalities: Worse after eating and loss of sleep. Better for lying down in bed

Coffea

Trivial name: Unroasted coffee (coffea cruda)

Source: The whole unroasted green bean of the coffea plant, *Coffea arabica*

Constitutional: Tall, lean, stooping people with dark complexions and sanguine disposition

Mental: Extreme sensitivity; intolerance of pain. Nervous excitement

Physical: Insomnia; vivid dreams. Neuralgia. Toothache in nervous patients

Modalities: Worse for excessive motion. Better for warmth and lying down

Colocynth

Trivial name: Bitter cucumber

Source: Prepared from *Citrullus colocynthus*, the bitter cucumber

Constitutional: Irritable persons who are easily angered; persons of stocky build; fair complexion

Mental: Very irritable; becomes angry – and feels humiliated – when questioned

Physical: Diarrhoea brought on by emotional state. Abdominal pain (colic) causing patient to double up. Neuralgia and sciatica

Modalities: Worse from anger. Better from warmth, pressure and lying with head bent forward

Conium

Trivial name: Common hemlock

Source: Whole plant of *Conium maculatum*

Constitutional: Dull and uninspiring

Mental: Depressed, timid, takes little interest in anything. Weak memory

Physical: Difficult gait associated with trembling and stiffness. Severe ache around liver region, jaundice. Nausea and insomnia in pregnancy

Modalities: Worse from lying down, mental or physical exertion. Better without food and with motion

Crataegus

Trivial name: Hawthorn berries
Source: The remedy is made from fresh ripe berries obtained from *Crataegus oxycanthus* (and similar species) of the hawthorn bush
Constitutional: None obvious
Mental: Nervous, apprehensive and despondent
Physical: Chronic heart disease; hypotension; giddiness, lowered pulse rate, insomnia
Modalities: Worse in warm room. Better from fresh air and rest

Drosera

Trivial name: Sundew
Source: Whole flowering plant of *Drosera rotundifolia*, a leafy insectiverous plant that lives in boggy areas. The remedy may also be derived from *D. intermedia* and *D. angelica*
Constitutional: None obvious
Mental: None obvious
Physical: Dry spasmodic barking cough (whooping cough?), hoarse. Retching and vomiting may follow attempts to bring up phlegm
Modalities: Worse in the evening and after midnight; when lying down

Euphrasia

Trivial name: Eyebright
Source: Remedy made from the whole fresh plant of *Euphrasia officinalis*
Constitutional: None obvious
Mental: None obvious
Physical: Copious watering of the eyes. Fluent bland coryza. Conjunctivitis, and sensitivity to light. Acrid burning eye discharges (cf. Allium cepa, where bland and Arsen alb where all discharges acrid). Hot red cheeks. Early stages of measles. Yawning when walking in the open air
Modalities: Worse in the evening, indoors, and from touch. Better in the dark

Ferrum phosphoricum

Trivial name: Phosphate of iron (Ferrum phos)
Source: The remedy is prepared from hydrated ferric phosphate (one of the tissue salts)
Constitutional: Nervous, sensitive and anaemic patients respond well to this remedy. Susceptibility to chest problems and colds
Mental: None obvious
Physical: First stages of head colds; inflamed tonsils. Croup. Stiff neck. Flushed appearance. Headache that improves with application of cold to forehead. Whitlows
Modalities: Worse at night and on right side. Better for application of cold

Gelsemium

Trivial name: Yellow jasmine

Source: Root of the fresh plant of *Gelsemium sempervirens*

Constitutional: Dull, uninteresting people with limited intelligence seem to respond well

Mental: Listless and wish to be left alone. Stage fright. Anxiety about passing exams; feelings of inadequacy; subject paces up and down, trembles (cf. Aconite, terror, and Argent nit, unable to move). Embarrassment

Physical: Symptoms of influenza becoming worse over several days. General feeling of 'heaviness'. Sneezing. Also useful in measles and measle-like skin rashes. Hangovers

Modalities: Worse in damp weather and for excitement. Better for motion and in the open air

Graphites

Trivial name: Black lead, plumbago

Source: The remedy is made from naturally occurring graphite, a compound containing carbon, iron and silica

Constitutional: Overweight subjects, with a sad temperament and a tendency for constipation and skin problems. Also, coarse-featured people with labouring or other similar manual jobs

Mental: Timidity, indecision. Subjects weepy and seek sympathy

Physical: Rough, hard skin with weeping eruptions, characteristically behind the ears (cf. Hepar sulph). Cold sores. Tendency for abrasions to turn septic very quickly

Modalities: Worse for warmth and at night; also during and after menstruation. Better in the dark and for wrapping up

Hamamelis

Trivial name: Witch-hazel

Source: The remedy is made from the bark, wood parts and roots of *Macrophylla virginia*

Constitutional: None obvious

Mental: Depression, restlessness, irritability

Physical: Haemorrhages of a slow passive type (e.g. nose-bleeds), varicose veins, bleeding haemorrhoids, leg ulcers. Aching and tiredness in different parts of the body. Phlebitis

Modalities: Worse in warm moist air and with movement

Hepar sulphuris

Trivial name: Hahnemann's calcium sulphide

Source: According to Hahnemann's original instructions, the remedy is prepared from calcium sulphide, made by combining material from the interspaces of oyster shells with pure flowers of sulphur

Constitutional: Subjects who are overweight, weak, sensitive and depressed; typically they collapse into an armchair with a sigh. Blonde subjects are also said to respond well

Mental: Hypersensitive to touch, dejected and sad. Irritable with self and others. Impulsive

Physical: Profuse perspiration. Sensitive cold sores. Sore, ulcerated nose. Abscesses, suppurating lesions. Acne (cf. Graphites and Sulphur)

Modalities: Worse from dry cold winds, cool air and draughts. Better in damp weather and from warmth and wrapping up

Hypericum

Trivial name: St John's wort

Source: Whole fresh flowering parts of *Hypericum perforatum*

Constitutional: None obvious; useful for subjects with a craving for wine

Mental: Melancholy. Depression

Physical: Blood and crush injuries, especially those involving tissues rich in nerve endings (e.g. digits). Deep cuts and lacerations with severe pain (cf. Calendula for superficial abrasions). Painful puncture wounds. Concussion

Modalities: Worse in the cold and with pressure. Better with application of warm compresses

Ignatia

Trivial name: St Ignatius' bean

Source: Derived from the seed pods of *Ignatia amara*

Constitutional: Subjects with tendency to mood swings from pleasure to tears. Bright precocious children

Mental: Stress and strain especially after emotional episode (e.g. grief after bereavement). Inability to work

Physical: 'Nervous' headaches. Hiccoughs

Modalities: Worse in the morning and after meals; also worse from strong odours. Better while eating and changing position

Ipecacuanha

Trivial name: Ipecac root

Source: Dried root of *Psdychotria ipecacuanha*

Constitutional: Fat children and adults seem to respond well to this remedy

Mental: Irritability, anxiety, sulky. Complaining. Impatient

Physical: Extreme and persistent nausea with little or no thirst. Asthma; wheezing cough. Croup

Modalities: Worse in winter, with lying down and emotional upset

Kali bichromicum

Trivial name: Dichromate of potash (Kali bich)
Source: Made by combining the potassium carbonate with chromic acid
Constitutional: Chubby persons (especially children) with a fair florid complexion and who are susceptible to catarrh
Mental: None obvious
Physical: Inflammations of mucous membranes. Snuffles in children. Nasal catarrh: stringy thick greenish yellow discharge. 'Bunged up' feeling – sinuses 'blocked'. Headache. Acne
Modalities: Worse in the morning, in hot weather and after drinking beer. Better for heat

Kali carbonicum

Trivial name: Carbonate of potassium, salt of tartar (Kali carb)
Source: Potassium carbonate
Constitutional: Weak, sallow-skinned, dark haired. Irritable, easily frightened. Dogmatic people with a strong belief in what is right for society (e.g. lawyers or policemen)
Mental: Despondent; does not wish to be left alone. Hypersensitive to pain. Feels cold intensely
Physical: Vertigo. Stuffed-up nose in warm room. Dry hoarse cough. Exhaustion, low back pain and sweating. Large difficult stools
Modalities: Worse for hot drinks, sleep and on left side. Better in warm weather and for movement

Ledum

Trivial name: Marsh tea, wild rosemary
Source: Whole fresh plant, or dried leafy tips of shoots, of *Ledum palustre*
Constitutional: None obvious
Mental: Anxiety, timidity, impatience
Physical: Aching in the eyes. Black eyes. Puncture wounds with small point of entry (rusty nail in the foot or insect bites) that are cool to the touch (cf. Apis, histamine reaction)
Modalities: Worse at night from heat of the bed and touch. Better from application of cold

Lycopodium

Trivial name: Club moss
Source: The remedy is made from the crushed spores of *Lycopodium clavatum*
Constitutional: A stooping posture, sallow complexion, skin often with wrinkles. Tend to be apprehensive, distrustful or intellectual. Often teachers, politicians or religious ministers

Mental: Anxiety, impatient. Poor concentration. Hypochondria. Active brain that prevents sleep at night. Afraid to be alone

Physical: Neuralgia. Eczema behind the ears; acne. Dyspepsia; bloated abdomen. Diarrhoea. Tickling cough. Numbness in extremities. Hives

Modalities: Worse on right side, and between 4 p.m. and 8 p.m. Also worse in stuffy rooms and with tight clothing. Better with motion and uncovering

Magnesium phosphoricum

Trivial name: Magnesia phos (Mag phos)

Source: Prepared from magnesium monohydrogen phosphate

Constitutional: Especially suited to thin dark subjects who are exhausted

Mental: Complains about illness, unable to think logically

Physical: Minor aches and pains including headaches, toothache, earache, etc. Cramp and colic; period pains. Hiccoughs. Abdominal pain and wind; bloated feeling

Modalities: Worse at night, on right side and with touch. Better for warmth and for bending double

Mercurius solubilis

Trivial name: Mercurius sol (Merc sol)

Source: The remedy is derived from a mixture of mercuric amidonitrates and metallic mercury obtained by dissolving mercury in nitric acid

Constitutional: Persons with slow reactions and slow speech

Mental: Confused, depressed and discontented

Physical: Halitosis, offensive greenish discharges from ear, eyes or nose. Mouth ulcers, painful unhealthy gums, metallic taste in the mouth and extreme thirst. Increased salivation

Modalities: Worse for heat and cold and for lying down. Better for rest and wrapping up

Natrum muriaticum

Trivial name: Sodium chloride (Natrum mur, Nat mur)

Source: The source for this remedy is common salt

Constitutional: Typical subject is withdrawn, moody and sullen. Difficult to please. Often with dark hair, greasy skin and a cracked lower lip. Takes much salt on food; frequently constipated

Mental: Impatience, anger. Easily upset. Aggravated by consolation

Physical: Blinding headaches. Colds. Dry hacking cough. Heartburn

Modalities: Worse with lying down and noise. Better from fresh air and lack of food

Natrum sulphuricum

Trivial name: Glauber's salts, Sol mirabile (Nat sulph, Natrum sulph)
Source: The source of this remedy is sodium sulphate
Constitutional: Most patients are fat and undersized. They tend to change from enthusiasm to disinterest in what they are doing and are sensitive, tense and fidgety. They have greasy florid skins
Mental: Bad temper, loss of memory. Emotional confusion
Physical: Bursting headaches at back of the head. Occipital pain. Concussion. Dry mouth with cracked lips. Mouth ulcers, Nasal catarrh with thick yellow discharge
Modalities: Worse with cold and noise. Better in dry weather and from changing position

Nux vomica

Trivial name: Poison nut (Nux vom)
Source: The remedy is made from the dried ripe seeds of *Nux vomica*
Constitutional: These patients are excessively irritable, both mentally and physically, although they seem to like hard work – usually of a mental type (managers, supervisors, etc.). They tend to keep late hours and like to eat rich food
Mental: Irritable, fussy, pompous, fault finding and impulsive
Physical: Hangovers. Headache. Indigestion and vomiting. Sour taste in the mouth. 24-hour influenza with shivering and stiffness. Insomnia (business worries?). Constipation
Modalities: Worse in morning and from mental exertion. Better with sleep and warmth

Phosphoric acid (Acid phosphoricum)

Trivial name: Phosphoric acid (Acid phos)
Source: The remedy is made from phosphoric acid
Constitutional: The remedy benefits those who are 'under the weather' as a result of concentrated studying, illness or loss of body fluids, or by grief or depression
Mental: Apathy, impaired memory. Despair. Homesickness
Physical: Exhaustion; interrupted sleep pattern; headaches
Modalities: Worse with noise, bad news, cold draughts. Better with sleep, movement and fresh air

Phosphorus

Trivial name: Phosphorus
Source: The remedy is made from yellow phosphorus
Constitutional: The remedy is most appropriate for tall, slim, intelligent subjects with a fair freckled skin, red hair and a fiery disposition that causes them to explode if provoked. They are sensitive and can blush, or even burst into tears, easily. Drink milk

Mental: Nervous, excitable, with a vivid imagination. Reluctance to talk about problems

Physical: Headaches. Dry niggling cough that seems to go on for weeks (viral, after flu?). Nosebleeds, and persistent bleeding after tooth extraction

Modalities: Worse for hot food or drink, touch. Better with cold food, fresh air, lying on right side and sleep

Pulsatilla

Trivial name: Wind flower (meadow anemone, pasque flower)

Source: The remedy to which the proving refers is made from the whole fresh flowering plant of *Pulsatilla pratensis* (syn *Pulsatilla nigricans*) and has a monograph in the German *Pharmacopoeia* (see Ch. 4)

Constitutional: Adults (especially women) who are fair-skinned, fair-haired, plump, affectionate, with changeable contradictory disposition. Children who are of similar physical appearance, and who blush easily

Mental: Depressed; tendency to be led by others. Requirement for others to show affection and attention

Physical: Headaches accompanied by yellow bland catarrh. Cough – loose in the morning and dry in the evening. Premenstrual syndrome; pain in back, tired feeling. Heartburn, colic

Modalities: Worse from heat, rich food. Better in the open air and with motion

Rhus tox

Trivial name: Poison ivy (poison oak, sumach), icodendron (Rhus tox)

Source: The remedy is prepared from the fresh leaves of a mixture of North American *Rhus* species, collectively called *Rhus toxicodendron*

Constitutional: Chilly people who hate the cold

Mental: Sad, listless; burst into tears for no apparent reason. Irritable, restless (pain or emotional)

Physical: Rheumatic conditions. Red itching skin; urticaria? Swollen red eyes

Modalities: Rheumatics worse at night, with application of cold, and initial movement. Better with gentle continued movement, application of heat and keeping dry (cf. Bryonia)

Ruta grav

Trivial name: Rue (bitter wort)

Source: The remedy is made from the whole fresh aerial parts of *Ruta graveolens* just before it flowers

Constitutional: None obvious

Mental: Anxiety, dissatisfaction with own performance
Physical: Headaches and eyestrain, as with studying. Muscular sprains and strains. Injuries to tendons and periosteum
Modalities: Worse for rest and cold. Better for movement

Sepia

Trivial name: Cuttlefish ink
Source: The remedy, Sepia officinalis, is made from the ink of the cuttlefish
Constitutional: Female patients who are tall, slim, with a dark waxy skin tend to benefit from this remedy. They have a rather 'offhand' manner and are said to be unresponsive to affection
Mental: Indifferent, irritable and easily offended. Emotional outbursts
Physical: Premenstrual syndrome. Headaches with nausea; low back pain. Constipation, insomnia
Modalities: Worse in forenoon and evenings in damp atmosphere especially when sweating. Better with warmth in bed

Silicea

Trivial name: Silica
Source: The remedy is made from pure flint, mainly silicon dioxide or silica
Constitutional: Intellectual adults and frail but lively children are the two groups that benefit from this remedy
Mental: Anxious, excitable and obstinate – even spiteful. Witty
Physical: Boils and abscesses; unhealthy skin. Has the ability to expel foreign bodies (e.g. splinters, grit, etc. in the skin). Migraines on right side. Tinnitus. Styes
Modalities: Worse in the morning and from washing. Better for warmth and wrapping up

Staphysagria

Trivial name: Stavesacre or palmated larkspur
Source: The remedy is prepared from the dried seeds of *Delphinium staphysagria*
Constitutional: These patients are often secretly battling with some private emotional problem
Mental: Suppressed anger; extreme sensitivity. Impatient and spiteful
Physical: Facial neuralgia. Recurrent styes. Painful lacerations and wounds. Eczema
Modalities: Worse from touch and emotional upset. Better for warmth and rest

Sulphur

Trivial name: Flowers of sulphur

Source: The remedy is made from sublimed flowers of naturally occurring sulphur

Constitutional: Traditionally sulphur is associated with people of unkempt appearance who have an aversion to washing. Lean body and stooping shoulders. Likes fresh air and hates tight clothes. Cold feet and warm head. Hot sweaty hands. 'Absent-minded professor' image (see mentals)

Mental: Forgetful, selfish, lazy, self-centred. Irritable and depressed. Sluggish

Physical: Dry, scaly, itchy red skin and scalp. Nasal herpes; snuffles. Burning sensation at margins of eyelids

Modalities: Worse at rest and in bed with warmth. Better in dry warm weather

Symphytum

Trivial name: Knitbone (comfrey)

Source: The remedy is made from the fresh root of the herb *Symphytum officinale*

Constitutional: None obvious

Mental: None obvious

Physical: Eases the pain and speeds up union of fractured bones. Painful injuries resulting from blow to the eye. Gastric and duodenal ulcers

Modalities: Worse for touch

Thuja

Trivial name: White cedar

Source: Fresh green twigs and 1-year-old leafy shoots of *Thuja occidentalis*

Constitutional: The Thuja patient tends to have a greasy skin and to perspire freely from exposed parts. They often have an unkempt appearance

Mental: Fixed ideas; emotions stirred easily

Physical: In OTC environment use should be restricted to treatment of warts, verrucae, carbuncles and polyps; adverse affects of vaccination

Modalities: Worse with damp and cold

Urtica

Trivial name: Stinging nettle

Source: The remedy is made from the fresh flowering plant of *Urtica urens*

Constitutional: None obvious

Mental: None obvious

Physical: Urticaria, hives. Burns and scalds (cf. Cantharis). Gout

Modalities: Worse from cool moist air and touch

REFERENCES

Sources used for this chapter include:

Boericke's Materia Medica with Repertory

Murphy, R (2000) *Homeopathic Remedy Guide*, 2nd edn. HANA Press, Blacksburg, VA.

Vermeulen, F (2002) *Prisma: The Arcana of Materia Medica Illuminated*. Emryss bv, Haarlem.

Appendices

APPENDICES CONTENTS

Appendix 1 Some useful addresses   357

Appendix 2 Further reading   361

Appendix 1

Some useful addresses

UK associations and resources – professional

Faculty of Homeopathy,
Hahnemann House, 29 Park Street West, Luton
LU1 3BE
Tel: 0870 444 3955; *Fax:* 0870 444 3960
www.trusthomeopathy.org

Faculty of Homeopathy in Scotland,
Glasgow Homeopathic Hospital, 1053 Great
Western Road, Glasgow G12 0XQ
Tel: 0141 211 1617; *Fax:* 0141 211 1610
hom-inform@dial.pipex.com

Society of Homeopaths,
11 Brookfield, Duncan Close, Moulton Park,
Northampton NN3 6WL
Tel: 0845 450 6611; *Fax:* 0845 450 6622
www.homeopathy-soh.org

British Holistic Medical Association,
39 Lansdown Place, Hove, East Sussex BN3 1EL
Tel: 01273 725951
www.bhma.org

Homeopathic Medical Association – UK,
6 Livingstone Road, Gravesend, Kent DA12 5DZ
Tel/Fax: 01474 560336
www.the-hma.org

Hom-Inform and British Homeopathic Library,
Glasgow Homeopathic Hospital, 1053 Great
Western Road, Glasgow G12 0XQ
Tel: 0141 211 1617; *Fax:* 0141 211 1610
hom-inform@dial.pipex.com

Prince of Wales Foundation for Integrated Health,
12 Chillingworth Road, London N7 8QJ
Tel: 0207 619 5140
www.fihealth.org.uk

UK associations – patients

British Homeopathic Association,
Hahnemann House, 29 Park Street West, Luton
LU1 3BE
Tel: 0870 444 3950; *Fax:* 0870 444 3960
www.trusthomeopathy.org

Patients' Association for Anthroposophical Medicine,
St Lukes Medical Centre, 51 Cairns Cross Road,
Stroud GL4 4EX

Institutions offering qualifications in homeopathy

The University of Westminster, London,
Department of Complementary Studies, offers
BSc (Hons) Health Sciences courses in herbal
medicine, homeopathy, nutritional therapy,

therapeutic bodywork and Traditional Chinese Medicine: www.wmin.ac.uk/sih/page-85.

Information on postgraduate qualifications in complementary and alternative medicine including homeopathy may be found at www.rccm.org.uk/static/Links_Courses.aspx?m=7.

A comprehensive and current listing of colleges offering homeopathic training may be found online at the Homeopathy home page (www.homeopathyhome.com).

Overseas institutions

Australia
Australasian College of Hahnemannian Homeopathy
http://users.netconnect.com.au/~i_golden/apphom.htm
Other details at
http://www.archibel.com/links/Homeopathy/Schools/Australia/
The UK Faculty of Homeopathy provides training for health professionals in Australia.

Ireland
Details at http://www.abchomeopathy.com/l.php/8

New Zealand
Auckland School of Classical Homeopathy
http://www.homeopathynz.co.nz/
Bay of Plenty College of Homeopathy
http://www.homeopathycollege.com/

South Africa
The only training recognised for registration as a professional homeopath in South Africa is the Masters Degree in Homeopathy – M.Tech(Hom) – offered at the Durban Institute of Technology (www.dit.ac.za) and the University of Johannesburg (www.ujhb.ac.za) with which the Technikon Witwatersrand (TWR) has merged, or SA Qualifications Standards Authority (SAQA) and Allied Health Professions Council of SA (AHPCSA) approved equivalent. The M.Tech(Hom) consists of a 5 year full-time medico-scientific course in classical/clinical/modern/conventional homeopathy as well as homeopharmaceutics, which is a legal requirement for registration. Graduates are

registered as homeopathic practitioners only after having completed their postgraduate internship. Medical practitioners registered with the Health Professions Council of SA (HPCSA) may also opt for the course offered by the SA Faculty of Homeopathy. Further details at http://www.homeopathy.org.za/.

Part time training leading to the award of MFHom from the UK Faculty of Homeopathy is currently available in South Africa. Details www.trusthomeopathy.org.

USA
Details at
http://www.homeopathyhome.com/directory/usa/training_colleges.shtml
And at
http://www.wholehealthnow.com/homeopathy_info/weblinks2.html

Hospital and clinics

Hospitals providing treatment in the UK under the NHS
Bristol Homeopathic Hospital,
Cotham Road, Cotham, Bristol BS6 6JU
Tel: 01179 731231
http://www.ubht.nhs.uk/homeopathy/

Dept of Homeopathic Medicine,
Mossley Hill Hospital, Park Avenue, Liverpool L18 8BU
Tel: 0151 724 2335

Glasgow Homeopathic Hospital,
1053 Great Western Road, Glasgow G12 0XQ
Tel: 0141 337 1824; *Fax:* 0141 211 1610

Royal London Homeopathic Hospital (RLHH),
60 Great Ormond Street, London WC1N 3HR
Tel: 0207 391 8891; *Fax:* 0207 391 8869
Patient Services: 0207 391 8888
http://www.uclh.org/about/rlhh.shtml

Tunbridge Wells Homeopathic Hospital,
Church Road, Tunbridge Wells, Kent TN1 1JU
Tel: 01892 542977

Clinic not NHS, but a registered charity

Manchester Homeopathic Clinic,
Brunswick Street, Ardwick, Manchester M13 9ST
Tel: 0161 273 2446

Suppliers of homeopathic remedies

Ainsworths Homeopathic Pharmacy,
36 New Cavendish Street, London W1G 8UF
Tel: 0207 935 5330; *Fax:* 0207 486 4313
www.ainsworths.com (also supply books)

Freeman's Homeopathic Pharmacy,
18–20 Main Street, Busby, Glasgow G76 8DU
Tel: 0141 644 1165/0845 22 55 1 55;
Fax: 0141 644 5735/0845 22 55 2 55
www.freemans.uk.com (also supply books)

Helios Homeopathic Pharmacy
97 Camden Road, Tunbridge Wells, Kent
TN1 2QR
Tel: 01892 537254; *Fax:* 01892 546850
www.helios.co.uk (also supply books)

Nelsonbach,
Broadheath House, 83 Parkside, Wimbledon,
London SW19 5LP
Tel: 0208 780 4200; *Fax:* 0208 780 5871
www.nelsonbach.com

New Era Laboratories, Seven Seas Ltd,
Hedon Road, Marfleet, Hull HU9 5NJ
Tel: 01482 375234; *Fax:* 01482 374345
www.seven-seas.ltd.uk

Weleda UK,
Heanor Road, Ilkeston, Derbyshire DE7 8DR
Tel: 0115 944 8200; *Fax:* 0115 944 8210
www.weleda.co.uk

Pascoe, Kern complex products
Noma (Complex Homeopathy) Limited,
Unit 3, 1–16 Hollybrook Road, Southampton,
SO16 6RB
Tel: 01703 770513; *Fax:* 01703 702459

Reckeweg complex products
Complex Homeopathy (Bolton) Limited,
Carne House, Markland Street, Bolton BL1 5AP
Tel: 01204 848835; *Fax:* 01204 841233

UK suppliers of books

British Homeopathic Association Book Service,
20 Main Street, Busby, Glasgow G76 8DU
Tel: 0845 22 55 492; *Fax:* 0845 22 55 493
www.bhabooks.com

Minerva Homoeopathic Books,
173 Fulham Palace Road, London W6 8QT
Tel: 0207 385 1361; *Fax:* 0207 385 0861
minervabks@aol.com

Suppliers of equipment, vials, storage boxes, etc.

Homeopathic Supply Company,
4 Nelson Road, Sheringham, Norfolk NR26 8BU
Tel: 01263 824683
http://www.homeopathicsupply.com/

Other UK homeopathic pharmacies

Buxton & Grant,
176 Whiteladies Road, Bristol, BS8 2XU
Tel: 01272 735025

Galen Pharmacy,
Lewell Mill, West Stafford, Dorchester, Dorset
DT2 8AN
Tel: 01305 263996; *Fax:* 01305 250792

Gould's,
14 Crowndale Road, London NW1 1TT
Tel: 0207 388 4752

Nelson's Homeopathic Pharmacy,
73 Duke Street, London, W1M 6BY
Tel: 0207 629 3118

Major European suppliers

Boiron France and subsidiaries
http://www.boiron.com/index_en.asp

Dolisos France and subsidiaries
http://www.dolisos.com/index.asp
DHU Germany and subsidiaries http://www.dhu.de
Heel Germany and subsidiaries
http://www.heel.com/
Staufen-Pharma Göppingen
http://www.staufen-pharma.de/stphd.html

Major US suppliers

Boericke and Tafel, California
Boiron – Bornemann Inc http://www.boiron.com/
Dolisos http://www.dolisos.com
Hahnemann Laboratories (Mike Quinn)
http://www.hahnemannlabs.com/
Standard Homeopathic Company, Los Angeles
(Hyland's products)
http://www.hylands.com/
Washington Homeopathic Products
http://www.homeopathyworks.com/
Other supplier details at:
http://www.homeopathyhome.com/directory/usa/
pharmacies.shtml

Major Australasian suppliers

Brauer Australia http://www.heel.com/about/?smid=4
Naturo Pharm New Zealand
http://www.naturopharm.co.nz/main.asp
Weleda Australia and New Zealand
http://www.weleda.co.nz/

Major South African Suppliers

Natura Homeopathic Laboratories (Pretoria,
Cape Town and Durban) http://www.natura.co.za
W Last Pharmacy http://www.wlast.co.za
Weleda Pharmacies
http://www.weledapharmacies.co.za

Appendix 2

Further reading

Family guides

Gibson, D (2005) *First Aid Homoeopathy in Accidents and Ailments*, 18th edn. BHA Book Service, Glasgow.

Hammond, C (1988) *How to use Homoeopathy*. Element, Blandford, Dorset.

Hunter, F and Kayne, S (1997) *People are Pets*. BHA Book Service, Glasgow (Human and Veterinary).

Lockie, A (1998) *Family Guide to Homeopathy*. Hamish Hamilton, London.

Lockie, A and Geddes, N (1992) *A Woman's Guide to Homoeopathy*. Hamish Hamilton, London.

Speight, P (1977) *Before Calling the Doctor*. CW Daniel, London.

Speight, P (1984) *Homeopathy for Emergencies*. CW Daniel, London.

General reading

Blackie, M (1976) *The Patient, not the Cure*. Macdonald, London.

Carlston, M (2003) *Classical Homeopathy*. Churchill Livingstone, Philadelphia.

Handley, R (1997) *In Search of the Later Hahnemann*. Beaconsfield Publishers, Beaconsfield, UK.

Wood, M (1992) *The Magical Staff: The Vitalist Tradition in Western Medicine*. North Atlantic Books, Berkeley, CA.

Wright-Hubbard, E (1990) *Homeopathy as Art and Science*. Beaconsfield Publishers, Beaconsfield, UK.

History

Babington-Smith, C (1986) *Champion of Homoeopathy: The life of Margery Blackie*. John Murray, London.

Cook, TM (1981) *Samuel Hahnemann*. Thorsons, Wellingborough, UK.

Haehl, R (1926) (trans. M Wheeler). *Samuel Hahnemann – His Life And Work*. Homoeopathic Publishing Company, London.

Hobhouse, RW (1984) *Life of Christian Samuel Hahnemann*. World Homoeopathic Links, New Delhi (various editions).

Practice of homeopathy

Bodman, F (1990) *Insights into Homeopathy*. Beaconsfield Publishers, Beaconsfield, UK.

Borland, D (1982) *Homeopathy in Practice*. Beaconsfield Publishers, Beaconsfield, UK.

Clarke, J (1973) *The Prescriber*. Homeopathic Book Service, Sittingbourne, UK.

Detinis, L (1994) *Mental Symptoms in Homeopathy*. Beaconsfield Publishers, Beaconsfield, UK.

Gibson, D (1981) *Elements of Homeopathy*. BHA Book Service, Glasgow.

Jack, R (2001) *Homeopathy in General Practice.* Beaconsfield Publishers, Beaconsfield, UK.

Kaplan, B (2002) *The Homeopathic Conversation.* Natural Medicine Press, London.

Lessell, C (2004) *Companion to Homeopathic Studies.* CW Daniel, Saffron Walden, UK.

Morrison, R (1993) *Desktop Guide.* Hahnemann Clinic Publishing, Albany, USA.

Morrison, R (1998) *Desktop Companion.* Hahnemann Clinic Publishing, Albany, USA.

Paterson, J (2002) *Bowel Nosodes.* Jain Publishers, New Delhi.

Pratt, N (1985) *Homeopathic Prescribing.* Beaconsfield Publishers, Beaconsfield, UK.

Shepherd, D (1993) *Physician's Posy.* CW Daniel, Saffron Walden, UK.

Swayne, J (1997) *Homeopathic Method.* Churchill Livingstone, Oxford.

Swayne, J (2000) *International Dictionary of Homeopathy.* Churchill Livingstone, Oxford.

Tyler, M (2003) *Homoeopathic Drug Pictures.* Homeopathic Book Service, Sittingbourne, UK.

Tyler, M (2003) *Pointers to the Common Remedies.* BHA Book Service, Glasgow.

Tyler, ML and Jollyman, NW (1988) *Homoeopathic Drug Pictures Index and Repertory.* CW Daniel, Saffron Walden, UK.

Vannier, L (1992) *Typology in Homeopathy.* Beaconsfield Publishers, Beaconsfield, UK.

Vermeulen, F (2002) *Prisma.* Emryss Publishers, Haarlem, Netherlands.

Vithoulkas, G (1979) *Homeopathy: Medicine for the New Man.* Arco, New York.

Watson, I (2004) *Guide to the Methodologies of Homeopathy.* Cutting Edge Books, Kendal, UK.

Materia medica and repertories

Boericke, W (1993) *Homoeopathic Materia Medica with Repertory.* Homoeopathic Book Service, Sittingbourne, UK (various editions available).

Boyd, H (1982) *Introduction to Homoeopathic Medicine,* 2nd edn. Beaconsfield Publishers, Beaconsfield, UK.

Candegabe, E (1997) *Comparative Materia Medica.* Beaconsfield Publishers, Beaconsfield, UK.

Clarke, JH (1952) *The Prescriber,* 9th edn. Homoeopathic Publishing Company, London.

Clarke, J (1991) *Dictionary of Practical Materia Medica.* CW Daniel, Saffron Walden, UK.

Julian, OA (1979) *Materia Medica of New Homoeopathic Remedies.* Beaconsfield Publishers, Beaconsfield, UK.

Kent, JT (1986) *Repertory of the Homeopathic Materia Medica.* Homeopathic Book Service, Sittingbourne, UK.

Kent, JT (2000) *Materia Medica of Homeopathic Remedies.* Homeopathic Book Service, Sittingbourne, UK.

Phatak, SR (1988) *Phatak's Materia Medica of Homoeopathic Medicines.* Foxlee-Vaughan, London.

Scholten, J (2004) *Repertory of the Elements.* Stichting Alonnissos, Utrecht, Netherlands.

Schroyens, F (2004) *Synthesis Repertorium 9.1.* Homeopathic Book Publishers, London.

Vermeulen, F (2000) *Concordant Materia Medica.* Emryss Publishers, Haarlem, Netherlands.

Vermeulen, F (2003) *New Synoptic Materia Medica I.* Emryss Publishers, Haarlem, Netherlands.

Vermeulen, F (2003) *New Synoptic Materia Medica II.* Emryss Publishers, Haarlem, Netherlands.

Mother and children

Borland, D (1981) *Homeopathy for Mother and Infant.* BHA Book Service, Glasgow.

Borland, D (1997) *Children's Types.* BHA Book Service, Glasgow.

Castro, M (1992) *Homoeopathy for Mother and Baby.* Macmillan, London.

Fergie-Woods, H (1981) *Homoeopathic Treatment in the Nursery.* BHA Book Service, Glasgow.

Pinto, G and Feldman, M (2000) *Homeopathy for Children.* CW Daniel, London.

Smith, T (1993) *Homeopathy for Babies and Children.* Insight Editions, Romsey, UK.

Smith, T (1993) *Homeopathy for Pregnancy and Nursing Mothers.* Insight Editions, Romsey, UK.

Smith, T (1994) *Homoeopathy for Teenager Problems.* Insight Editions, Romsey, UK.

Speight, P (1991) *Homoeopathic Remedies for Children.* CW Daniel, Saffron Walden, UK.

Webb, P (1999) *Homoeopathy for Midwives (And All Pregnant Women).* BHA Book Service, Glasgow.

Wynne-Simmons, A (2004) *Children's Toybox*. BHA Book Service, Glasgow.

Research topics

Bellavite, P and Signorini, A (1995) *Homeopathy: A Frontier in Medical Science*. North Atlantic Books, Berkeley, CA.

Dean, ME (2004) *The Trials of Homeopathy*. KVC Verlag, Stuttgart, pp 245–246.

Lewith, GT and Aldridge, D (eds) (1983) *Clinical Research Methodology for Complementary Therapies*. Hodder and Stoughton, London.

Specific treatments

Borland, D (1983) *Digestive Drugs*. BHA Book Service, Glasgow.

Logan, R (1998) *Homeopathic Treatment of Eczema*. Beaconsfield Publishers, Beaconsfield, UK.

Smith, T (1993) *Homoeopathy for Everyday Stress Problems*. Insight Editions, Romsey, UK.

Smith, T (1994) *Homoeopathy for Psychological Illness*. Insight Editions, Romsey, UK.

Speight, P (1985) *Overcoming Rheumatism and Arthritis*. CW Daniel, Saffron Walden, UK.

Speight, P (1990) *Homoeopathic Remedies for Ears, Nose and Throat*. CW Daniel, Saffron Walden, UK.

Speight, P (1990) *Tranquillisation: The Non-Addictive Way*. CW Daniel, Saffron Walden, UK.

Speight, P (1992) *Coughs and Wheezes*. CW Daniel, Saffron Walden, UK.

Sport

Morgan, LW (1990) *Treating Sports Injuries the Natural Way*. Thorsons, Wellingborough, UK.

Speight, L (1989) *Sports Injuries*. CW Daniel, Saffron Walden, UK.

Subotnick, S (1991) *Conventional, Homeopathic and Alternative Treatments – Sports and Exercise Injuries*. North Atlantic Books, Berkeley, CA.

Thomas, E (2000) *Homeopathy for Sport, Exercise and Dance*. Beaconsfield Publishers, Beaconsfield, UK.

Theory of homeopathy

Blackie, M (1986) *Classical Homoeopathy*. Beaconsfield Publishers, Beaconsfield, UK.

Bodman, F (1990) *Insights into Homeopathy*. Beaconsfield Publishers, Beaconsfield, UK.

Boyd, H (1989) *Introduction to Homeopathic Medicine*. Beaconsfield Publishers, Beaconsfield, UK.

Foubister, D (1989) *Tutorials on Homoeopathy*. Beaconsfield Publishers, Beaconsfield, UK.

Gaier, H (1991) *Encyclopaedic Dictionary of Homoeopathy*. Thorsons, London.

Gemmell, D (1997) *Everyday Homeopathy*. Beaconsfield Publishers, Beaconsfield, UK.

Gibson, D (1981) *Elements of Homeopathy*. BHA Book Service, Glasgow.

Gibson, D (1987) *Studies of Homoeopathic Remedies*. Beaconsfield Publishers, Beaconsfield, UK.

Hahnemann, S (1998) *Chronic Diseases*. Homeopathic Book Service, Sittingbourne, UK.

Lessell, C (1994) *The Infinitesimal Dose: The Scientific Roots of Homoeopathy*. CW Daniel, Saffron Walden, UK.

Livingston, R (1991) *Homoeopathy: Evergreen Medicine*. Asher Press, Poole, Dorset.

O'Reilly, WB (ed) (1996) *Organon of the Medical Art by Samuel Hahnemann*. Birdcage Books, Redmond, WA.

Paschero, T (2000) *Homeopathy*. Beaconsfield Publishers, Beaconsfield, UK.

Roberts, HA (1972) *Principles and Art of Cure by Homeopathy*. Homeopathic Book Service, Sittingbourne, UK.

Sankaran, R (1993) *Spirit of Homeopathy*. Homoeopathic Medical Publishers, Mumbai, India.

Sankaran, R (1994) *Substance of Homeopathy*. Homoeopathic Medical Publishers, Mumbai, India.

Sankaran, R (1997) *Soul of Remedies*. Homoeopathic Medical Publishers, Mumbai, India.

Sankaran, R (2000) *System of Homeopathy*. Homoeopathic Medical Publishers, Mumbai, India.

Sankaran, R (2002) *Insight Into Plants.* Homoeopathic Medical Publishers, Mumbai, India.

Scholten, J (2000) *Homeopathy and Minerals.* Stichting Alonnissos, Utrecht, Netherlands.

Scholten, J (2000) *Homeopathy and the Elements.* Stichting Alonnissos, Utrecht, Netherlands.

Vithoulkas, G (1980) *The Science of Homoeopathy.* Grove Press, New York.

Travel

Lessell, C (1999) *World Travellers' Manual of Homeopathy.* CW Daniel, Saffron Walden, UK.

Speight, P (1989) *Travellers' Guide to Homoeopathy.* CW Daniel, Saffron Walden, UK.

Dental

Kayne, S (2001) *Complementary Therapies for Pharmacists.* Pharmaceutical Press, London.

Lessell, C (1993) *Dental Prescriber.* BHA Book Service, Glasgow.

Lessell, C (1995) *Textbook of Dental Homeopathy.* CW Daniel, Saffron Walden, UK.

Veterinary

Allport, R (2000) *Heal Your Cat the Natural Way.* Mitchell Beazley, London.

Allport, R (2000) *Heal Your Dog the Natural Way.* Mitchell Beazley, London.

Allport, R (2001) *Natural Healthcare for Pets.* Harper Collins (Element), Glasgow.

Ball, S and Howard, J (1999) *Bach Flower Remedies for Animals.* CW Daniel, Saffron Walden, UK.

Biddis, K (1987) *Homeopathy in Veterinary Practice.* CW Daniel, Saffron Walden, UK.

Chapman, BM (1991) *Homoeopathic Treatment for Birds.* CW Daniel, Saffron Walden, UK.

Day, C (1990) *Homoeopathic Treatment of Small Animals.* CW Daniel, Saffron Walden, UK.

Day, C (1995) *Homoeopathic Treatment of Beef and Dairy Cattle.* Beaconsfield Publishers, Beaconsfield, UK.

Hunter, F (2004) *Everyday Homeopathy for Animals.* Beaconsfield Publishers, Beaconsfield, UK.

Hunter, F and Kayne, S (1997) *People are Pets.* BHA Book Service, Glasgow.

Macleod, G (1981) *Treatment of Cattle by Homeopathy.* CW Daniel, Saffron Walden, UK.

Macleod, G (1989) *Veterinary Materia Medica and Clinical Repertory.* CW Daniel, Saffron Walden, UK.

Macleod, G (1991) *Treatment of Horses by Homeopathy.* CW Daniel, Saffron Walden, UK.

Macleod, G, (1992) *Dogs: Homeopathic Remedies.* CW Daniel, Saffron Walden, UK.

Macleod, G (1994) *Pigs: Homoeopathic Approach to Treatment.* CW Daniel, Saffron Walden, UK.

Macleod, G (1997) *Cats: Homeopathic Remedies.* CW Daniel, Saffron Walden, UK.

Macleod, G (2000) *Goats: Homeopathic Remedies.* CW Daniel, Saffron Walden, UK.

Saxton, J and Gregory, P (2005) *Textbook of Veterinary Homeopathy.* Beaconsfield Publishers, Beaconsfield, UK.

Wolff, HG (1994) *Homoeopathic Medicine for Dogs.* CW Daniel, Saffron Walden, UK.

Flower remedies and tissue salts

Bach, E (1986) *Twelve Healers.* CW Daniel, Saffron Walden, UK.

Bach, E (1996) *Heal Thyself.* CW Daniel, Saffron Walden, UK.

Boericke, W and Dewey, WA (2003) *The Twelve Tissue Remedies of Schüssler.* Homeopathic Book Service, Sittingbourne, UK.

Chancellor, PM (1971) *Handbook of the Bach Flower Remedies.* CW Daniel, London.

Gilbert, P (1984) *A Doctor's Guide to the Biochemic Tissue Salts.* Thorsons, Wellingborough, UK.

Harvey, CG and Cochrane, A (1995) *The Encyclopaedia of Flower Remedies.* Thorsons, London.

Isbell, W (1995) *Christchurch Flower Essences Handbook.* Lighthouse, Christchurch, NZ.

Mansfield, P (1995) *Flower Remedies.* Optima, London.

Ramsell, NM (1991) *Questions and Answers on Bach Flower Remedies.* CW Daniel, Saffron Walden, UK.

Vlamis, G (1994) *Rescue Remedy.* Thorsons, Wellingborough, UK.

Wheeler, FJ (1996) *Bach Flower Remedies Repertory.* CW Daniel, Saffron Walden, UK.

Online sources of information

Alternative Medicine Foundation http://
www.amfoundation.org/homeopathinfo.htm

British Homeopathic Library http://www.
hom-inform.org/

Elixirs.com – theory and practice newsletters
http://www.elixirs.com/newsletter.htm

Homeopathic education services
http://www.homeopathic.com/

Homeopathic internet resources http://www.
holisticmed.com/www/homeopathy.html

Homeopathic sites and useful links

Kent Homeopathic Associates
http://www.repertory.org/links.html

HI Links http://
www.homeoint.org/lienamis.htm#english

Homeopathy home – general resource http://
www.homeopathyhome.com/reference/
index.shtml

Homeoweb – general resource
http://www2.antenna.nl/homeoweb/

Index of Remedies

Note: Figures in bold refer to figures and tables/boxed material.

A

ABC remedy, 236
Acid nitric *see* Nitric acid (Acid nitric)
Acid phos *see* Phosphoric acid (Acid phos)
Acid sulph, first aid/acute applications, 242
Aconite napellus (Acon), **112**, 186, 327, 338
    adolescent problems, 238
    antenatal treatments, **235**
    anthroposophical medicine, 256
    antidotes, **207**
    anxiety, 244
    cold/flu treatment, **217**
    complementary/incompatible remedies, **191**
    cough remedy, **218**
    cystitis, 230
    dental applications, **245**
    earache treatment, **219**
    fear/terror, **222**, 246
    first aid/acute applications, 183, 214, **215**
    Glasgow Acute Kit, **331**
    keynotes, **168**
    prescription, **124**
Actaea racemosa (Cimicifuga), 111
Aesculus, antenatal treatments, **235**
Agaricus muscarius (Agar, Ag mus), **112**, 186, 243
AGE complex, 182, **217**
Agrimony, 258
Allium cepa (Allium c, All-c), **112**, 338
    allergies/allergic disease, 228, **229**
    antidotes, **207**
    cold/flu treatment, **217**
    complementary/incompatible remedies, **191**
    conjunctivitis treatment, **220**
    cough remedy, **218**

keynotes, **168**
Aloe, **235**
Alumina
    antenatal treatments, **235**
    constipation, **218**
Ambra grisea, 87, **191**
Ammonium bromatum, **124**
Ammonium carb, **191**
Ammonium muriaticum, 240
Anacardium, 241
Anthracinum, 174
Antimonium crudum, 338
    adolescent problems, 238
    complementary/incompatible remedies, **191**
    headache, **194**
Antimonium tartaricum, 339
    complementary/incompatible remedies, **191**
    cough remedy, **218**
    indigestion/colic, **221**
    prescription, **124**
Apis mellifica (Apis), 51, **86**, 111, **112**, 186, 243, 339
    allergies/allergic disease, 228
    basophil granulation effects, 304
    complementary/incompatible remedies, **191**
    conjunctivitis treatment, **220**
    cystitis, **232**
    first aid/acute applications, **215**
    folk medicine, 85
    frostbite, 243
    Glasgow Acute Kit, **331**
    prescription cost, **21**
    runner's knee, 241
    'scrumpox,' 243
    traveller's kit, **247**
    whole insect *vs.* venom, 83
Aqua crystalisata, 88
Argent nitricum (Argent nit), 10, 186, 327, 339
    adolescent problems, 238

antenatal treatments, **235**
anthroposophical medicine, 256
anxiety, **222**, **224**, 244
complementary/incompatible remedies, **191**
conjunctivitis treatment, **220**
dental applications, **245**
diarrhoea, 138, **219**, 244
dosage/dose regimens, 182
foreboding, **222**
Glasgow Acute Kit, **331**
keynotes, **168**
preparation, 92
tennis/golfer's elbow, 241
traveller's kit, **247**
Arnica montana (Arn), **112**, 339
    administration, 133
    adolescents, 237
    antenatal treatments, **235**
    antiinflammatory effects, 293
    clinical research, 282, 291–3
    combinations, 214
    delayed onset muscle soreness (DOMS), 241–2
    dental applications, 244, 245, **245**
    dosage/dose regimens, 182
    eye injuries, **220**, 240
    first aid/acute applications, 183, 214, **215**, 225, 240, **240**, 241, 242
    fractures, 240
    Glasgow Acute Kit, **331**
    keynotes, **168**
    market for, 26
    mastitis, 311
    mixtures, 226
    mother tincture use, 92
    NMR analysis, 108, **109**
    pain control, 292
    postoperative bruising, 292
    postpartum, 236
    prescription, 128, **128**, 129, 130
    runner's knee, 241

source material, 85
topical, 225, 226, 241, 293
traveller's kit, **247**
veterinary uses, **251,** 311
Arsenic, 59
agricultural research, 310
performance-enhancing remedy, 244
prescription, **124**
toxicity, 200
Arsenicum album (Arsen alb, Ars),
112, 174, 340
adolescent problems, 237, 238
allergies/allergic disease, **229**
antidotes, **207**
clinical trials, 293
cold/flu treatment, **217**
complementary/incompatible
remedies, **191**
constitutional remedy, **177**
diarrhoea, 138, 244, **246**
gastrointestinal diseases, 243, **246**
Glasgow Acute Kit, **331**
headache treatment, **221**
keynotes, **168**
prescription, **124**
prescription cost, **21**
skin conditions, **223**
traveller's kit, **247**
veterinary uses, **251**
Arsenicum iodium (Arsen iod), 182
allergies/allergic disease, **229**
cold/flu treatment, **217**
Arundo, **229**
Astacus fluviatilis, **86**
Atropa belladonna *see* Belladonna
Atropine, prescription, **124**
Aurum, 53, 91
Aurum metallicum (Aurum met), **112,**
156

B

Bach flower remedies, 237, 238, 258–61
Bach Rescue Cream, 261
Bacillinum, 171, **190**
Bacillus no. 7, **179**
Badiaga (Spongilla fluv), **86**
Bambusa, 256
Baryta carb, 74, **191**
Baryta mur, **21**
Bee glue (propolis), 88
Belladonna (Bell), **139,** 340
acute response, **185**
adolescent problems, 238
anthroposophical medicine, 256
antidotes, **207**
clinical research, 282
cold/flu treatment, **217**

complementary/incompatible
remedies, **191**
dental applications, **245**
dosage/dose regimens, 182
earache treatment, **219**
first aid/acute applications, **215**
Glasgow Acute Kit, **331**
headache, **221, 224**
heat exhaustion, 243
keynotes, **168**
mastitis, 311
peculiars, 187
prescription, **124,** 128, **128,** 129
prescription cost, **21**
scarlet fever treatment, 48
skin conditions, **223**
sore throat, **224,** 230
traveller's kit, **247**
Bellis perennis
first aid/acute applications, **215,**
226, 241, 242
postpartum, 236
Berberis, 230
Berlin wall, 88
Betula
allergy/allergic disease, 298–9
NMR analysis, 108
Blatta orientalis, **86**
Bonnet, 89
Borax
dental applications, **245**
foot and mouth outbreak, **252**
Boron, 308
British Homeopathic Journal, 62, 63, 332
see Homeopathy
Bromatums, 111, **124**
Bryonia, 186, 340
cold/flu treatment, **217**
complementary/incompatible
remedies, **191**
constipation treatment, **218**
constitutional remedy, **177**
cough remedy, **218**
Glasgow Acute Kit, **331**
headache treatment, **221**
indigestion/colic, **221**
keynotes, **168**
mastitis, 311
muscle/tendon injuries, 241
Burn ointment, 226, **247**

C

Cactus grandiflorus (Cercus
grandiflorus), 111, 243
Calcium (calcarea) carbonicum (Calc
carb), 87, 186, 341
complementary/incompatible
remedies, **191**

constitutional remedy, **177**
keynotes, **168**
miasmatic remedy, **156**
Calcium (calcarea) fluorica (Calc
fluor), 111, 245, **264,** 311
Calcium (calcarea) phosphoricum
(Calc phos), **264,** 341
dental applications, 245, **245**
keynotes, **168**
Calcium (calcarea) sulphoricum (Calc
sulph), 187, **264**
Calendula, 243, 327, 341
abrasions, **223**
blisters, 240
dental applications, **245**
eye drops, 106
first aid/acute applications, 214,
215, 225
mother tincture use, 92
topical, 92, 225, 226
traveller's kit, **247**
variations in source material, 84
Calendula cream
nappy rash, 237
postpartum, 236
Calendula talc, 227
Camphora (Camphor), 341–2
as antidote, 206
hypothermia, 243
Cantharis vesicator (Canth), **86,** 111,
112, 342
antenatal treatments, **235**
antidotes, **207**
blisters, 240
burn ointment, 226, 247
complementary/incompatible
remedies, **191**
cystitis, 230, **232**
first aid/acute applications, **215,**
216
Glasgow Acute Kit, **331**
keynotes, **168**
skin conditions, **223**
Carbo veg
adolescent problems, 238
antenatal treatments, **235**
complementary/incompatible
remedies, **191**
constitutional remedy, **177**
first aid/acute applications, **215**
indigestion/colic, **221**
keynotes, **168**
Carcinosin, miasmatic remedy, **156**
Carcinosinum, 111
Caulophyllum, 201, 234–6, 342
Causticum, 342
antenatal treatments, **235**
blisters, 240
cystitis, **232**

Centaury, 258
Cerato, 258
Cercus grandiflorus (cactus grandiflorus), 111
Chamomilla, 343
    clinical research, 282
    complementary/incompatible remedies, 191
    Glasgow Acute Kit, 331
    indigestion/colic, 221, 224, 236
    keynotes, 168
    prescription, 128, 129
    teething, 224, 236
Charcoal, 53
Chelidonium, 343
Chicory, 258
China (Cinchona officinalis), 343
    antenatal treatments, 235
    diarrhoea treatment, 219
    Hahnemann's work, 46–7
Chocolate, 88
Cimex lectularoius, 86
Cimicifuga (Actaea racemosa), 111
Cinchona officinalis see China (Cinchona officinalis)
Cineraria, eye drops, 106
Clematis, 258
Cobalt, performance-enhancing remedy, 244
Coca, 243
Cocculus, 343–4
    morning sickness, 234, 235
    prescription, 124
    traveller's kit, 247
Coccus cacti (Cocc cact, Coc-c), 86, 112
Coffea, 51, 344
    antenatal treatments, 235
    complementary/incompatible remedies, 191
    insomnia, 244
    prescription cost, 21
    traveller's kit, 247
Colchicum, prescription, 124
Colocynth, 344
    complementary/incompatible remedies, 191
    Glasgow Acute Kit, 331
    indigestion/colic, 221, 224, 236
Comudoron®, traveller's kit, 247
Conium, 235, 311, 344
Cortisone, 173
Crataegus, 345
    anthroposophical medicine, 256
    prescription, 128, 130
    source material, 85, 327
Croton tiglium
    diarrhoea, 244
    prescription, 124

Cuprum metallicum (Cuprum met, Cu met), 112

D

Damiana (Turneria), 111
Digoxin, 51
Diphtherinum, 172
Disci comp, 256
DNA, 83
Drosera, 218, 345
'Dr Vogel' range, 182
Dulcamara
    cold/flu treatment, 217
    cystitis, 232
Dysentery Co, 179

E

Echinacea tincture, 190, 226, 230
Electricity, 88
Equisetum, 237
Eupatorium perf, 182, 217, 230
Euphrasia officinalis (Euphr), 112, 345
    adolescent problems, 238
    allergies/allergic disease, 227, 227–8, 229
    antidotes, 207
    conjunctivitis treatment, 220
    eye drops, 106, 243
    Glasgow Acute Kit, 331
    keynotes, 168
    traveller's kit, 247
'Eyebright,' 106

F

Ferrum metallicum (Ferrum met), 92, 186, 244
Ferrum phosphoricum (Ferrum phos), 219, 264, 345
Flower remedies, 237, 257–63
Fluoratums, 111, 245
Fluorine, 245
Folliculinum, prescription, 124
Formica rufa, 86, 256

G

Gaertner, 179
Gelsemium sempervirens (Gels), 112, 182, 346
    adolescent problems, 238
    allergies/allergic disease, 229

anxiety, 244
    cold/flu treatment, 217, 224, 230
    complementary/incompatible remedies, 191
    diarrhoea, 138, 219
    Glasgow Acute Kit, 331
    headache, 221
    keynotes, 168
    prescription, 124
    worry/stage fright, 222
Gentian, 258
Glonoinum, heat exhaustion, 243
Gold see Aurum
Graphites, 346
    adolescent problems, 238
    complementary/incompatible remedies, 191
    constitutional remedy, 177
    skin conditions, 223

H

Haemorrhoid ointment, 226
Haloperidol, 173
Hamamelis, 346
    antenatal treatments, 235
    first aid/acute applications, 225
Hecla lava, 87
Helix tosta, 86
Hepar sulpharis (Hepar sulph), 346–7
    abrasions/wounds, 239
    adolescent problems, 238
    boils, 230
    complementary/incompatible remedies, 191
    skin conditions, 223
Histamine, 301
Holly, 260
Homarus, 86
House dust mite, 189
Household fluids, 88
Hydrastis, source material, 85
Hydrogen, 88
Hyoscymus, prescription, 124
Hypercal, 226
Hypericum perforatum (Hyp, Hyper), 112, 186, 347
    200c, anaesthesia, 74
    abrasions, 223
    blisters, 240
    dental applications, 245
    first aid/acute applications, 214, 215, 216, 225
    Glasgow Acute Kit, 331
    keynotes, 168
    peculiars, 187
    postpartum, 236
    topical, 225, 226

traveller's kit, **247**
veterinary uses, **251**

I

Ignatia, 347
  complementary/incompatible
    remedies, **191**
  constitutional remedy, **177**
  Glasgow Acute Kit, **331**
  grief, **222, 224**
  keynotes, **168**
  peculiars, 188
  prescription, **124**
Impatiens, 258
Influenzinum, 171, **172**
Insecticides, 88
Iodatums, 111
Iodum, **229**
Ionising radiation, 51
Ipecacuanha (Ipecac, Ipec, Ip), **112,**
    186, **190,** 347
  adolescent problems, 238
  complementary/incompatible
    remedies, **191**
  coughs, 162, **218**
  diarrhoea treatment, **219**
  Glasgow Acute Kit, **331**
  influenza, **224**
  keynotes, **168**
  mastitis, 311
  morning sickness, **235**
  prescription cost, **21**

K

Kali arsenicum, **124**
Kali bichromium (Kali bich), 348
  cold/flu treatment, **217**
  complementary/incompatible
    remedies, **191**
  earache treatment, **219**
  mustard gas research, 174
Kali bromatum (Kali brom), **124**
Kali carbonicum (Kali carb), 348
Kali muriaticum (Kali mur), **264**
Kali permanganicum (Kali perman),
    92
Kali sulphuricum (Kali sulph), **264**
Kernpharma®, 182
Kreosotum, 245

L

Lachesis (Lach), **112,** 171
  constitutional remedy, **177**

frostbite, 243
  premenstrual syndrome, 233, **233**
Lactrodectus mactans, 51, 85, **86,**
    111
Lapis alb, **156**
Larch, **260**
Ledum pal (Ledum), 348
  complementary/incompatible
    remedies, **191**
  eye injuries, **220,** 240
  first aid/acute applications, **215,**
    216, 226
  Glasgow Acute Kit, **331**
  insect bites, 243
  jellyfish stings, 243
  keynotes, **168**
  tetanus prevention, 239
  traveller's kit, **247**
Leuticum *see* Syphilinum
Luna, 88
Lycopodium, 348–9
  adolescent problems, 238
  complementary/incompatible
    remedies, **191**
  constitutional remedy, **177**
  ultraviolet (UV) spectroscopy, 107

M

Magnesium phosphoricum (Mag
    phos), **221, 264,** 349
Mag pol Aust, 88
Matricaria chamomilla *see*
    Chamomilla
Medorrhinum, 13, 111, **156,** 177
Melissa Co, traveller's kit, **247**
Merc cyantus (Merc cyan), 92
Mercurius solubilis (Merc sol), 186,
    349
  agricultural uses, 249
  complementary/incompatible
    remedies, **191**
  dental applications, **245**
  miasmatic remedy, **156**
Mercury, 47
Mimulus, 258
Mistletoe, injection, 106, **106**
Morbillinum, **172**
Morgan Gaertner, **179**
Morgan pure, **179**
Mullein (verbascum oil), 226
Mutabile, **179**

N

Natrum arsenicum (Nat arsen), **124**
Natrum bromatum (Nat brom), **124**

Natrum carbonicum (Nat carb), 243
Natrum fluor, dental applications,
    245
Natrum muriaticum (Natrum mur,
    Nat mur, Nat-m), 53, 87,
    112, 186, **264,** 349
  adolescent problems, 238
  allergies/allergic disease, **229**
  antidotes, **207**
  complementary/incompatible
    remedies, **191**
  constipation treatment, **218**
  constitutional remedy, **177**
  constitutional types, 158
  headache treatment, **221**
  keynotes, **168**
  premenstrual syndrome, 233, **233**
  skin conditions, **223**
Natrum phosphoricum (Nat phos), 53,
    264
Natrum salts, 53
Natrum sulphuricum (Nat sulph), 53,
    264, 350
New Era Tissue Salt range, 180
Nitric acid (Acid nitric)
  NMR analysis, 108
  verucca/warts, 244
Noctura®, traveller's kit, **247**
'No-Jet-Lag,' 180
Nux vomica (Nux vom, Nux-v), 74,
    112, 350
  allergies/allergic disease, **229**
  antenatal treatments, **235**
  cold/flu treatment, **217**
  complementary/incompatible
    remedies, **191**
  constipation treatment, **218**
  constitutional remedy, **177**
  cystitis, **232**
  gastrointestinal diseases, 243
  Glasgow Acute Kit, **331**
  headache, **194, 221**
  indigestion/colic, **221, 224**
  keynotes, **168**
  prescription, **124**
  prescription cost, **21**
  source material, 85
  succussation studies, 95
  traveller's kit, **247**

O

Odor Off®, 250
Olive, **260**
Opium, 49, **218**
Oscillococcinum (Oscillo), 180
Osteoarthritic nosode (OAN), 111,
    171

P

Paeonia, 226
Parotidinum, **172**
Pascoe range, 181–2
Passiflora
  insomnia, 244
  prescription cost, **21**
  traveller's kit, **247**
Penicillin, **124**
Perhexiline maleate, 173
Pertussin, 86, 171, **172**
Pertussis, 86
Petroleum, 87, **247**
Phosphoric acid (Acid phos), 350
  adolescent problems, 238
Phosphorus, 186, 350–1
  antidotes, **207**
  complementary/incompatible
    remedies, **191**
  constitutional remedy, **177**
  constitutional types, 158
  cough remedy, **218**
  miasmatic remedy, **156**
Phytolacca, 226, 311
Plantago major, 170
Plumbum metallicum (Plumbum met),
    91, **218**
Podophyllum
  antenatal treatments, **235**
  diarrhoea, **219**, 244
Powell PX range, 181
Prednisolone, prescription, **124**
Propolis (bee glue), 88
Proteus, **179**
Psorinum, 111, **156**, 177
Pulex irritans, **86**
Pulsatilla nigricans (puls), 75, **112**, 186,
    351
  adolescent problems, 238
  antenatal treatments, **235**
  antidotes, **207**
  catarrh, **224**
  cold/flu treatment, **217**
  complementary/incompatible
    remedies, **191**
  constitutional remedy, **177**
  constitutional types, 158
  cough remedy, **218**
  diarrhoea treatment, **219**
  emotional state, **222**
  Glasgow Acute Kit, **331**
  headache treatment, **221**
  keynotes, **168**
  peculiars, 188
  premenstrual syndrome, 233, **233**
  styes, **220**
  succussation study, 94
  veterinary uses, **251**

Pulsatilla pratensis, 111
Pulsatilla vulgaris, 111
Pyrethrum, 227, 248
Pyrethrum spray, traveller's kit,
    247

R

Radium bromide, 88
Reckeweg range, 181
Rescue Remedy, 238, 260–1
ReVet®, 250
Rhododendron, 186, 241
Rhus toxicodendron (Rhus tox), **112**,
    186, 351
  antenatal treatments, **235**
  antidotes, **207**
  chickenpox, 237
  clinical trials, 293
  complementary/incompatible
    remedies, **191**
  first aid/acute applications, 214,
    215, 225, 241
  fungal infections, 244
  Glasgow Acute Kit, **331**
  injection, 106
  keynotes, **168**
  mustard gas research, 174
  prescription cost, **21**
  runner's knee, 241
  'scrumpox,' 243
  topical, 225, 226, 241
  veterinary uses, **251**
Ricin, 174
RNA, 83, 89
Rock rose, 258, **260**
Rubella, 171, **172**
Ruta graveolens (Ruta grav), 351–2
  administration, 133
  adolescent problems, 237, 238
  complementary/incompatible
    remedies, **191**
  eyestrain, **220**
  first aid/acute applications, 214,
    215, **216**, 225, 240, **240**,
    241
  Glasgow Acute Kit, **331**
  injection, 106
  keynotes, **168**
  runner's knee, 241
  tennis/golfer's elbow, 241
  topical, 225

S

Sabadilla, allergies/allergic disease,
    228, **229**

Salt (sodium chloride), 53
Sanicula, 87
  bedwetting, 237
  traveller's kit, **247**
Scarletinum, **172**
Scleranthus, 258, **260**
Scorpion, 85, 89
Secale cornutum, 86
Sepia, 186, 352
  antidotes, **207**
  complementary/incompatible
    remedies, **191**
  constitutional remedy, **177**
  constitutional types, 158
  depression treatment, 48
  fungal infections, 244
  keynotes, **168**
  lotion, 226
  morning sickness, **235**
  premenstrual syndrome, **233**, 234
Sequoia sempervirens, 89
Silicea (Silica), 53, 256, **264**, 352
  boils, 230
  complementary/incompatible
    remedies, **191**
  constitutional remedy, **177**
  mastitis, 311
Silver, 53
Skookum chuck, 87
Sol, 88, 248
Solanum tuberosum aegrotans, 86–7
Spider, 88, 89
Spongia, cough remedy, **218**
Sportenine (Boiron), 242
Staphylococcus, 86
Staphysagria, 352
  abrasions/wounds, 239
  dental applications, **245**
  eye injuries, 240
  first aid/acute applications, **215**
  styes, **220**
Strychnine, prescription, **124**
Sulphur, 87, 91, 353
  abrasions/wounds, 239
  adolescent problems, 238
  agricultural research, 308
  antidotes, **207**
  chickenpox, 237
  complementary/incompatible
    remedies, **191**
  constitutional remedy, **177**
  constitutional types, 158
  diarrhoea treatment, **219**
  first potency, 92
  fungal infections, 244
  headache treatment, **221**
  'itch,' 154
  miasmatic remedy, **156**
  modalities, 187

NMR analysis, 108
prescription, 128, **128**
scabies, 153–4
skin conditions, 153–4, **223**
skin rashes due to, 200
styes, **220**
veterinary uses, **251**
Sulphuratums, 111
Sulphur D4, NMR analysis, 108
Sulphuric acid, first aid/acute
    applications, 242
Sycotic Co, **179**
Symphoricarpus, 234, **235**
Symphytum officinale (Symph), **112,**
    353
    dental applications, **245**
    eye injuries, 240
    first aid/acute applications, **215**
    fractures, 240
    keynotes, **168**
Syphilinum, 87, 111, **156**

T

Tabacum (Tabac, Talc), **112**
    agricultural uses, 249
    traveller's kit, **247**
Tamus
    first aid/acute applications, 225,
        227
    skin conditions, **223**
    topical, 225

Tarantula hispanica, **86**
Tela aranearum, 88
Tellurium, fungal infections, 244
Thuja occidentalis (Thuja), **112,** 353
    adolescent problems, 238
    complementary/incompatible
        remedies, **191**
    first aid/acute applications, 225,
        227
    miasmatic remedy, **156**
    prescription, **128,** 130
    topical, 225, 227
    verucca/warts, 244
Thyroid, prescription, **124**
Traumee, 243
Tuberculinum, 111, **156,** 177
Turneria (Damiana), 111
Typhoidinum, **172**

U

Urtica, 353
    allergies/allergic disease, 228,
        229
    blisters, 240
    first aid/acute applications, **215,**
        225, 227
    HPLC analysis, 84, **84**
    skin conditions, **223**
    topical, 225, 227
    traveller's kit, **247**
Ustilago maydis, 86

V

Vaccine derivatives, prescription, **124**
Vanadium, performance-enhancing
    remedy, 244
Varicella, **172**
Variolinum, 87
Veratrum album
    constipation treatment, **218**
    diarrhoea, 244
    prescription, **124**
Veratrum viride, prescription, **124**
Verbascum oil (Mullein), 226
Vervain, 258, **260**
Vespa cabro (Vespa, Vesp), 111, **112**

W

Water violet, 258
Whitfield's ointment, 243
Wyethia, allergies/allergic disease, **229**

X

X-ray, 88

Z

Zincum metallicum (Zinc met, Zinc
    m.), 91, **194**

General Index

Note: Entries in **bold** *refer to figures and tables/boxed material, common abbreviations used in subentries include: CAM, complementary and alternative medicine; OTC, over-the-counter; RCT, randomised controlled trial.*

A

Abbreviation systems, 110–13, **112**
Abrasions, **215, 223,** 226, 239
Absorption, 133
Accreditation, 62
Achilles tendon injuries, 241
Acne, **223, 238**
Acupuncture, 4, 25, 33
Administration methods
  Bach flower remedies, 259
  first aid/acute treatments, 214
  frequency, 105, 127
  method, 133–4
  multiple remedies, 189
  see also Dosages/dose regimens
Adolescents, 237–8, **238**
Adulteration, 43
Adverse reactions, 140
  CAM, 31, 162
  homeopathic remedies, 53, 200–1
    see also Aggravations
  orthodox drugs, 14, 15, 160
  placebos, 147
  reporting, 201, **202–3**
Advertising, 17
Advice, 133–4, **134**
  administration, 133
  aggravations, 133, 204
  immunisation fact sheet, 172
  inappropriate treatment, 200
  pharmacists, 29–30, 329
  point-of-sale, 17
  storage, 134
Advisory Board on the Registration of
    Homeopathic Products,
    116
Aesculapius in the Balance, 42
Africa, homeopathy in, 68–9
Aggravations, 49, 53, 133, 162, 199,
    200, 201–4
  complexes (complex remedies),
    182

incidence, 204
labour, 234
management of, 204
skin conditions, 200, 201–2
types, 203
Agricultural homeopathy, 249
  Bach flower remedies, 261
  research, 308, 310
AIDS *see* HIV infection/AIDS
Ainsworth, John, 62
Alaskan essences, 262
Alcohol
  medication process role, 104
  in remedy composition, 101
  use in remedy preparation, 90, 127
Alcoholism, 51, 326
Allergens, 87, 168, 228
Allergies/allergic disease, **223**
  allergic reactions, 227, **227**
  lactose sensitivity, 127, 201
  observational studies, 298
  paint fumes, 10
  RCTs, 294
    placebo effect, 288–9
  treatment, 227–30, **229**
    CAM response, 227
    constitutional, 228, 230
    evidence base, 228
    homeopaths *vs.* GPs, 11
    isopathic, 228
    placebo effect *vs.* homeopathy,
      148
  see also specific conditions
Allergodes, 88, 170
Allopathic drugs, 160
  adverse effects, 14, 15, 160
  caffeine-containing, 205
  CAM interactions, 20, 31, 123, 142,
    204–5
  dose–response curves, 160, **161**
  effects, **163**
  efficacy, 147–8
    reduced, 20, 142

OTC remedies as substitute, 122
prescription costs, 20–3, **21**
properties, **162**
remedies, complementary to,
    205
risks
  perception of, CAM 'push
    factor', 18
  risk:benefit ratio, 140
  thalidomide, 14
  solid dose forms, 101
  tautopathic remedies, 86, 88, 328
  see also specific drugs/drug types
Allopathy, 13
  decision to use, 141–2
  homeopathy similarities, 161–3
  homeopathy *vs.,* 159–61
  origin of term, 49
  symptomatic treatment, 156
  see also Allopathic drugs
Alternative medicine, 4, 13, 327
  see also Complementary and
    alternative medicine
    (CAM)
Altitude sickness, 243
Amazon flower essences, 262
American Foundation for
    Homeopathy, 76
American Homeopathic
    Pharmaceutical
    Association, 26
American Institute of Homeopathy, 75
Anaemia, 13, 232
Anaesthesia, homeopathic, 74
Analgesia, 244
Anecdotal evidence, 33–4, 149, 299
  see also Case studies
Angina, 51
Animal material, 85, 86, **86,** 87
*Annals and Transactions of the British
    Homeopathic Society,* 62
Antenatal treatments, 234, **235**
Anthrax, 174

Anthroposophical medicine, 255–7
  evidence, 256–7
Antibiotics, 22, 232
Antidiarrhoeal preparations, 10, **219, 244**
Antidotes, 206–7, **207**
Antihistamines, 10
Anti-IgE antibodies, Benveniste controversy, 302–4
Antimalarials, 46–7
Antitussives, 147–8
Anxiety, 138, **219, 222, 224,** 244
  dentistry, 244
  holistic approach, 10
  miasm hypothesis, 154
Apothecaries, Hahnemann's views of, 42–3
Apothecaries' Lexicon, 43
Argentina, homeopathy in, 73–4
Argentine School of Homeopathic Medicine, 73–4
Arndt Schultz Law, 54
Aromatherapy, 4
  interactions, 123
Arrhythmias, 51
Arsenic poisoning, 43, 174
Asia, homeopathy in, 70–1
Aspirin, homeopathy *vs.* in RA, 286–7
Assimilated model of integrated CAM delivery, 28
Asthma, 12, 227
  Hering's Law and, 156, **157**
  homeopathic treatment models
    evidence base, 228
    homeopaths *vs.* GPs, 11
    vibrational resonance, 151
  see also Allergies/allergic disease
Athlete's foot (tinea pedis), 243
Attitudes and awareness studies, 307–8, **309**
Australia
  educational institutions, 358
  homeopathy in, 71
  suppliers, 360
Australian bush essences, 262
Autonosodes, 87
Avogadro limit, 54
Avogadro's number, 54, 152
Ayurveda, 5

B

Bach, Edward, 258
  bowel nosodes, 178
  flower remedies *see* Bach flower remedies
Bach flower remedies, 258–61, 329
  administration, 259

adolescent problems, 237
  clinical uses, 259–60, **260**
  evidence, 261
  groups, 260
  'original healers', 258
  preparation, 259
  rescue remedy, 260–1
Back pain, 15
Bacteria
  bowel, 178–80
  infections, treatment, 230–1
  miasm hypothesis, 154
  source material, 86
  see also specific infections
Bailey flower essences, 262
Baillieston Clinic, 67
Basophils, Benveniste controversy, 302–4
Bedwetting, 237
Bee stings, 51, **215**
Behaviour
  adolescent, 237
  animal, 250
  experimental proving, 52
Belgian Homeopathic Compendium for Pharmacists, 190
Beliefs, illness/health, 308
Benveniste, Jacques, **305**
  death, 306
  editorial censorship, 276
  interview with, 304–6
  Nature controversy, 302–4
Bias, publication, 275–6
Bioassays, 108
Biochemic tissue salts, 263–5, **264**
Biodynamic farming, 256
Biological materials, 85–7
Biological warfare, 174
'Biophysical paradigm', 301
Bioterrorism, 174
Bites, **215**
Black eye, **220**
Blackie Foundation Trust, 63
Blackie, Margery, 61, 63
Blank carriers, 131
Blisters, 239–40
Blood and crush injuries, **216**
Blushing, **238**
Body odour, **238**
Boericke's *Materia Medica,* 178, 192, **193**
'Boiling method', 259
Boils, 230, **238**
Boots Company, homeopathic training, 324
Botanical experiments, 308
Botanical names, 111
'Bowel' nosodes, 178–80, **179**
Brazil, homeopathy in, 73

Bristol Eye Hospital, 68
Bristol Homeopathic Hospital, 68, **69**
British Holistic Medical Association, 357
British Homeopathic Association (BHA), 62–3, 322, 332, 357
  information, 328
  recommendations and, 136
British Homeopathic Journal, 62, 63, 332
  see also Homeopathy
British Homeopathic Library, 332, 357
British Homeopathic Manufacturers' Association (BAHM), 82
British Homeopathic Pharmacopoeia, 82
British Homeopathic Society, 12, 62
  laws/regulations, 62
  pharmacies supplying CAM, 16
  publications, 62
  Royal family support, 23
British National Formulary (BNF), 147–8
British Pharmaceutical Conference, homeopathy debate, 61
Broken bulk dispensing, 131
Bronchoconstriction, 146
Bronchodilation, 146
Bronchospasm, 146
Bruising, **215**, 226, 242–3
  RCTs, 292
Burns, **215, 216, 223,** 226, 227

C

Caffeine, remedy interactions, 205
Californian essences, 262
Canalisation, 190
Cancer, placebos/placebo effect, 146
Candegabe, Eugenio, 74
Cara software package, 198
Carbo, Dr, 73
Carpal tunnel syndrome surgery, RCTs, 292
Case studies, 33–4, 299–300
  quality criteria, 299
Catarrh, **217, 224**
Cellular repair, 155
Censorship, homeopathy research, 276
Centers for Disease Control and Prevention (CDCs), CAM user profile, 15
Centesimal potency, 95–6, **96,** 126
Centre for Continuing Pharmacy Education, 324
Chemical names, 111
Chemicals
  low dose/ultralow dose exposure, 173–5
  source materials, 87

Chemical terrorism, 174
Chemical warfare, 173–4, 174–5
Chi, 150
Chickenpox, **172**, 237
Chilblains, **223**, 227
Children
    bedwetting, 237
    bee stings, **215**
    Borlands classification of types, 159, **159**
    constitutional remedies, 158–9
    diseases of, 172, 237
    isopathic vaccines, 172
    randomised controlled trials (RCTs), 294
    see also Adolescents; Infants
Chinese medicine, 33
Chiropractic, 5
Cholera
    homeopathic treatment, 60–1, 76
        Hahnemann's, 43–4
    nosodes, 171, 172, 246–7
    orthodox treatment, 60
Chondromalacia, 241
Christchurch flower essences, 262
Chromatographic analysis
    quality control, 107, 108
    Urtica analysis, 84, **84**
Chronic Diseases, their Nature and Homeopathic Cure, 43, 153
Cicero, holism concept, 7
Classification systems, 5–6
    House of Lords' Report (2000), 5–6
        groupings, 6
    NCCAM, 6
    by system of therapy, 5
Climate, 243
Clinical audit, 33, 307–8
Clinical proving, 52
Clinical therapeutic observation, proving, 52
Cochrane Collaboration, CAM classification, 4
Cochrane Library, CAM meta-analyses, 32–3
Coffee, 133
Colds, 214, **217**, 244
Colic, **222, 224,** 236–7
Companies Act (1929), 62
Competence to treat, 140–1, 200
Complementary and alternative medicine (CAM), 3–38
    availability, 135
    classification, 5–6
    common applications, 24–5, 30, 122
    competence, 140–1, 200
    current interest in, 14–15
    definitions, 4, 14
    demand for, reasons, 18–23

    pull factors, 18, 20–3
    push factors, 18–20, 308
    diagnosis in, 19
    first UK chair in, 324
    'green' association, 14, 23
    healthcare integration, 27–8
        models, 28
        research role, 312
    healthcare professional's views, 27
    holistic approach see Holism/holistic approach
    information sources, **29,** 29–31
    markets, 25–7
    misconceptions, 23
    national differences, 24–5, **25**
        see also Global development
    national regulatory bodies, 6, 82, 136
        see also individual organisations
    perception of, 23
        pharmacy staff, **29**
        risk, 18, 122
    recent developments, 34
    research see Research
    risk:benefit ratio, 24, 140
    Royal support, 23
    types, 4–5
    user profiles, 15–17
    see also specific types/procedures
Complementary medicine, 4, 13, 14, 327
    see also Complementary and alternative medicine (CAM)
Complexes (complex remedies), 55, 81, 180–2
    aggravations, 182
    criticism, 182
    first aid/acute treatments, 214
    licensing/registration, 114
    nomenclature, 111, 129
    polypharmacy vs., 189
    popularity, 180
    prescribing, 126, 129
    prescription/prescribing, 181
    tissue salts, 265
    topical, 226
    utility, 182
    veterinary, 311
    see also Polychrests; Remedies
Complexity theory, 151
Computerised repertorising, 196–8
Concentration, **238**
Concomitants, 187
Confidence, **260**
Conjunctivitis, 106, **220**
Consensus statements, 34
Constipation, **218,** 326

Constitutional remedies, 158–9, 176–7, **177**
    allergies/allergic disease, 228, 230
    antenatal, 234
    premenstrual syndrome, 233–4
Constitutional Type Questionnaire (CTQ), 158
Constitutional types, 157–9
Consultations
    CAM practitioners
        initial questions, 7
        patient input, 330
        placebo effect and, 148
        time taken, 19, 20, 175
    orthodox medicine
        factors affecting, 18–19
        time taken, 18, 19, 20
Consumerism, healthcare, 19
Contamination, 109
    eye drops, 106
    packaging and, 110
Controversies in Health Care Policies, 23
Cooperation, homeopathy research, 275, 313
Costa Rica, homeopathy in, 74
Coughs, 123, 147–8, 162, 214, **218,** 244
Counselling see Advice
Creams, 105, 225–6
Crush injuries, **216**
Crystals, 101–2
    medicating process, 101, 131–2
    prescription/dispensing, **128,** 129–30
Cuba, homeopathy in, 74
Cullen, William, 46, 325
Cultural factors, CAM pull factors, 23–4
Cure, healing vs., 145
Cystitis, 230, 232, **232**

D

Dead leg, 240
Decimal potency, 96, **97,** 126
Deficiencies, 13, 232, 263
Delayed onset muscle soreness (DOMS), 241–2
    RCTs, 294
Delphi project, 300
Dentistry, homeopathic, 74, 244–6, **245**
    training, 323
Depression, 48, 91, 325
    miasm hypothesis, 154
Desktop Companion (Morrisson), 196
Detwiller, Henry, 75
D'Hervilly-Gohier, Melanie, 44–5
Diabetes, 13
    dose form and, 127

Diagnosis
    CAM practitioners, 19
    iridology/iridiagnosis, 5
    orthodox medicine, 19
    self-diagnosis, dangers, **138,** 138–9,
        139
Diarrhoea, 138, 244
    childhood, RCTs, 294
    first aid treatment, **219**
    holistic approach to treatment, 10
    'traveller's', **246**
Dilution, 53–5
    centesimal, 92, 95–6, **96**
    decimal, 92, 96–7, **97**
    Hahnemann method, 92–3, 98
    Korsakovian, 95, 97–8
    potentisation, 54, 92–3
    terminology, 95–7
    theories of, 94–5
Diphtheria, **172,** 230–1
Diploma level training, 323
Diploma of the Faculty of
        Homeopathy (DFHom),
        323
Disease, 145–65
    anthroposophical approach to,
        256
    constitutional types, 157–9, 176
    environmental factors, 8
    genetic factors, 8
    Hering's law and, 155–7
    miasmatic view, 43–4, 153–5
    nosodes, 86–7
    totality of symptoms, 185–6
    vital force and, 149–53, 156
Disease aggravations, 203
Dispensing, 130–2
    broken bulk, 131
    extemporaneous, 131–2
    liquid forms, 130
    original pack, 130
    solid dose forms, 127–30
    written protocols, 131
    see also Medicating process;
        Prescription/prescribing
DNA, 155
DNA repair, 155
'Dope testing', 142, 239, 244
Dosages/dose regimens, 127–30, **128,**
        182–91
    changing, 200
    chronic conditions, 185–8, **189**
    first aid/acute conditions, 183–5,
        185, 214
    isopathic vaccines, 171–2, 228
Dose–response curves, 160, **161**
Drainage therapy, 190
Drink, remedy inactivation, 133
'Dr Jack's kit', 190, 330

Drug abuse, 13
Drug interactions, 20, 31, 123, 142,
        204–5
    research, 313
Drug pictures, 51, 168, 178, 179, 327
    learning, 330
    veterinary, 251
    see also Repertories/repertorising
Drugs (orthodox) see Allopathic drugs
Dudgeon, Robert, 64
Dynamisation see Potentisation
Dysrepair, 155

E

Earache, **219**
Economic factors
    as CAM pull factor, 20–3
    CAM research, 32, 271
    OTC preparations, 22–3
    prescription costs
        CAM *vs.* allopathic drugs, 20–2,
            21
        cost savings/patient, 21
    remedy packaging, 110
Eczema, 156, **157, 223**
Editorial censorship, homeopathy
        research, 276
Education, 321–33
    homeopathy in South Africa, 69
    institutions, 357–8
    lectures, 324–9
        audience, 324
        content, 324–5
        example, 325–9
        influencing factors, 325
        tips, 328–9
    medical education and
        CAM acceptance, 28
        in UK, 322
        in USA, 76
    pharmacists and, 61, 322, 323
        starting up, 329–33
    provision, 323
    training courses, 321–4
Education Development Officer of the
        Faculty of Homeopathy,
        324
Effectiveness, 280–1, **281,** 298, 307,
        312
Efficacy, 31, 280–1, **281**
    perceptions of, 25, 30
    prescription drugs, 18, 20
Elderly patients, 205
The Emergence of Homeopathy, 47
Emotional factors
    Bach remedies, 260, **260**
    in disease, 146, 156

allergies/allergic disease, 230
    PMS, 233
Emotional states, **222**
Energy, lack of, **260**
Entanglement theories, 306
Environmental factors, 8
Envy, **260**
Epidemics, homeopathic treatments,
        43–4, 60, 75–6
'Essences' see Flower remedies
Ethical issues, placebos, 147
European Coalition on Homeopathic
        and Anthroposophic
        Medicinal Products
        (ECHAMP), 82, 116–17
European Commission, placebo
        studies, 288
European Committee for Homeopathy
    nomenclature confusion, 111
    Pharmacy Subcommittee, 117,
        201
European countries
    CAM usage, 25, **25**
    homeopathy in, 72–3
    research, 31
    see also European Union Directives;
        specific countries
European pharmacopoeia, 117
European Union Directives
    Directive for Medicinal Products
        (1992), 82
    EU Directive 92/73 EEC, 17,
        113–17
        article 7, 114, 116
        article 9, 114–15
        implementation, 116
    EU Directive 2001/82, 116
    EU Directive 2001/83, 116
    EU Directive 2004/27/EC, 116
    EU Directive 2004/28/EC, 116
European Union Pharmaceutical
        legislation reform, 116–17
European Union Regulation 2309/93,
        116
Evidence based research, 31, 53
Examination fear, **238**
Examinations, South Africa, 69
Expectorants, 147–8, 162
Experimental proving (pathogenesis),
        52
Experimental studies, 279
Explanatory studies, 280
Export control, 113
Extemporaneous dispensing, 131–2
Extraction process, 90–2, 327
Eye drops, 105–6
Eye problems, 105–6, **238**
    injury, **220,** 240
Eye strain, **220, 238**

F

Faculty Certificate in Basic
Homeopathic Pharmacy,
322
Faculty of Homeopathy, 62, 332, 357
Diplomas, 323
education role, 322–4
Fellowships, 324
immunisation fact sheet, 172
membership (MFHom), 62, 322,
323
Scottish branch, 67
veterinary homeopathy, 250, **252,**
323
Fainting, **215**
Farming, 116, 249, 256
see also Agricultural homeopathy;
Veterinary homeopathy
Fear, **222, 238**
of flying, 246
see also Anxiety
First aid/acute applications, 182,
183–5, 213–54
acute self-limiting conditions,
216–24, **224**
common applications, 214
dental uses, 244–6, **245**
keynote (three-legged stool)
approach, 183–4, 214
principles, 214
record keeping, 198, **199**
response, 184, **185**
sporting injuries, 239–43
topical preparations, 225–7
travel and, 246–8
useful treatments, 214–16, **215,**
216
see also specific applications/injuries
First Aid Homeopathy, 214–15
'Five flower remedy', 261
Flatulence, **222**
Flower remedies, 257–63
see also Bach flower remedies
Fluorescence graph imaging, quality
control, 107
Fluorine, 246
Flying, fear of, 246
Folk medicine, 168
Food and Drug Administration (FDA)
chocolate production, 88
remedy licensing, 117
Food, remedy inactivation, 133, 206
Foot and mouth disease, 251
Foreboding, **222**
Foundation courses, 323
Foundation for Integrated Health, 28
Fractures, **215,** 240
French Homeopathic Pharmacopoeia, 82

Friends, as information source, 29
Frog metamorphosis, succussation
studies, 95
Frostbite, 243
Fungal infections, 243–4
Furunculosis, 310, **311**

G

Galen, 150
Gastroenteritis, **138**
Gels, 105
Gender issues, 19
General practitioners (GPs)
CAM acceptance, 28
CAM integration, 27
homeopathy services, 22
consultation times, 18, 19, 20
'Generals', 185, 194
General sales list classification, 17
Genes, 155
Genetic factors, disease, 8, 154
German Homeopathic Pharmacopoeia, 82
German measles (Rubella), **172**
Germany, homeopathy in, **40,** 72
see also Hahnemann, Samuel
Gibson's rheumatoid arthritis trials,
286–8, **287**
Glasgow Acute Kit, 330, **331**
Glasgow Homeopathic Hospital, 66–7,
67, 358
children's, 236
Glasgow Homeopathic Hospital
Outcome Scale (GHHOS),
33, **282,** 282–3, **283**
VAS hybrid, 283, **284**
Glass containers, 127
plastic *vs.,* 109–10
Global development, 59–78
training courses, 324
see also individual countries/regions
Globules, 102
Globuli, 102
Golfer's elbow, 241
Gonorrhoea ('sycotic' miasms), 153,
154
miasmatic remedies, **156**
GP10/FP10 forms, 20
Gram, Hans Burch, 74–5
Grants, 271
Granules, 102
medicating process, 131–2
prescription/dispensing, **128,**
129–30
GRECO, 294
Green Man group, 262
'Green revolution', 14, 23
Grief, **222, 224**

Guidelines, 34, 198
Guiding Symptoms, 83
Gum disease, 13

H

Haematoma, 241
Haemorrhoids, 226
Hahnemann dilution method, 92–3, 98
Hahnemann Medical College, 75, 76
Hahnemann, Samuel, 39–46, **46,** 326
apothecaries, views of, 42–3
birthplace, 39, **40**
criticism of, 43, 50
death, 45
education, 42
employment, 43
family, 39, **41,** 44
global influence, 60, 64
'half homeopaths', 12
marriages, 44–5
memorabilia, 45–6, **46**
memorials/commemoration, **41,**
45, **72,** 77–8
multiple prescribing, 188–9
preparation methods, 90
publications, 42, 43, 46, 50–1, 54,
55
translation into English, 64
studies/homeopathy development,
46–9
Cinchona experiments, 46–7
Law of Cure, 47–8
Law of Similars, 49, 51
miasm hypothesis, 43–4, 153
the *Organon,* 50–1
self-experimentation, 47, 48–9
see also Provings
serial dilution, 53
simplexes, 43, 55
see also Homeopathic principles
veterinary homeopathy, 249
vitalism, 150
Hangover, **224**
Hawaiian essences, 262
Headache, **221, 224**
Boericke's repertory entries, **193, 194**
Kent's repertory entries, **195**
observational studies, 298
Healing, 145–6
anthroposophical medicine, 255
'art' *vs.* 'science', 160–1, 328
Hering's observations, 155–6
Health
beliefs, 308
statistics, 60
WHO definition, 4
Health and Homeopathy, 63, 332

Healthcare
  alternative *vs.* complementary
      approaches, 12–14
  budgets, 19
  CAM integration into, 27–8
    research role, 312
  consumerism, 19
  patient-centred approach, 15
  United Kingdom, 15
    see also National Health Service
      (NHS)
Healthcare professionals
  CAM views, 27
  homeopathy training, 321–4
  as information source, 29
  OTC requests, 122
  prescribing, 125
  recommendation of, 136
Heat exhaustion, 243
Helios Homeopathic Pharmacy, 98
Herbalism, 5
  homeopathy distinction/confusion,
    18, 83, 327
  perceived risk, 18
  safety issues, 31
Hering, Constantine, 83, 96, 156
  Hering's Law, 155–7
  Psorinum investigation, 178
Hering's Law, 155–7
Herpes simplex infections, 243
High-performance liquid
      chromatography (HPLC)
  quality control, 108
  Urtica analysis, 84, **84**
Himalayan tree and flower essences,
    262
Hippocrates, 47, 150
HIV infection/AIDS, 13, 24
  steroid interactions, 205
  tautopathic treatment of skin
      reactions, 174
Hoenigsberger, Julian Martin, 70
Holism/holistic approach, 7–12, 160
  concept of, 7
  debate, 4
  definitions, 7
  factors affecting, 8–11
  individualised treatment, 8, 9
  linear treatment approach *vs.*, 8–9,
    9
  normal state of wellbeing, 156
  normal state of well-being, 7–8
  origin of term, 7
  orthodox medicine and, 11–12
  vital force and, 151
HomeoNet, 330
Homeopathic aggravations, 203
Homeopathic anaesthesia, 74
Homeopathic Children's Hospital, 67

'Homeopathic drops', 100
'Homeopathic elixir', 100
Homeopathic hospitals, United
      Kingdom, 63–8, 358–9
Homeopathic immunotherapy, 228
  RCTs, 288–91
Homeopathic Medical College of
      Pennsylvania *see*
      Hahnemann Medical
      College
Homeopathic Medical Repertory
      (Murphy), 196
Homeopathic medicating potency,
    101
Homeopathic medicine *see* Remedies
Homeopathic pharmaceutical
      industry, United States,
      76
Homeopathic Pharmacopoeia
      Convention of the United
      States (HPCUS), 117
Homeopathic Pharmacopoeia of the USA
      (HPUS), 82
Homeopathic pharmacopoeias, 81–3
  variations, 82, 84, 90, 96
  see also specific publications
Homeopathic principles, 50–5, 326
  Hering's Law, 155–7
  Law of Cure, 47–8, 55
  Law of Similars, 49, 51, 151–3
  like-cures-like, 51–3, 160, 326
  minimal dose (serial dilution),
      53–5
  provings *see* Provings
  simplexes (single remedies), 43, 55,
      225, 326
  theory of disease and treatment,
      145–65
  vibrational planes, **150,** 150–1
  see also Homeopathy, theories of
Homeopathic Society, 63
Homeopathic treatment
  allopathic *vs.* homeopathic
      approaches, 159–63
  chronic illness, 152, 182, 185–8
    concomitants, 187
    modalities, 186–7
    peculiars, 187
    totality of symptoms, 185–6
  facilities, 137–8
  first-aid/acute *see* First aid/acute
      applications
  follow-up/patient review, 198–200
    guidelines, 198
    possible actions, 199–200
  healing *vs.*, 145
  holistic approach to *see*
      Holism/holistic approach
  inappropriate, 200

levels of, 182–93
  see also Dosages/dose regimens
  linear *vs.* holistic approach, 8–9, **9**
  provision *see* Treatment provision
  record keeping, 139, 197, **199**
  theory of disease and, 145–66
  see also Prescription/prescribing;
      Remedies
Homeopathic Trust, 63
  research grants, 271
Homeopaths
  lack of, 271
  training, 321–4
  see also Non-medically qualified
      professional practitioners
Homeopathy, 5, **134**
  academic/medical resistance, 73
  allied therapies, 255–66
  availability, 135
  common applications, 24–5, 30,
      122, 330
  criticisms, 160
  decision to use, 141–2
  direction of cure, 155–7
  GP-based services, 22
  herbalism distinction/confusion,
      18, 83, 327
  historical background, 39–58, 325–6
    global development, 59–78
    Hahnemann's contribution *see*
        Hahnemann, Samuel
    Kent, James T., 64
    see also individual
        countries/regions
  markets, 26–7
  mechanisms *see* Homeopathy,
      theories of
  media reporting, 12
  origin of term, 49, 326
  orthodox medicine and, 12, 13
  orthodox medicine *vs.*, 159–63
  patient information, 133–4, **134**
  perceived efficacy, 24
    by healthcare professionals, 30
  popularity, 270
  principles *see* Homeopathic
      principles
  remedies *see* Remedies
  theoretical basis *see* Homeopathy,
      theories of
  treatment using *see* Homeopathic
      treatment
  user profiles, 16–17
  variations in response, 157
  women, 231–6
Homeopathy, 62, 63, 332
  see *British Homeopathic Journal*
Homeopathy and the Elements, 72
Homeopathy and the Minerals, 72

Homeopathy, theories of, 94–5, 328
    Benveniste controversy, 302–4
    disease, 146–65
    entanglement theories, 306
    local causality, 300–1
    non-local causality, 301–6, **305**
    placebo effects *see*
            Placebos/placebo effect
    research, 300–8
    vital force, 149–53
    see also Homeopathic principles
'Homeotherapeutics' *see* Homeopathy
Homeo-Web, 330
Home sickness, **238**
Hopelessness, 146
Hormesis, 51, 173
Hormonal imbalance, 232
Hormone replacement therapy (HRT),
    13, 234
Houldsworth Homeopathic Hospital,
    66
House of Lords' Report (2000)
    CAM research funding, 32
    classification of CAM, 5–6
Hypnosis, 24
Hypothermia, 243

I

Immune responses, 85
Immunotherapy, 228
    RCTs, 288–91
Import control, 113
India, homeopathy in, 70
Indian Homeopathic Pharmacopoeia, 82
Indigestion, **222, 224**
Individualised treatment plans, 326
    Hahnemann's views, 49
    holistic approach and, 8, 9, 160
    RCT problem, 297
Infants, 236–7
    colic, **224,** 236–7
    nappy rash, 237
    teething, 149, **224,** 236–7
Infection(s), 230–1, 243–4
    miasm hypothesis, 154
    nosode vaccines, 171, 172, **172**
    wounds, 239
    see also specific infections
Inflammatory conditions, 85, 293
Influenza, **172, 217, 224,** 230
    RCTs, 294
    vaccination, 171
Information sources, 29–31, 328, 330
    useful addresses, 357–60
Injections, 106, **106**
Insect bites/stings, 51, **215,** 243, 248
Insect material, 85, **86,** 88

Insect repellents, 227
Insomnia, 51, 244, 326
Institutional censorship, homeopathy
        research, 275
Integrative medicine, 27–8
    Foundation for Integrated Health,
        28
    models, 28
Integrative Medicine Data Collection
        Network (IMDCN), 283
Integrative Medicine Outcomes Scale
        (IMOS), 283
Interactions, 204–7
    allopathic drugs, 20, 31, 123, 142,
        204–5
    aromatherapy oils, 123
    foodstuffs, 133, 206
    other remedies, 190, **191,** 206
    research, 313
International Directory of Homeopathy,
        113
International Hahnemann Association
        (IHA), 75
International Olympic Committee
        (IOC) drug controls, 239,
        244
Internet, 330
Ireland, educational institutions, 358
Iridology/iridiagnosis, 5
Iron deficiency anaemia, 13, 232
Ischaemic heart disease, 146
ISIS software package, 198
Isopathic remedies, 87, 168, 170
    allergies/allergic disease, 228
    allergodes, 88, 170
    nosodes *see* Nosodes
    sarcodes, 85, 86, 170
    tautopathic (tautodes), 86, 88, 170,
        173–5
    as vaccines, 171–3, **172,** 246–7, 251,
        310
Israel, homeopathy in, 70–1

J

Jealousy, **260**
Jellyfish stings, 243
*Journal of the British Homeopathic
        Society,* 62
Journals, publication bias, 275–6

K

Kent Homeopathic Associates Inc.,
        197
Kent, James Tyler, 64, 66, 75–6, 156
    constitutional types, 158

Kent's *Repertory of the Homeopathic
        Materia Medica,* 192, 194,
        195
Keynote (three-legged stool)
        prescribing
    classical remedies, 175
    'first aid'/acute, 183–4, 214
    polychrests, 168, **169**
    research role, 313
Ki, 150
Kleijnen's meta-analysis of RCTs,
        294–6, **295**
Knee surgery, RCTs, 292
Korsakovian dilution methods, 95
Korsakovian potentisation method,
        97–8
Korsakov, Simeon Nicolaevich, 97

L

Labelling, 132, **132**
    EU Directive 92/73 EEC article 1,
        113
    mislabelling, 201
Labour, 201, 234–6
Lacerations, 214
La Chimie Royale et Pratique, 168
Lactose, 127
    intolerance/sensitivity, 127, 201
    powders, 102
    trituration with, 91–2
Lancet, 'death of homeopathy', 296
Latin America, homeopathy in, 73–4
Law of Contraries, 49
Law of Cure, 47–8
    minimal dose, 53–5, 326
    placebo effect and, 148
Law of Similars, 49, 51, 151–3
Lectures, 324–9
Licenced Associates of the Faculty of
        Homeopathy (LFHom),
        323
Licensing, 17, 113–17
    national rules, 114–15
    routes, **115**
    see also European Union Directives
Lifestyle factors
    holistic approach and, 8
    responsibility, 19
Like-cures-like, 51–3, 160, 326
Linctus, 100
Liniment, 105, 226
Liquid potency, 100, 101, 104, 127
    dispensing, 131, 132
Liquids, 100
    medicating, 132
    prescription/dispensing, 130,
        131

Liquid state, 301
Liverpool, homeopathy in, 68
LM potentisation method, 99–100
LOAD acronym, 141, 183
Local causality theories, 300–1
London Homeopathic Hospital *see*
    Royal London
    Homeopathic Hospital
Lotion, 105, 226
'Luetic' miasms (syphilis), 153
    miasmatic remedies, **156**
Lux, Joseph Wilhelm, 249

M

MacRepertory Classic, 197
MacRepertory Pro, 197
Malaria, 46–7, 246–7
    nosodes, 171, 172
Malaysia, homeopathy in, 71
Manufacturers, 136
    special licences, 117
    United States, 76
    see also Suppliers
Market model of integrated CAM
    delivery, 28
Marsh fever, 46–7
Massage, 5
Mastitis, 226, 311
Materia medica, 46, 52, 75, 337–54
    nomenclature and, 110, 125
    prescribing remedies, 125
    see also Repertories/repertorising;
      specific publications
Materia Medica (Boericke), 178
    with Repertory, 192, **193**
Materia Medica of New Homeopathic
    Remedies, 173
Materia Medica Pura, 54
Measles, **172**
Media reporting
    Benveniste controversy, 304
    as CAM pull factor, 23
    homeopathy, 12
    information source, 29
    'natural' medicine, 23
Medical Act, 61
Medical education, homeopathy and,
    28, 76, 322
Medical records, 139
Medicating process
    oral dose forms, 132
    solid dose forms, 101, 102, 103–5,
      104, 131–2
    topical dose forms, 132
Medicinal aggravations, 203
Medicinal herbalism *see* Herbalism

Medicines
    allopathic *see* Allopathic drugs
    homeopathic *see* Remedies
Medicines Act (1968), amendments,
    117
Medicines and Healthcare products
    Regulation Authority
    (MHRA), 82, 116
Membership of Faculty of
    Homeopathy (MFHom),
    62, 322, 323
Meningitis, 13
Menopause, 234
Mental concomitants, 187
'Mentals', 185, 194
'Mercurial fever', 47
Mercury, syphilis, 47
'Meridians', 4
Mexico, homeopathy in, 73
Miasmatic remedies, 155, **156,**
    177–80
Miasm hypothesis, 43–4, 153–5
    constitutional types and, 159
    controversy, 154
    definitions, 154
    DNA level, 155
    genetic traits, 154
    new interpretations, 155
    types of miasm, 153–4
Miccant Ltd., 198
Microbial material, 87
Migraine, RCTs, 294
Minimal dose, 53–5, 326
Mislabelling, 201
Misleading content, homeopathy
    research, 276
Mixtures *see* Complexes (complex
    remedies)
Modalities, 186–7
Morning sickness, 14, 234, **235**
Morrisson's *Desktop Companion,* 196
Mother tinctures, 101
    definition, 81–2
    dilution transfer, 93
    direct use, 92
    extraction, 90–2, 327
    prescription/dispensing, 130,
      132
    quality control, 107–9
    strengths, 90
    supplier variations, 108–9
    topical use, 105, 226–7
Mumps, **172**
Murphy's *Homeopathic Medical*
    Repertory, 196
Muscular problems, 226
    sport-related, 240–2
Mustard gas, 173–4

N

Nappy rash, 237
Nasal congestion, **217**
Nasal sprays, 106
National Center for Complementary
    and Alternative Medicine
    (NCCAM), 76–7
    areas of focus, 77
    CAM classification, 6
    CAM research funding, 32
    CAM user profile, 15
    Strategic Plan (2005–2009), 77
National Center for Health Statistics
    (NCHS), CAM user
    profile, 15
National Health Service (NHS)
    CAM provision within, 134–5
      access to, 135
      audit, 307
      House of Lords' report (2000), 6
      prescriptions/prescribing, 14,
        20–2, 125, 135, **135**
      see also Prescription/prescribing
    CAM research funding, 32
    healthcare delivery in, 14
    homeopathic hospitals in, 64–8,
      358–9
    patient records, 139
National Institutes for Health (NIH),
    76
    see also National Center for
      Complementary and
      Alternative Medicine
      (NCCAM)
National licensing rules, 114–15
National School of Medicine and
    Homeopathy (Mexico),
    73
Natrum mur person, 158
Nature, Benveniste controversy, 302–4
Naturopathy, 5
Nausea, 14, **222**, 234, **235**
NCCAM, classification systems, 6
Nelson, educational material, 322,
    329
Neuberger, Julia, 23
'Neurotic' symptoms, 19
The 'new perception', 263
Newspaper reporting, 23
New Zealand
    educational institutions, 358
    homeopathy in, 71–2
    licensing in, 117
    suppliers, 360
New Zealand flower essences, 262–3
New Zealand Homeopathic Society, 72
Nigeria, homeopathy in, 69

NMR spectroscopy, variations in production and, 84
Nomenclature, 110–13, **112**, 125–6, 129
  biochemic tissue salts, 263
Non-lactose fermenting bacteria, 178–9
Non-local causality theories, 301–6
Non-medically qualified professional practitioners
  consultations
    initial questions, 7
    time taken, 19, 20
  diagnosis, 19
  OTC requests, 122
  patient–practitioner relationship, 27
  recommendation, 136
  training courses, 321–4
Non-pareils, 102
Non-professional customers, 122
Nosodes, 170, 171
  animal, 76
  autonosodes, 87
  'bowel', 178–80, **179**
  cystitis remedies, 232
  definition, 86
  miasmatic remedies, **156**, 177–80
  nomenclature, 111
  plant, 86
  uses, 86–7
  as 'vaccines', 171, **172**, 246–7, 251
  veterinary, 251, 310
Nuclear magnetic resonance (NMR), quality control, 107, 108, **109**

O

Observational studies, 279, 298–300
Observer Patient Interactive Chart (OPIC), 33, 283, 285, **285**
Office of Complementary Medicine see National Center for Complementary and Alternative Medicine (NCCAM)
Oils, 226
Ointment, 105, 225–6
Oncotic miasms, 154, **156**
Online information sources, 330
Oral preparations, 100–1
Oral solution, 101
Organic farming, 116, 249
Organisations, 332, 357–60
  see also individual bodies
Organon, 50–1, 55, 75
Organophosphates, 52
Original pack dispensing, 130

Orthodox medicine
  accountability, 14
  approach to healthcare, 12–14
  CAM integration, 27–8
    homeopathy and, 12, 13
    research role, 312
  as CAM 'push factor', 18–20, 308
  constitutional response, 158
  consultation time, 18–19
  disenchantment with, 18–20, 328
  failure, 18
  historical aspects, 42, 325
    cholera epidemic, 60
    empirical vs. rationalist views, 49
    vitalism, 150
  holistic approach, 11–12
  homeopathy similarities, 161–3
  homeopathy vs., 159–61
  perceived risk, 18
  placebos, 147
  vaccination risk, 171
  women and, 231–2
  see also Allopathic drugs; Allopathy
Osteopathy, 5, 24, 33
Otalgia, 226
Outcome measures, 33, 272, 281–5
  clinical response, 274
  lack of validated, 272
  misleading, 276
  placebo RCTs, 289
  pooled results, 282, **283**
  'well being' response, 274
  see also specific measures
Outlines of Veterinary Homeopathy, 249–50
Overall Progress Interactive Chart (OPIC), 33, 283, 285, **285**
Over-enthusiasm, **260**
Over-the-counter (OTC) preparations, 16–17
  acute illness, 152, 183–5, 188
  allergodes, 170
  causes for concern, 123
  chronic illness, 188
  economics of, 22–3
  efficacy, 147–8
  guidelines for use, 142
  homeopathy user profiles, 16
  interventions, 122–3, 138
  length of use, concern, 17
  markets, 25–7
  point-of-sale advice, 17
  problems of providing, 137–9
  record keeping, 197, **199**
  request characteristics, 122
  requests for, 122
  research, 313

retail outlets, 25
  sources of requests, 122
  sports injuries, 243
  supply, 121–3
  see also Pharmacies; Pharmacists

P

Packaging, 109–10, 127
  EU Directive 92/73 EEC article 1, 113
Paediatric homeopathy, 236
  see also Children; Infants
Pain, 214, 242–3
  dental, 244
  holistic approach and, 8
  RCTs, 292
  rheumatic conditions, 186
Paracelsus, 47
'Particulars', 194
Pathological material, nosodes, 86–7
Patient(s)
  associations, 357–8
  expectations/attitudes, 139
    placebo effect and, 146
    research, 307–8
  follow-up, 198–200
  information, 133–4, **134**
    see also Advice
  'patient power', 23
  selection for RCTs, 296–7
Patient-centred healthcare, 15
  integrated CAM delivery, 28
  see also Individualised treatment plans
Patient–doctor relationship, factors affecting, 19
Patient Medication Records (PMR) systems, 139
Patient–practitioner relationship, 27
Patient's Association for Anthroposophical Medicine, 357
Peculiars, 187
Peer review, homeopathy research, 276
Percolation, 90, **91**
Performance-enhancing remedies, 244
Personality factors, 10–11
Perspiration, **238**
Pharmaceutical industry, homeopathic in US, 76, 360
Pharmacies
  homeopathic treatment provision, 137–42
    addresses, 359–60
    facilities, 137–8
    problems, 137–9

homeopathy user profiles, 16
Mexico, homeopathic remedies, 73
patient records, 139, 198, **199**
staff perceptions, **29**
see also Over-the-counter (OTC)
    preparations; Pharmacists
Pharmacists
    CAM knowledge/advice, 17, **29,**
        29–30, 329
    changing roles, 137–8, 333
    competence, 140–1, 200
    Hahnemann's views of, 42–3
    homeopathy organisations, 332
        see also individual bodies
    information on preparation, 117
    responsibility for customer safety,
        123, 140
    setting up homeopathy practice,
        329–33
        gaining knowledge, 329
        publicising interest, 333
        setting up stocks, 330–2
        stock control, 332–3
    training, 61, 322, 323
        see also Education
    veterinary homeopathy, problems,
        251
Pharmacy, homeopathy in UK, 59–60
Pharmacy Subcommittee of the
        European Homeopathic
        Committee, 117
Phosphorus person, 158, 176
Physical concomitants, 187
Pills, 102, 131
Pillules, 102, **128,** 128–9
Placebos/placebo effect, 10, 30, 146–9
    definitions, 146
    duration of effect, 149
    ethical issues, 147
    experimental proving, 52
    homeopathic research
        enhanced response, 286
        errors, 273
        quantification of, 275
        RCT studies of, 288–91, 295, 296
    homeopathy *vs.*, 148–9
    pain relief, 146
    as part of dose regimen, 129–30
    passive *vs.* active placebos, 148
    pharmacodynamics, 148
    side-effects, 147
Plant material, 83–5, 86, 327
    anthroposophical medicine, 256
Plastic containers, 127
    glass *vs.*, 109–10
Pneumonia, 190
Point-of-sale advice, 17
Poisoning, 43
Poisoning by Arsenic, 43

Poisons, supply, 121, 123
Polychrests, 11, 168, 327
    constitutional remedies, 176
    'first aid', 183
    first aid/acute treatments, 214
    keynotes, **169**
    OTC requests, 122
    OTC user profiles, 16
    rationale, 152
Polypharmacy, 123, 188–91
Polyvinyl chloride contamination, 110
Postgraduate courses, 323
Postoperative bruising, RCTs, 292
Postoperative ileus, RCTs, 294
Potency, 95
    50 millesimal (LM), 99
    centesimal, 95–6, **96,** 126
    changing, 200
    decimal, 96, **97,** 126
    high potencies, preparation, 98
    homeopathic medicating, 101
    OTC preparations and, 123
    prescriptions, 126
    vibrationary resonance, 152
Potentisation, 54, 92–100, **93,** 326
    allopathic vaccines, 162
    dilution, 54, 92–3
    Korsakovian method, 97–8
    LM method, 99–100
    mechanical, 98
    Skinner method, 98–9, **99**
    succussion, 93–5
    theories of *see* Homeopathy,
        theories of
Potentiser, 98
Powders, 102, **103,** 127
    medicating process, 102, 131–2
    prescription/dispensing, **128,**
        129–30
Pragmatic studies, 280
Prayer, 15
Pregnancy, homeopathy in, 142, 234–6
    antenatal/preconception, 234, **235**
    labour, 234–6
Preliminary Certificate in Veterinary
        Homeopathy (PCVH),
        323
Premenstrual syndrome (PMS), **233,**
        233–4
Preparation (of remedies), 81–120, **100,**
        326
    Bach flower remedies, 259
    definitions, 81–2
    extraction, 90–2, 327
    high potencies, 98
    homeopathic pharmacopoeias, 81–2
    information for pharmacists, 117
    nomenclature issues, 110–13, **112**
    packaging/storage, 109–10, 127

    labelling, 113, 132, **132,** 201
    patient information, 134
    research, 313
    potentisation *see* Potentisation
    processes, 89–100
    quality control, 107–9
    sources of materials, 83–9, 327
        animal/insect, 85, **86**
        biological, 85–7
        chemical, 87
        collection, 85
        control, 107
        controversies, 83
        miscellaneous, 87–8
        new sources, 88–9
        plant, 83–5
        variations in, 84, **84**
    terminology, 95–7
    topical preparations, 105
    yields, 90
    see also specific methodologies
Prescription-only medicines (POMs),
    125
Prescription/prescribing, 20, 123–30,
    128
    acute illness, 152, 168
    allopathic *vs.* CAM remedies, 20–2,
        21
    anthroposophical medicine, 256
    chronic illness, 152, 182, 185–8
    clarification, 126
    complexes, 181
    constitutional, 176
    contacting prescriber, 126
    dosages/dose regimens, 127–30,
        128, 182–91
        complicated, 129
        granules/crystals/powders,
        129–30
        isopathic vaccines, 171–2
        liquids, 130
        tablets/pillules, 128–9
    dose form, 126–7
    first aid/acute applications, 182,
        183–5, 213–54
    inconsistencies, 128–9
    keynote (three-legged stool), 168,
        175
    multiple, 123, 188–91, **190**
    NHS prescriptions, 14, 125, 134–5
        as CAM pull factor, 20–2
        charges, 135, **135**
        format, 125
        GP10/FP10 forms, 20
    potency, 126
    prescription-only remedies, 123, **124**
    pricing/charges, **135,** 135–6
    private prescriptions, 125
        pricing, 135–6

quantity, 127
remedy details, 125–30
name, 125–6
sources of request, 125
see also Dispensing; Remedies
Primary Care Certificate (PCC), 323
Primary Health Care Examination
(PHCE), 323
Prince of Wales
CAM support, 23
Foundation for Integrated Health,
28, 357
report into cost of complementary
medicines, 22
Problem-based learning, 300
Professional competence, 140–1, 200
Progress reviews, 198–200
Prophylactic healthcare, 14, 184
bacterial infections, 231
isopathic remedies as, 171–3, **172**
veterinary, 310
Provings, 51–3
chemicals, 87
chocolate, 88
clinical therapeutic observation,
52
clinical/toxological, 52
clinical verification, 53
experimental, 52
Hahnemann's work, 47, 48–9
mixtures, 55
new/alternative protocols, 53
patient follow-up as, 200
'Psora' miasms, 153, **156**
Psychological effects
first aid treatment, **222**
placebos, 146
Psychophysical effects, placebos, 146
Publication issues, homeopathy
research, 275–7
Public Health Act, 60
Public health, isopathic remedies, 173,
247
Public, OTC requests, 122
Pulled muscle, 240
Pulsatilla person, 158
Puncture wounds, **215, 216,** 226
Purity measures, 107

Q

Quality control, 107–9
EU directive 92/73/EEC, 113
Queen Mother, homeopathy
patronage, 23, 63
Quin, Frederick Hervey Foster, 59–60
homeopathy and orthodox
medicine, 12

London Homeopathic Hospital, 60,
63–4
Quinine, 162
Quinquaginatamillesimal (LM)
potentisation method,
99–100

R

Rabies, 168
RADAR program, 197
Radiation, 51
Randi, James, 303
Randomised controlled trials (RCTs),
32–3, 270, 285–91
Arnica, 291–3
Arsenicum album, 293
children, 294
criticisms, 286, 288, 289
delayed onset muscle soreness
(DOMS), 241–2
difficulties/problems, 33, 275–7,
296–8
bias, 287
blinding, 297
patient selection, 296–7
quality of evidence, 297–8
randomisation, 297
response, complexity of, 297
early trials, 286
Gibson's rheumatoid arthritis
trials, 286–8, **287**
meta-analysis, 294–6, **295**
methodology, 272
observational studies vs., 298
placebos, 147, 288–91
place in homeopathy research, 285
quality, 32
Rhus tox, 293
systematic reviews, 296
see also Outcome measures
Record keeping, 139, 198, **199**
Referrals, 141, **141**
Reflexology, 5
Registered Malaysian Homeopathic
Medical Practitioners
Association, 71
Registration, 63, 71
EU directive 92/73/EEC, 113, 114
EU pharmaceutical legislation and,
116–17
Regulated model of integrated CAM
delivery, 28
Regulatory bodies, 6
competence, 141
definitions, 82
practitioner recommendations, 136
see also individual organisations

Relatives, as information source, 29
Remedies, 11, 167–209, 328
absorption, 133
administration frequency, 105, 127
administration method, 133–4, 189
adverse reactions, 53
aggravations, 49, 53, 133
antidotes, 206–7, **207**
biochemic tissue salts, 263–5, **264**
choice of/choosing, 167–212
acute conditions, 183–5
chronic conditions, 185–8
computerised repertorising,
196–8
concomitants, 187
grading, 194–6, **196**
like treats like, 51–3, 160, 326
modalities, 186–7
peculiars, 187
repertories/repertorising, 192–6,
193, 194, 195, 196
research purposes, 273
symptoms/disease aetiology,
185–6
see also Homeopathic principles
'classical', 175–6
complementary, 190, **191**
definitions, 81–2, 113
'drug pictures' see Drug pictures
effects, 163
'essence of', **175,** 175–6, 184
experimental proving see Provings
GSL classification, 17
identification, 125
interactions see Interactions
kits
'Dr Jack's kit', 190, 330
Glasgow Acute Kit, 330, **331**
legal status, 113–17
'unlicensed products', 117
see also European Union
Directives; Licensing
long-term use, 17, 123
market for, 25–7
multiple prescribing, 123, 188–91
new uses, 81, 328
nomenclature, 110–13, **112,** 263
confusion, 110–11, 125–6, 129
standardisation, 113
own label, 61
patient expectations, 139
potentisation, 54
preparation see Preparation (of
remedies)
prescription costs, 20–2, **21**
presentations/preparations, 100–6,
160
see also specific types
primary vs. secondary actions, 49

properties, **162**
safety *see* Safety issues
setting up stocks, 330–2
storage, 109–10, 134
supply (of named), 121–36
    dispensing, 130–2
    OTCs *see* Over-the-counter
        (OTC) preparations
    patient information, 133–4
    prescription-only, 123, **124,**
        125–30
    product availability, 136
    self-diagnosis and, 138–9
    suppliers, 332, 359
    third-party requests, 138
    see also Prescription/prescribing
types, 168–82
X-ray exposure and, 248
see also Flower remedies;
        Repertories/repertorising;
        Treatment; *specific*
        indications; specific types
Repertories/repertorising, 192–6
    Boericke's, 192, **193**
    computerisation, 196–8
    Kent's, 192, 194, **195**
    remedy grading, 194–6, **196**
    veterinary homeopathy, 250
Repertorising chart, **196**
Repertory of the Homeopathic Materia
        Medica (Kent), 192, 194,
        195
Reporting cards, 201, **202–3**
Rescue remedy, 260–1
Research, 31–4, 269–319
    agricultural homeopathy, 308, 310
    aims, 272
    anecdotal evidence, 33–4, 149
    anthroposophical medicine, 256–7
    assessment scales, 274, **274**
    attitudes/awareness studies, 307–8,
        309
    Bach flower remedies, 261
    case studies, 33–4, 299–300
    cholera, 60–1
    classification, 32–4, 271
    clinical audit, 33, 307–8
    in Cuba, 74
    current position, 313–14
    emphasis, time for change, 311–13
    European, 31
    evidence-based, 31, 271–7
    experimental studies, 279
    explanatory studies, 280
    homeopathy efficacy/effectiveness,
        279–300, 311–13
        early work, 279–80
        measures, 280–1, **281**
    homeopathy mechanisms, 300–8

interactions, 313
meta-analyses, 32–3, 276, 288,
    294–6, **295**
methodology, 272
    data collection, 307
observational studies, 279, 298–300
ongoing work, 277
OTCs, 313
outcome measures *see* Outcome
    measures
pragmatic studies, 279, 280
problems
    funding difficulties, 32, 271
    interactions with colleagues, 275
    methodological, 272, 276
    placebo error, 273
    publication issues, 275–7
    test materials, 273
protocol design, 277–9
    advice, 278
    categories, 279
    checklists, 279
    headings, 277
quality of, 32
randomised controlled trials *see*
        Randomised controlled
        trials (RCTs)
recording data, 273–4
systematic reviews, 296
techniques, 272–5
'three-legged stool approach', 313
validity, 273–4
    external, 278, **279**
    internal, 278, **278**
veterinary homeopathy, 310–11
Respiratory tract infections, 230
    RCTs, 294
Rheumatic conditions
    anthroposophical medicine, 256–7
    Gibson's rheumatoid arthritis
        trials, 286–8, **287**
    pain, 186
Ricin, 174
Risk:benefit ratio, 140
    CAM, 24, 31
    women and, 231
Risk perception, 18, 31, 122
Risk, vaccination/immunisation, 171
Royal family, CAM support, 23, 63
Royal London Homeopathic Hospital,
    63–6, **66**, 358
    children's ward, 236
    diversification, 65
    extension, 64, **65**
    foundation, 60, 63–4
    HCLH merger, 66
    NHS reorganisation, 65–6
Rubella, 171, **172**
Runner's knee, 241

Russia, homeopathy in, 72–3, 97
Russian Homeopathic Association, 73

S

Safety issues, 31, 200–7
    allopathic drugs, 18
    EU directive 92/73/EEC, 113
    inappropriate treatment, 200
    intervening in OTC sales, 122–3,
        138
    see also Adverse reactions;
        Aggravations;
        Interactions
Salmon, furunculosis, 310, **311**
Sankaran, P., 70
Sankaran, Rajan, 70
Sarcodes, 170, 171
    definition, 85
    uses, 86
    as vaccines, 171–3, 246–7
Scabies, 139, 153
Scarlet fever, 47, **172**
Schollz, Albert, 71
Scholten, Jan, 72
Schroyen's *Synthesis*, 196
Schüssler salts, 263–5, **264**
Schüssler, Wilhelm Heinrich, 263
Scientific fraud, 304
Scorpion bites, 168
Scotland, homeopathy in, 61, 63, 66–7
Scottish Homeopathic research and
        Educational Trust
        (SHRET), 63, 271
Scrumpox, 243
Securitainer®, 110
Self-diagnosis, dangers of, **138**, 138–9,
        139
Sepia person, 158
Shiatsu, 5
Shock, 214, **215**
Shyness, **238**
Side-effects *see* Adverse reactions
Silica glass, potentisation and, 97
Similima, 332
Simplexes (single remedies), 43, 55,
    225, 326
Skin conditions, 20, 214, **223**, 226
    aggravations, 200
Skinner potentisation method, 98–9, **99**
Skinner, Thomas, 98
Skin tests, 228, **229**
Smallpox, 168, **172**
Smuts, Jan Christian, holism, 7
Sneezing, **217**
Social factors, holistic approach and, 8
Society of Homeopaths, 63, 332, 357
    vaccination views, 172

Socio-economic groups
    homeopathy user profiles, 16
    orthodox medicine and,
            consultation and, 19
Soda glass, 110
Soft tablets, 103
Soft tissue injuries, **215, 216,** 226, 240
Software packages, repertorising, 197
Solid dose forms, **101,** 101–5, **103,**
            127
    medicating process, 101, 102,
            103–5, **104,** 131–2
    prescription/dispensing, **128,**
            128–30, 131
    terminology confusion, 102
Sore throat, **224,** 230
Source materials *see under* Preparation
            (of remedies)
South Africa
    educational institutions, 358
    homeopathy in, 68–9
    suppliers, 360
Special Manufacturing Licenses, 117
Spectroscopy, quality control, 107
Sports medicine, 239–44
    advantages of using homeopathy,
            239
    common illnesses and treatment,
            243–4
    common injuries and treatment,
            239–43
    performance-enhancing remedies,
            244
    see also specific injuries/ailments
Sprains, **215,** 240
Stage fright, **222**
Starting up, 329–33
Steiner, Rudolf, 255–6
Sterile preparations, eye drops, 105–6
Steroids, homeopathy interactions, 20,
            142, 205
Stings, 51, **215,** 243
Stocks, 82
Storage, 109–10, 134, 313
Strains, **215,** 240
Stress, 146, **215,** 325
Strong spirit (ss) *see* Liquid potency
Styes, **220**
Succussion, 93–5, 327
    emulsification of vaccines, 162
    hand *vs.* machine, 93–4
    number, 93
    theories of, 94–5
    variations in, 93
Sucrose, 127
'Sugar pill', 147
Sulphur person, 158
'Sun method', 259
Sun, reactions to, 248

Suppliers, 332, 359
    mother tinctures variations, 108–9
    see also Manufacturers
Suppositories, 106
Swelling, 242–3
'Sycotic' miasms (gonorrhoea), 153,
            156
Symptoms, 326
    depth, 155–6
    'generals', 185, 194
    'guiding', 175
    holistic approach to, 7–12, 160
    Law of Similars and, 151–3
    'mentals', 185, 194
    'particulars', 194
    totality in chronic prescribing, 185–6
    treatment of, 150
    see also Drug pictures
Synonyms, 111
Synthesis (Schroyen), 196
Syphilis
    'luetic' miasms, 153, 154, **156**
    mercury, 47
Systematic reviews, 296

T

Tablets, 103, 127
    medicating process, 103, 131–2
    prescription/dispensing, **128,**
            128–9, 131
    trituration, 92, 103
Tautodes *see* Tautopathic remedies
Tautopathic remedies, 86, 88, 170,
            173–5, 328
Tea, 133
Teenagers, 237–8, **238**
Teething, 149, **224,** 236–7
Temperature modalities, 186
Tennis elbow, 241
Terror, **222, 260**
Terrorism, 174
Tetanus, 239
Thalidomide, 14
Third-party requests, 138
Three-legged stool prescribing *see*
            Keynote (three-legged
            stool) prescribing
Time modalities, 186–7
Tinea pedis, 243
Tobacco mosaic virus, 310
Topical preparations, 105, 130, 132,
            225–7
    first aid/acute applications, 225–7,
            241
    mixed, 226
    mother tinctures, 105, 226–7
    single remedy, 225

Toxins, low dose exposure, 173–5
Toxological proving, 52
Traditional therapies, 4
Training courses, 321–4
    locations, 323
Trauma, 214, **215**
Traveller's kit, 246, **247**
Traveller's medicine, 246–8, **247**
Treatment provision, 135, 137–42
    deciding to treat, 139–42
        competency, 140–1, 200
        homeopathy or allopathy?,
            141–2
        referral, 141, **141**
    guidelines, 140–1
    NHS *see* National Health Service
            (NHS)
    problems, 137–9
        facilities, 137–8
        obtaining information, 138
        records/recording, 139, 198, **199**
        self-diagnosis, **138,** 138–9, **139**
        veterinary homeopathy, 251
Trituration, 90–2
    biochemic tissue salts, 263
    Korsakovian, 97
    lactose, 91–2
Trituration tablets, 103
Tubercular miasms, 154
Tunbridge Wells Hospital, 67–8, 358
Twain, Mark, 76
Typhoid, Hahnemann's treatment of,
            43

U

Ultraviolet (UV) spectroscopy, quality
            control, 107
Uncertainty, **260**
Unio Homeopathica Belgica, 22
United Kingdom
    associations/resources, 357–8
    CAM research funding, 32
    CAM usage, 24, 26–7
    healthcare delivery, 15
    homeopathy in, 59–68
        historical aspects, 59–61
        homeopathic hospitals, 63–8
        organisations/publications,
            63–4
        pharmacy, 61–2
    pharmacists' views on CAM, 30
    product licensing, 113–17
    Statutory Instrument SI 1995/308,
            82
    training courses, 321–4
    see also National Health Service
            (NHS)

United Kingdom Homeopathic
       Medical Association
       (UKHMA), 357
United States
    CAM usage
        markets, 26
        user profiles, 15
    educational institutions, 358
    homeopathic pharmaceutical
        industry, 76, 360
    homeopathy in, 74–8
        Hahnemann memorial, 77–8
        history, 74–6
        NCCAM *see* National Center for
            Complementary and
            Alternative Medicine
            (NCCAM)
    pharmacists' views on CAM, 30
    product licensing, 117
University College London Hospitals
    Trust (UCLH), 66
University of Exeter Centre for
    Complementary Studies,
    324

V

Vaccines
    isopathic remedies as, 171–3, 246–7
        human, 171–3, **172**
        veterinary, 173
    isopathy, 168
    'succussation', 162
    tautopathic remedies, 86, 328
Verruca, 139, 244

Veterinary homeopathy, 159, 236,
    249–52
    Bach flower remedies, 261
    isopathic vaccines, 173, 247, 310
    popular remedies, 250–1, **251**
    research, 310–11
    revival of interest, 250
    training courses, 322, 323
Veterinary medicines, 116, 117, 250
Veterinary Surgeon's Act (1966), 251
Vibrational planes, 150–1, **151**
Vibrationary resonance, 151–3
Viral infection
    miasm hypothesis, 154
    treatment, 230–1
    see also specific infections
Visual Analogue Scale (VAS), 33, **274,**
    281–2
    GHHOS hybrid, 283, **284**
    observational studies, 299
    placebo RCTs, 289, 290
Vital force, 149–53, **151,** 156
    levels (planes), 150–1
Vitamin deficiency, 232
Volunteers, experimental proving, 52
Vomiting, **222, 246**

W

Waldorf School Movement, 256
Warts, 227, 244
Water polymers
    homeopathy theories, 95, 301–2, **302**
    'memory', Benveniste controversy,
        302–4

Weir, John, 61
Weleda, educational material, 322,
    329
Wessekhoeft, William, 75
Wholesalers, 136
Whooping cough, **172**
Women
    homeopathic physicians, 64
    homeopathy and, 231–6
        advantages, 231–2
        cystitis, 230, 232, **232**
        menopause, 234
        PMS, **233,** 233–4
        pregnancy, 142, 234–6
World Health Organization, health
    definition, 4
World Pharmacy Conference (FIP), 31
Worry, **222**
Wounds, **215, 216,** 226, 239
W-WHAM process, 141, **141**

X

X-rays, effects on remedies, 248

Y

Yellow card scheme, 201, **202–3**
Yellow fever, 76

Z

Zoological names, 111